THE DR. MILTON D. QUIGLESS, SR. Story

A Memoir of Race, Medicine, and Purpose in the Segregated South

COMPILED BY CAROL QUIGLESS

The Dr. Milton D. Quigless, Sr. Story:
A Memoir of Race, Medicine, and Purpose in the Segregated South
- REMARKS - NOTES - OBSERVATIONS –
Second Edition

Printed in the United States of America
Paperback ISBN: 978-1-963732-14-6
Hardback ISBN: 978-1-963732-15-3

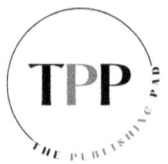

The Publishing Pad
www.thepublishingpad.com

A great read. I'm proud to be of Quigless lineage.

– Dr. Charles R. Quigless, Jr.

This autobiography is a poignant, fascinating, and uplifting story of human achievement. It should serve as an example for young African American males today, providing them with a fine role model for success. Dr. Quigless was an ordinary person who did ordinary things extraordinarily well. He was truly the exemplary "Renaissance man" with a tremendous zest for working and living. This memoir is a "must read" for African American and Southern history scholars and enthusiasts.

– C. Rudolph Knight
a.k.a. "Baby Knight," born May 2, 1947,
Quigless Clinic-Hospital

Dr. Quigless's lively account of his personal and professional life allows readers to enter the world of a Black physician who practiced during most of the 20th century. He and the African American medical profession grew up together. Dr. Quigless knew many of the greats in Black medical history but also knew and worked with the ordinary physician of color trying to practice as best he could in the segregated and racist South. We meet white doctors and white citizens who helped Dr. Quigless at various stages of his life and other whites who threw roadblocks in his way. We also learn about Black physicians and citizens who helped and hindered him. He, like most African American physicians of the early and mid-20th century, had to overcome the distrust of Black patients toward physicians of their own race who believed that Black doctors were not as good as white doctors. Throughout this memoir, Dr. Quigless maintains his humor and equanimity, telling the stories as he saw them, never with vindictiveness or meanness. Though Dr. Quigless practiced in eastern North Carolina, his story could have taken place anywhere in the South. Dr. Quigless represents all Black physicians growing up and practicing in that region during the early and mid-20th century.

– Todd L. Savitt, PhD, Historian of Medicine Brody School of Medicine, East Carolina University

CONTENTS

FOREWORD

I t has been fourteen years since my father's memoir, *Looking Back: The Way It Was*, was first published. Now, I feel it is time to reintroduce my dad's story to a new generation of readers, so they can look back through his eyes to view a different time and a different version of America than most of us know today.

It amazes me that Dr. Milton D. Quigless, Sr., is still so widely remembered for his skill, smarts, and wit. On what would have been his 116th birthday on August 16, 2022, over 700 local people wished him well on Facebook. Some of the people were babies or children when he touched their lives. Like my dad, many people he knew have passed on, but the stories live on through their children and grandchildren. His story continues to be fascinating and relevant.

New material was found that begged to be brought to light, such as his handwritten diary from when he was a resident at City Hospital No. 2 in St. Louis, Missouri in the early 1930s. Complete with a new title—*The Dr. Milton D. Quigless Story: A Memoir of Race, Medicine, and Purpose in the Segregated South*—this edition has been streamlined, reorganized, and reformatted for easier reading, but without losing my dad's distinctive voice and enduring spirit.

Acknowledgment and thanks are in order to Michele Cruz and her mother, Mary Carpenter, who made sense out of the thousands of manuscript pages they combed through to create the first edition; the typists who transcribed volumes of cassette tapes—I wish I knew your names to thank you personally; Quincy Robinson who got the ball rolling with early editing for this edition; the current editor, Angela Frazier, who did a massive editing job and provided me with endless encouragement and support, and Doris Stith who proofread the manuscript. I offer deep gratitude to Lynn Murray, BSN and Richard Pantalone, MD for transcribing my Dad's handwritten diary which I found next to impossible to read. For keeping my dad's story alive and recognized, I give thanks to the Phoenix Historical Society: African American History of Edgecombe County, particularly Mavis Stith and James W. Wrenn; David C. Dennard, PhD, the first African American Professor of History at East Carolina University and Todd L. Savitt, PhD, Historian of Medicine, Brody School of Medicine, East Carolina University; The Country Doctor Museum; Laupus Library at Brody School of Medicine, East Carolina University; Duke University Library; and the North Carolina Museum of History.

My heartfelt thanks go to the many patients from up and down the east coast and State of North Carolina that travelled to be treated by my dad. He could not have done his work without his staff that supported him over the years – nurses, pharmacy staff, cooks, orderlies, administrative staff, some of which were whole families. Although too many to list here, please know that you are remembered with gratitude.

The biggest thanks must go to my sister, Helen G. Quigless, Jr., without whose insistence my dad never would have embarked on recording his story; my brother Milton D. Quigless, Jr., for his participation and unwavering belief in our dad; and our mother, Mrs. Helen G. Quigless, who stood by our dad, the love of her life, through thick and thin, straight to the end.

– *Carol Quigless*

INTRODUCTION

My father was quite a humorist. This was one of his favorite jokes: "The bedridden old man was dying. He asked that his lawyer and his doctor be brought to his room. He had the doctor stand to his left and the lawyer stand to his right. The old man then closed his eyes and folded his hands across his chest. After a while someone asked him what he was doing. He said, 'I am dying like sweet Jesus, between two thieves.'"

I worked for him the summer between my junior and senior years of medical school.

During this time, I learned more about him than at any time that we were both living. One of his techniques was to find common ground with any patient and then build a doctor-patient relationship. With an elderly patient he might open with something like, "Do you remember how cold it was in the winter of '45?" After a while, he would let the patient get around to what was ailing him, but not until the patient was emotionally comfortable.

One day a child was brought in with right lower quadrant abdominal pain. As the boy was whisked past his office in a wheelchair, Daddy told me to check on the patient and let him know what was wrong. Very quickly, I made the diagnosis of acute appendicitis. He laughed and said that the child had right lower lobe pneumonia because in the brief glimpse my father got as the child went by his office he noticed flaring nostrils, which with abdominal pain and elevated white blood count meant lower lobe pneumonia on the side that was tender due to referred pain.

Another lesson that summer was about asthma. He gave large doses of intravenous (IV) Solu-Cortef, which always stopped the asthma attack in just a few minutes. A few months later, back at Meharry Medical College, I saw a child in the ER with status asthmaticus and gave the IV Solu-Cortef, which quickly normalized the patient. The pediatric department chairman was furious when he found out about this, saying that surely, I had caused adrenal insufficiency. My understanding is that, presently, adrenocorticosteroids are usually included in the treatment of acute asthmatic attacks.

My father was undoubtedly the largest prescriber of Depo-Medrol in eastern North Carolina. He used it to great advantage for any skin rash that was not a fungus and also for rheumatoid arthritis.

I do not know where he got SIC from. This was salicylate, iodine, and colchicine given intravenously for rheumatoid arthritis.

I asked him, "How can you do a hysterectomy for large fibroid tumors with no blood bank?" He really laughed this time and said, "If you clamp before you cut, it will not bleed...dummy!" He also happily did C-sections, appendectomies, tonsillectomies, and other procedures with ether anesthesia.

My father gave digoxin and diuretics until either the pulse rate slowed, the patient could lie flat, or the ankle edema was gone. He never learned to read an electrocardiogram, but if the pulse was erratic, he sent the patient to Duke or Chapel Hill.

He never referred a patient to a doctor in Tarboro for anything, as he reasoned that the patient could have gone to that doctor initially, and my father did not want the patient to get the idea that any doctor short of Duke or UNC could treat him as well as he did.

Some illustrative personal history—when he was working summers as a dining car waiter and sleeping car porter on the

Milwaukee Railroad out of Chicago to pay his way through medical school, the Depression hit, and many people, including him, got laid off. He told me that he continued to go to work, even though he was not scheduled to be paid, because he had nothing else to do, the work was fun, and the cars needed to be made up. He never missed a paycheck.

Also, while railroading in the summer of 1932 during Prohibition, his group was buying liquor in Canada and selling it in Chicago. In August, one of his associates got caught. Everybody in the group had to pay into the pot to get the fellow out of jail, so my father had no money for medical school that fall and had to stay out of school for that year. By working a whole year, he was quite well-to-do for a senior! He graduated a year late in the class of 1934 with Matthew Walker and other luminaries.

Walter Plemmer came to my father in the late 1930s. He was a thirteen-year-old boy dying of hemophilia, with many of his cousins already dead. My father's reasoning was very clear. No females ever got hemophilia, so he gave Plemmer massive injections of estrogens, which stopped the bleeding and eradicated all traces of the disease. These injections continued periodically for the rest of his life. Plemmer became a regionally famous pianist and bandleader in eastern North Carolina. An amateur quartet he directed won the competition to appear on the Ed Sullivan Show in the late 1950s. He played the piano at my father's funeral in 1997.

Most hemophiliacs were treated with pooled plasma after this became available in the 1950s. However, most hemophiliacs caught AIDS from the plasma, and many of them died in the mid to late '80s. Plemmer lived a long, happy, and productive life, and died in 2000 at about age 77 of causes having nothing to do with hemophilia. Undoubtedly, he was the longest-living hemophiliac at the time of his passing.

My father and I were riding on West End Avenue past Vanderbilt Hospital when I was a student at Meharry in about 1970. As we rode by, I asked him if he ever went to the Grand Rounds presentations at Vanderbilt Medical School. He pointed out a door and said, "That is the door I went in to wash pots in the Vanderbilt kitchen. All I ever saw of Vanderbilt was greasy pots." He also, later that same day, pointed to the Tennessee State Capitol building and told me that inside that building, he took the Tennessee State Medical Licensure exam and scored the highest in the state for that year...including among the students from Vanderbilt!

– Dr. Milton D. Quigless, Jr., FACS
from the 2009 *Journal of the National Medical Association*

CHAPTER 1

BEGINNINGS

Although I am by no means a writer, I got some notes together to tell my life's story. Four or five years ago, I promised my oldest daughter, Helen, that I would write about my life. She finally ran me into a corner until I said, "I've got to write up this thing."

It's going to take the hours I usually spend dozing in front of the television, sipping beer, driving slowly through the countryside, or playing with the kids, but I'm going to go through with it. In thinking back over the past, I believe it will give me a chance to re-live all those moments, days, weeks, months, and years during which I achieved some successes—and chalked up some dismal failures—in the things I set out to do.

I would like to ask you, "What would you say if someone were to ask what your earliest memory was? When did you first realize that you were a person?"

The first thing I remember is being awakened from a peaceful sleep to find big, round faces looking down and talking in my face. Everything was white, and I wondered what it was all about and wished they would let me go back to sleep.

The next thing I remember were those same people waking me, taking me out of a nice warm bed, and putting clothes on me. I felt more comfortable with nothing on. The clothes scratched my skin. I was carried out of this peaceful, quiet, comfortable, cool place I liked, and into the sunshine.

One particular day, I was dressed in all those clothes that scratched my body, taken out into the bright sunshine, and then inside another building where the light was not so bright. I went to sleep again. I didn't sleep long before I was awakened by a loud noise. I looked around; all I could see were ceiling boards up above. I was taken to that building at regular intervals and much later learned it was a church.

After some time, the loud noises were not irritating, but soothing. These noises were people singing. As I grew older and was able to sit alone in a seat, I'd take my nap and be awakened by the singing. Immediately, I'd leave my seat and go forward to find a person with a particularly loud, booming voice that was my father's. Once I found him, I'd crawl up in his lap and go back to sleep.

My existence was somewhat pleasant during that time, and there was always somebody to play with. One thing I particularly remember was my habit of looking at that ball of fire in the sky, trying to figure out what it was. Once, my sister caught me looking, yanked me around, gave me a whack on the bottom, and cautioned me to not look at the sun like that because it might affect my eyes.

What's the next thing I remember? A big, dark-brown, soft-spoken motherly person. She talked to me and took care of me almost completely. She dressed me, fed me, and walked me around. Whenever I felt irritated, she'd pick me up and soothe me. I later learned she was my Aunt Nora.

One day, when I was about one-and-a-half years old, Aunt Nora took me away from these people with whom I had identified. We left at night and went to a noisy place with large white flashing lights. There was a peculiar odor in the air that I didn't recognize. The next thing I knew, it was daylight, and we were moving. We were on a train to a distant city called Pine Bluff, in Arkansas.

Once there, I was among another group about whom I knew nothing. Everybody was pleasant, however. There seemed to be a lot of people who played with me, fed me, and carried me around. I vividly remember a man who'd pick me up, put me in the basket of his bicycle, and ride me all over town.

When Aunt Nora and I got home, I didn't remember my sisters or anybody else. The three months I had been away had blotted them all from my memory. I had to become re-acquainted with every member of my family.

For a while I wondered what I was doing with these people. I had been happy in Pine Bluff. Now I had to re-adjust to these children and to people coming to visit and calling me "Milton," a name I didn't remember. I became very interested in a tiny baby lying in a crib, crying most of the time. I was told she was my baby sister, Thelma.

I was born August 16, 1904, in the small southern town of Port Gibson, Mississippi. The town was located about fifteen miles from the Mississippi River and had a population of about two thousand. Though it was not much of a town, it was the whole world to me. That world extended anywhere from ten to twelve blocks in any given direction from my home.

Port Gibson was a beautiful little town. When Grant marched from Richmond, Virginia during the Civil War, he passed through Vicksburg, Mississippi, tearing it up. Port Gibson was about thirty-two miles below Vicksburg. When the Union Army got to Port Gibson, they found the quaint little town with all its churches and mild-mannered people so appealing that Grant decided it was too beautiful to burn. Racial relations were pretty good at that time, too, because everybody knew everybody else. Families living there were close-knit. Search the court records back two or three generations and you'll find that most of the residents were at least distant cousins.

My grandfather, whom everyone called "Papa Charlie," was well-known not only as a bricklayer but also as a liquor drinker. His first love was "trotting" horses; liquor was second; and the family ran about third in line. By the time I came along, Grandpa was about seventy-five years old and rather senile. His bricklaying days were over, and his drinking had slowed down, but he was still fond of his horses. He spent all his spare time around the livery stable.

Papa Charlie was the type of fellow you would stop and take a second look at. He was about five feet two inches tall with a light brown complexion, high cheek bones, and two plaits of straight black hair hanging to his waist. He talked with a very different southern drawl and could give you the genealogy of every horse that passed nearby.

He enjoyed telling stories about the days of the Civil War. The way I understood it, he was too young to be drafted as a soldier, so he was left on the plantation somewhere near Natchez. He often talked of the tense situation when Grant marched through the South. He told of how they tried to hide everything of value in caves and underground. The slaves worked day and night to accomplish this for their masters, while praying the Yankees would get close enough so they would not have to work so hard. When they heard the rumble of cannons, they started jumping up and down, yelling for joy. The master of the plantation, who was also too old to go to war, caught them celebrating. As a result, they ran off into the woods and waited for the Yankees to get there because they were afraid of the master.

Grandpa had several trotting horses. One was a beautiful mare called Pocahontas, of which he was especially proud and intended to breed to a famous stud. Without his knowledge or consent, some of the boys in the neighborhood put Pocahontas in a pit and bred her to a little white jackass. Grandpa bragged about how much he was going to be able to get for the foal when it was born. When Pocahontas delivered, instead of a fine-looking colt, all he got was a stunted white mule. Grandpa got his gun and went all over town trying to find out who had tricked him.

The little white mule was named Kate and became a member of the family. Believe it or not, Kate lived to be over forty years old. Old Kate was a gentle mule, and we became attached to her. Many days I would slip up on her back and then slide down her neck. She would not bother me at all. But if anyone tried to bother us, she would back up to them and raise her hind leg, just like Old Maude in the funny papers. She was as attentive to us as a watchdog. She was already a grown mule when I was born, and she died when I was thirty years old.

A funny thing happened once with old Kate. Pop needed some cash, so he took her to the stable and sold her. When we came home and found out what had happened, we raised so much sand that he had to go back and get Kate, paying ten dollars more than he'd received for selling her. He never tried to sell her again.

My father was John M. Quigless. I don't know a lot about his history except that he grew up in Port Gibson. When he was about eighteen, he decided to leave and go to New Orleans in hopes of finding a job. He was hired as a waiter. But after about a year, he decided he did not like city life and returned to Port Gibson, where he got a job as a mechanic's helper at Port Gibson Oil and Mill. This is when he met the fair lady, Agnes Brazand, who was to become my mother.

Pop said he loved her so much he didn't know what to do. I've heard him say many times, "When I first met her, I could have eaten her up." About thirty years later, he said he wished he had. It goes without saying that he'd laugh as he said that because Mama would be giving him "the mean eye."

Daddy was in his mid-thirties when he lost part of his right hand at the oil mill. It was his job to oil the machinery. He was oiling some gears, which operated the conveyor, and he had to climb a ladder to squirt some oil in between the gears. His foot slipped, and as he was falling, he threw out his hand, trying to catch himself. It got caught in the machinery. After an operation, he was left with only the thumb and index finger of that hand, thus ending his job at the mill.

Back in those days there were no such things as old age pensions, Social Security, or compensation insurance to take care of an injury on the job. Because we already had some horses and Old Kate, Pop decided to buy a two-horse wagon and begin making his living hauling freight from the railroad station to different stores in town. He tried to find freight to haul so we could all eat, but he wasn't doing a very good job of it. So, Mama had to step in and start managing the family's finances. She opened her first restaurant.

Everyone called my Mama "Miss Agnes." She must have been a beautiful young woman because she was still attractive at age eighty. She was the eldest of five children—she had two sisters and two brothers named Tanzy, Janie, Rufus, and Calvin. Mama was about eight or ten years of age when my maternal grandmother died, shortly after the birth of her fifth child. My maternal grandfather had a difficult time raising the children alone, so he later remarried. It was hard for him to feed his family, so Mama went to work at an early age babysitting for a white family named Jones.

Captain Jones had been in the Confederate Army. He and his wife lived in Port Gibson with their several children, all girls.

She must have been doing a good job at taking care of the family because it came to the attention of Captain Jones, who asked my grandfather to let them take Mama to live with them to look after their children.

Her primary duty was to care for the children, but they soon looked upon her as a member of the family. She was taught along with the Joneses' children by their tutor. She was also taught skills such as sewing and cooking and began going everywhere with the family. Captain Jones was a devout Episcopalian, and my mother went to church every Sunday with the family. She sat with them in their pew instead of being relegated to the balcony like all the other Blacks. My mother absorbed quite a bit of culture and was taught many skills. She became accustomed to having nice things around. As a result, she always made it a point to try and give our family some of the niceties that she enjoyed as a member of the Jones family. My mother stopped working for them when she married my father.

Mama had been well trained by the Jones family. Her expertise as a cook really came in handy when she had to help feed the family after my father's injury. She had the idea of opening a restaurant and of preparing dinners for some of the more affluent families in Port Gibson. Mama did not cook soul food for the whites; she cooked the types of food to which she knew they were accustomed. She cooked hot dinners for several different families in town, placed them in boxes, and my father would deliver them in time for their big dinners every day at noon.

Mama and Papa became very famous in Port Gibson, but the work became so heavy that Mama almost worked herself to death and had to close the restaurant. She developed symptoms of what, in this day and time, would be diagnosed as a peptic ulcer. Mama was so sick that she was put to bed. I became sick, too, and Mama put me into bed with her. When the doctor came to check on her, she asked him to take a look at me as well. He did and said, "Agnes, that boy has smallpox." She threw me out of the bed, and my sister, Virgie, threw me out of the house.

Mama rested and recovered and started looking around to see what else she could do to help my father support the family. She noticed a big, rambling house situated in the center of town, which had been built to serve as a boarding house. It was a place where those who had no family or permanent home could stay and get their meals, either on a weekly or monthly basis.

The people attempting to operate the boarding house earlier had failed miserably, but there were already men and teachers who ate their evening meals at our house, and students and professors from Alcorn College, the first Black land grant college in the country, about four miles from Port Gibson, would stop in too.

The two-story building had eight rooms on the second floor and six rooms on the first. The first floor had a dining room and ample kitchen space. Mama rented the entire building, intending to use six of the rooms on the second floor for rental and four of the rooms downstairs for the family. She contacted Mr. Frishman, who operated furniture and grocery stores, advertised as being the "poor man's friend." Mama bargained with him to outfit the house with used furniture and agreed to pay him the magnificent sum of twenty dollars per month on the outlay. In short order, the Quigless Boarding House was open for business.

During that time, the larger circuses like Ringling Brothers and Barnum & Bailey always had Vicksburg on their itinerary. However, the terrain there was so rough that the circus people had trouble managing the heavy circus wagons, which would get out of control and disrupt the parade, sometimes injuring the animals, especially the elephants. It was for that reason that the circus most often exhibited in a nearby smaller town such as Port Gibson. It was not so far from Vicksburg to prevent the audiences from taking a short drive to view the circus. Whenever circuses came to town, the performers always went throughout the town trying to find home-style cooking.

Mama noticed this and thought it a good idea to furnish the circus performers with the food they liked. Accordingly, she established a roadside stand as close to the circus grounds as possible. She baked several chickens, a couple of fresh hams, a cured ham, made potato salad, and added condiments such as mustard, mayonnaise, ketchup, dill and sweet pickles, and of course, lots of coffee. My father would set up these roadside stands, which Mama would cover with bed sheets.

It was usually early in the morning, most of the time before dawn, when the circus would come by the railroad station. Mama was eager to attract those circus employees who went to work early in the morning without breakfast but would stop long enough to buy a sandwich before starting to work. Their hunger was intensified by the aroma of fresh-brewed coffee. The circus employees stopping by would soon tell others about the good food, and the next thing you knew, there was a long line waiting to be served there at the roadside stand. As a rule, all the sandwiches were sold out by noon.

The stand had to be set up and the food out and ready to be served before dawn. This meant we left home about two o'clock in the morning. My brother, John, my younger sister, Thelma, and I were too young to help, however, we were hustled out with the others and slept on a pallet, which was prepared for us in the wagon. We three younger children made friends with the performers and were always given free tickets to the circus and sideshows.

The most terrifying part of all of this for my mother was the animals. The elephants would pass by our food stand, smell the brewing coffee and cooked food, and start toward the aroma. Using their big trunks to smell, they investigated everything along the highway, including the three of us lying asleep in the wagon. Mama almost had a fit each time; she was afraid they might hurt us, but they never did. Mama would regain her composure once the animals had moved on by.

There were six children in my family. I had three sisters and two brothers. My brother Johnny was four years older than I, born in 1900. My other brother Charlie came along before him, in 1898. Ruth was three years older than Charlie. Virgie, my oldest sister, was born in 1894. And Thelma, the youngest, was born in 1906.

Virgie was very energetic and eager to learn. The colored school only went to the ninth grade, and Virgie, in the eighth grade, did well with her studies. At that time there was a shortage of teachers for the country schools. Virgie decided to leave school and take a teaching job. She passed the exam and was assigned a school on the Mississippi River, near a little village called Grand Gulf, about fifteen miles from Port Gibson. The school was not located in the village but in the wilderness, far from civilization, about a quarter mile from the Mississippi River, surrounded by swamps. Her salary was thirty-five dollars a month, from which she paid ten dollars for room and board and sent from ten to fifteen dollars a month to Mama, leaving enough to spend on herself.

As a rule, schools back then were usually confined to one-room buildings with one teacher for all the different classes. I remember going to one of the schools where Virgie taught. The children sat around in different parts of the building on hard wooden benches. The lunches they brought were very interesting, consisting of a baked sweet potato, a type of molasses bread, or a mixture of cornbread and molasses.

The school supervisor thought that Virgie was doing well teaching the illiterate children in the county. But Virgie had become dissatisfied with her monthly salary. She somehow got in touch with a family in Vermont and went to work for them as a servant. She was there for two years and loved everything except the weather.

From Vermont she moved to Englewood, New Jersey, and got a job as a domestic servant, where the pay was much better. She was able to send money home to help us along. She later heard of another good opening for a domestic servant in Chicago and went to work for Dr. Skyles, a pioneer pediatrician in the "Windy City." Virgie died around 1935 from Graves' disease, or thyrotoxicosis.

My next eldest sister, Ruth, never had a music lesson but could play the piano from the time she was twelve years old. She played by ear and could learn anything she heard. She mystified people by the quality of music she played without ever having a lesson. Ruth finished the ninth grade and applied for a teaching job. At that time, anyone with a diploma could apply for a teaching job and go out into the rural areas to teach. The pay was forty-five to sixty dollars per month. A lot of the teachers taught long enough to make enough money to get away and go north to Chicago or St. Louis.

Ruth taught at a rural school about eight miles from Port Gibson, then later at Hollandale, Mississippi, up in the Delta. At that time, Virgie was working for Dr. Skyles, who lived in the suburbs near Dr. Lownesberry, the chief surgeon of the Chicago,

Milwaukee, and St. Paul Railroad. Dr. Lownesberry had several small children and needed a good helper in his home. Virgie recommended Ruth for the job. So, Ruth went to Chicago.

My oldest brother, Charlie, was a quiet sort of fellow who never had much to say. Charlie and I developed a special relationship. As far back as I can remember, I was very much underweight. I always wanted to play and do the things other children my age were doing. In view of my frail physical condition, my mother saw to it that I was accompanied by Charlie. Charlie was about eight years older and felt burdened by having to look after his little brother. Whenever he went out to play, I would tell Mama that I wanted to go, too. Mama would say, "Charlie, now you must take your little brother with you."

That would always make Charlie angry, and he'd say, "Ah shucks, Mama. I don't want to be bothered by looking after that little brat. Why can't you keep him home?"

Then Mama would repeat, "If you can't take your little brother with you, then you can't go." Charlie would relent and let me tag along. This scene repeated itself every afternoon after school. I think Charlie really began to hate my guts.

He hated school as much as I did, and he really loved hunting. With his single-barrel shotgun, Charlie became quite proficient at killing birds, adding to our menu from time to time. I got the idea that I wanted to go hunting with Charlie. He protested and complained that I'd get hurt if I followed him, but as usual, Mama insisted he take me along.

One day, Charlie got so exasperated with me for not listening to him that he turned on me and said, "Boy, I don't know what to do with you. I feel like knocking your brains out." He began hitting me on top of my head. I began feeling funny and blacked out. Sometime later I came to and found myself lying on the ground. Charlie was shaking me and calling my name over and over. When I finally was able to answer, he stood me up. Charlie said, "Promise me you won't tell Mama about this, and I'll take you hunting every time I go."

I was so glad to hear him say he would take me hunting without the customary argument that I readily agreed. From that day forward he routinely called me whenever he wanted to go hunting. I was no trouble to him. I followed his advice, and as long as we were in the woods and the gun was loaded, I stayed directly behind him.

After about six hunting seasons, when I was about eleven or twelve, Charlie said to me, "Milton, I think you're old enough to shoot this gun. I'm going to put a tin can on this stump, and I want you to shoot it off." I was ecstatic. I took the gun, cocked it, aimed it at the tin can, and pulled the trigger. When the shot fired, the shotgun kicked the hell out of me. Charlie decided then and there that it would be a long time before I could shoot the gun again. However, he persuaded my father to get me a single shot rifle and taught me how to load it and aim at the target. From that day on, whenever we went hunting, he had the shotgun, and I had my rifle.

When I got my rifle, I started hunting for birds with our dog, Old Top. With this rifle that only cost $7.50 new, I missed so many birds that one day my dog lay down in the field and refused to point any more of them. It was Charlie who discovered a way to remedy the dilemma. Again, he set a tin can on a stump so I could practice aiming. When I first pulled the trigger, the bullet struck a board three feet to the right of the can. About thirty shots later, Charlie showed me how to aim three feet to the left of the can. Gradually, I started hitting the bull's eye.

Mama always saw to it that Charlie was along when I went hunting. So, when Charlie got a job, I didn't have a chance to go hunting anymore. One day, I slipped out of the house, got the dog, and went alone. Old Top flushed a covey of quail, I singled out one, took aim, and shot. I winged the bird. When it fell to the ground, there was a mad scramble between me and Old Top. Finally, I caught it, and because it was out of season, I hid it in my shirt and tore out for home.

I was so excited about having killed a bird that I didn't slip back into the house. I ran in the front door and right into Mama. She was so mad at me for going hunting without Charlie that she bopped me across the head. It so happened that there was a cocklebur on my cap that stuck in her hand, which infuriated her even more. However, when I pulled the bird from my shirt, she too became elated. After all, I had killed a bird on my own. Old Top appeared to be elated also. I cleaned the bird, and Mama cooked it for me. She made some gravy, which she poured over some grits, and I had a sumptuous meal all by myself.

CHAPTER 2

INSPIRATION

Our family was never destitute nor hungry. We existed under circumstances whereby we could not splurge. We always had good Christmas holidays, and Santa Claus always came with fruits, nuts, and the like. We had the necessities because everyone worked and did so under the supervision of my mother, the real brains of the family.

I was very fond of my mother and followed her around all the time. One cool fall day she was raking leaves, and I was "helping," though not very well. A lady came to the fence, calling my mother over. "Mrs. Quigless, come here a minute. Get up to Mrs. Smith's house right away!" They had a whispered conversation, and then Mama said, "Okay, I'll be right there!" She told me to go into the house, but I wanted to go with her. When I argued, she simply repeated, "I said to go in the house." I protested, saying, "No, I want to go with you." She turned me around, whacked my bottom a couple of times, ran me into the house, and shut the door. I climbed out the window and ran up the street behind her.

At Mrs. Smith's house, Mama knocked on the door, and when it was opened, I ran around her, right into the room. What faced me was such a traumatic experience that even now I'm not able to recall it all. As I ran into the house, a lady cried, "Good God Almighty! What is that boy doing in here?" I looked around and saw a lady whom I knew real well, except now she was in the bed crying, grunting, and screaming, and her legs were propped open. There was a big round thing between her legs. She cried out again, "Good God Almighty! Get that boy out of here."

One woman threw me to another, with the second one throwing me out the door. At the same time, I heard Miss Lottie King telling them, "Don't do him like that! You're going to make him remember everything. Take it easy. Just ease him out the door."

I was lying out in the chicken yard when Miss Lottie came out and got me. She washed my face, gave me a piece of cake, took me in her arms, and asked, "Do you want to see the baby?"

I didn't know what she meant when she talked about seeing the baby. She took me into a room where there was a real baby that looked just like my sister had when she was much younger. This baby looked funny. It was quiet, real quiet. It wasn't fussing or kicking its heels up, and it looked slimy and greasy. Miss Lottie asked, "Do you like the baby? Isn't it a pretty baby?"

I didn't see anything pretty about it. Later, I realized I had been looking at a dead baby. The lady gave birth to twins. The first one had been born dead, and the mother was in the process of delivering the second when I barged in. I got hooked on medicine that very morning. From then on, I was inquisitive every time I saw anybody in pain. I had to see what was going on. If I saw anyone, or anything, bleeding, I'd try to stop it. I became very concerned whenever I found that somebody was ill.

About that time, I noticed that everyone seemed to be taking a special interest in me and trying to feed me. I was puny and very skinny but didn't know what all the fuss was about. From then until I was old enough to go to school, I got everything I wanted very easily. When I was six years old and the time came to go to school, my happy existence seemed to end abruptly. I didn't like getting up early, getting dressed, and getting out in the chilly wind to walk a mile to school. And after getting to school, I had to sit on a hard bench all day.

The only part of school I enjoyed was the opening hour when everybody came into the largest room in the school, and Mr. Addison, the principal, got up to say a few words and sing hymns. Then, we marched back to our respective rooms.

My first grade teacher was Mrs. Richardson. She taught first through third grades. As I think back on it now, I feel she gave all her students a good foundation. I was there to learn my ABC's. Mrs. Richardson pointed to a letter of the alphabet on the board, and we followed along in a sing-song manner. We learned our alphabet and then started putting simple words together on our slates. I was soon bored with all that stuff.

At the second-grade level, we had books. We were assigned one or two pages to study overnight and had to recite those pages the next day. After reciting the pages, I would sit and listen to the other classmates recite the same thing. I sat there listening for the bell to ring in the end of the school day. I was anxious to get back home and check on the chickens, dogs, cats, and Old Kate, the mule. Whenever I'd find an injured animal around, I would do whatever I could to bind their wounds or make them more comfortable. As a general rule, when you approach an injured animal, you have to be very careful, or they turn on you and bite. Oddly enough, they never did that to me.

We always had two or three dogs around. Once we had a female dog, Pup, that I noticed was getting very fat. One day I came home from school and called her but couldn't find Pup anywhere. I finally found her all curled up under the house. She wouldn't come to me. I soon found that my dog was having puppies. After a while, my father came looking for me. I called to him, "Come here and see what's happening to Pup." He came over and didn't snatch me up or try to run me away. Instead, he tried to explain what was happening.

First, I had seen the baby being born, and now I was watching puppies being born. I became even more interested in animals than before.

Once, between the ages of five and six, I was walking down the street and saw some larger boys chasing one another. One, Will Crawford, slipped and fell right in front of a horse-drawn buggy and was impaled on the buggy shaft. The shaft entered the right side of his chest, and he was just hanging there. A man came and pulled him off the shaft, which left a gaping hole in the boy's right side. The incident happened right in front of Dr. Sherrod's office. He ran out, bringing a towel which he stuffed into the gaping hole. The doctor then got out a needle and thread, and even though the boy was screaming, he began closing up the hole without the aid of anesthesia. That was the first operation I ever witnessed.

The nearest hospital to Port Gibson was in Vicksburg, and only the most serious injuries were transported there, most often by train—that is, if the injured or their families had enough money to pay for hospitalization. It goes without saying that most of the Blacks were unable to pay for hospital care, and unless the landowners agreed to pay for it, the Blacks had only the local physicians to take care of them. There were four white doctors in Port Gibson: Drs. Acker, May, Redus, and Bailey.

Dr. Acker didn't have much of a practice. To tell the truth, he was more interested in farming than practicing medicine. One day, while I was working in a department store, I had a wad of chewing tobacco in my mouth. Dr. Acker came in, saw me, and laughed, saying, "Hey, hey—chewing tobacco." I had so much in my mouth that I became dizzy. The next thing I knew, I was on the floor. That tobacco had made me drunk as a fish. I was later told that when I passed out, Dr. Acker reached a finger in my mouth and pulled the wad of tobacco out. Someone else dashed cold water over my head. I was taken home and put directly to bed where I stayed the remainder of the day. I was still dizzy the following day. Needless to say, that ended my tobacco chewing.

Another time, I was walking down the street and saw a boy I didn't particularly like. We fought every time we came near each other. This time when we started fighting, I had him on the ground. I looked around and saw one of his big brothers was coming up with a brick in his hand.

I got up and ran like the devil. He started after me and was gaining on me, so I ducked behind a tree. That was the worst thing I could have done because the tree was small. I threw out my arm to ward off the blow of the brick. It hit my forearm, causing severe pain in my elbow. I tried straightening my arm but couldn't. I went home crying.

Dr. May's office was less than two blocks from my house. Mama took me there, and Dr. May told me I had dislocated my elbow. He manipulated my arm until my elbow relocated. I had no further relationship with Dr. May until my little sister got a goiter, but Dr. May didn't know what was wrong with her.

While I was working in the drugstore, Dr. Redus would come in quite often and talk with the people gathered there while he sipped a Coke. From these conversations I learned that he had been trained at Johns Hopkins. He was the physician who took care of the more serious injuries in town. As I remember it, Dr. Redus was the best-prepared physician in the area. If a Black person was injured or seriously ill and, for one reason or another, could not be taken to the hospital in Vicksburg, Dr. Redus would be called in.

He was a tall, lanky man who talked fast. He didn't lose any time in treating patients. He would ask a few questions, pop a thermometer in their mouths, say "uh hum" two or three times, and start writing prescriptions.

Dr. Sherrod was the only Black doctor in Port Gibson. Nowadays you hear a lot about role models. I didn't know anything about the term "role model" when I was a kid, although as a child I heard a lot about Dr. Sherrod. I was about eight years old when I finally had a chance to meet and talk with him. From the first time I learned who he was, I noticed and watched him, because I already had thoughts of becoming a doctor. This tall, handsome, dignified gentleman greatly interested me.

Dr. Sherrod had brown skin, walked very erectly, and was immaculately dressed at all times. In the winter, he wore a black wrap coat, striped trousers, and black shoes with gray spats. He smoked a pipe and looked just like the man depicted on the Prince Albert tobacco can. He spoke slowly, his voice low and soothing, and his English was very good.

I took note of these characteristics with the idea that I had to walk, talk, and act exactly that way when I became a doctor. I also admired the high-spirited horse he had hitched to his polished ribbon-tied buggy as he drove to his office every morning. I admired the way he controlled his horse and his low, smooth-spoken commands. I never saw him use a whip on the horse. I even remember his first car. I was impressed with the idea of his having an automobile. I was sorry, however, that he got rid of his horse and buggy.

Dr. Sherrod was doing quite well in his practice when I spoke to him one day. He said, "Hello, my boy." I remember how good I felt with that greeting. I made it a point to cross the street, sit on his step, and ply him with questions while he sat in an easy chair waiting for his next patient. He didn't seem to mind my intrusions on his leisure time and always encouraged me to return the following day to talk. I wanted to ask him to give me a ride in his new car, but I never got the nerve.

Dr. Sherrod was dedicated to serving his people. If I had been made to suffer all the hardships he did during his lifetime, I know I would have left Port Gibson and all those Black people to their own fate.

Dr. Sherrod came to Port Gibson and started his business shortly after finishing medical school. His first office was in a two-room cabin. After a few years, he was able to get enough money together to build an office. He saw lots of patients, and most of them had little or no money. The white doctors in the community paid him little attention. Because he was the only Black doctor in town, they referred their Black patients to him. They did not want to treat them anyway and would send them to "their own doctor."

He employed a cleaning lady who worked with him for three or four years. She decided to marry and asked Dr. Sherrod to loan her enough money to buy furniture. He agreed to do it if she would sign a note, agreeing to pay him so much per month until the note was clear. She made monthly payments for about six months and then suddenly stopped working for Dr. Sherrod. She stopped making payments altogether, saying she had paid him all she owed. Dr. Sherrod looked for the note she signed but could not find it anywhere. He made a grave mistake at that point. He made another note and signed her name to it. When they went to court, he produced the note he had forged, and she then turned around and produced the original. He was charged with forgery.

It was felt that Dr. Sherrod was getting ahead too fast, much to the chagrin of many of the whites. The judge convicted him of forgery and sentenced him to one year in jail, which Dr. Sherrod served. During that time, he lost his building.

After being released from jail, he took up practice again in another two-room shack where he stayed until he was able to erect another office just off Main Street in the center of town. In his new office, he added a pharmacy and hired a pharmacist fresh out of school. His practice took off, and he was able to buy his first car.

Dr. Sherrod prospered despite all the roadblocks put in his way. He married a lady who was not from Port Gibson. She was very light-skinned. In fact, unless they were told, most folks did not know if she was white or colored. Mrs. Sherrod stood by him through everything, even when he was in prison. After resuming his practice, he was able to build a nice new modern home that even included a bathroom with a tub, which did not set too well with the white folks in town.

Later, Mrs. Sherrod became seriously ill and started having convulsions. Dr. Sherrod called in some white doctors to treat her. The white doctors suspected that Mrs. Sherrod was suffering from strychnine poisoning, which they believed had been administered by Dr. Sherrod. In spite of their treatment, Mrs. Sherrod died. The house was quarantined, and a pathologist was called in from the University of Mississippi Medical School to conduct an autopsy, which caused much talk. No strychnine was found in her body, and it was determined that she had died of meningitis. The funeral was arranged for the next day, a very cold and stormy day. I shall never forget it. I was shining shoes at Bo Watson's barbershop when all of this happened and had a hard time cleaning off that red cemetery mud.

Dr. Sherrod had a brother who also practiced medicine in another Mississippi town. When he heard of Dr. Sherrod's troubles, he came to Port Gibson to visit him. As he approached the house, which was under guard by the law, he was told he could not enter. He informed the police in no uncertain terms that he, too, was a doctor, that this was his brother's house, and he was going in. The guards did not put up any resistance. He had to have a place to stay while in Port Gibson, so he came to my mother's boardinghouse for food and lodging. He seemed quite upset about the way Dr. Sherrod was being treated. He did not seem the type to take insults kindly, and when he removed his coat, I noticed a big pistol strapped under his left arm.

I continued spending time talking with Dr. Sherrod until I left Port Gibson to attend Alcorn College. When I returned on holidays, I'd quote my progress to him. He always seemed interested in what I was doing. I was in pre-med school, working as a sleeping car porter and railroad employee, which enabled me to get free passes to travel on almost all railroads. It was then, as it is now, that most high schools and colleges observed spring break. As a rule, I would get a pass on the Illinois Central Railroad and go to Port Gibson to visit my folks. I would also visit Dr. Sherrod.

On one such visit, I got a disquieting report about Dr. Sherrod. I was told that he had been tricked out of a sum of money by a small group of white people who had come to Port Gibson. One of the white women went to Dr. Sherrod's office asking for treatment. He was talking to her when two white men broke through the door, accusing Dr. Sherrod of sexual molestation of the woman. They told him they would report him to the police if he did not give them five hundred dollars.

In view of the trouble that he'd had with the law before, Dr. Sherrod decided to give them the money and wrote a check.

The group left his office, and Dr. Sherrod immediately stopped payment on the check. In the meantime, the white men went to the hardware store and bought a plow for twenty-five dollars and presented Dr. Sherrod's check for payment. The merchant gave the men their change, and they left town. When the merchant presented the check for payment at the bank, he was told that Dr. Sherrod had stopped payment.

The merchant demanded that the bank cashier give him his money "because he was not going to let that nigger doctor cause him to lose five-hundred dollars." The cashier gave the merchant the money, and Dr. Sherrod lost his.

By that time, Dr. Sherrod was getting old in spirit and in health. I had been practicing in Tarboro, North Carolina about six years when my mother informed me that Dr. Sherrod had died in his sleep. When I think back over Dr. Sherrod's life as I knew it, I admire his dedication to treating Black patients and his determination to continue working under difficult circumstances.

I have often wondered if his difficulties subconsciously affected my activities in Tarboro, influencing me to go on with my work in spite of roadblocks. I wonder if the roadblocks which caused him to work harder had anything to do with my decision to operate on patients in tenant houses, to build a hospital without help, to run a pharmacy where indigent patients could buy medications at reduced prices, and to try to make living a little easier for the people I treated. I have, however, enjoyed one great advantage over Dr. Sherrod's own labors under difficult circumstances in Mississippi. I have had the sympathy, and even cooperation, from most of the people in North Carolina, Black and white.

CHAPTER 3

NO SCHOOL DAYS

lthough I wanted to become a doctor, I hated school and was always trying to figure out ways to keep from going. Mrs. McCloud taught fourth and fifth grades. She was very strict and demanded that we do our lessons. If we didn't, she had a way of stimulating us with a rattan switch. I liked her though because she took interest in each of us.

The sixth and seventh grades were taught by Mrs. Belgrave. I understood from other students that she was very tough. To tell the truth, one of the reasons I stopped going to school was to keep from going into her class. I figured that if I complained of headaches, stomachaches, or sore throats early enough in the morning, my parents would let me stay in bed. Being the skinniest thing already, I found I could hoodwink them very easily. My father seemed to know from the beginning that I was putting them on to keep from going to school. When he started to hit me, however, my mother would say, "No, don't hit him. Remember, he's very puny, and you might hurt him." So, I would get to stay home. I'd stay in bed until around 9 or 9:30 a.m., then get up and tell my mother, "I'm feeling much better, Mama."

"Okay, just eat your breakfast," she said. "Then if you feel like going back to bed, you may."

I'd go back and get a book and start reading. Sometimes I'd stay in bed all day long if I didn't have anything interesting enough to get me up and going. I began having throat trouble about that time and found that it wasn't necessary to make up an excuse to keep me from going to school. My parents took me to Dr. Bailey. He told them my sore throat needed to be treated. I went to see him three times a week, every other day.

While he treated me, I asked a lot of questions. I'd ask him what he was putting in my throat whenever he painted my tonsils with iodine. After a while, my throat got worse, and when he painted it, I'd almost choke. An old lady told my mother, "That doctor is going to kill that boy, when all he needs is to gargle with salt water, and he'll get along all right."

Well, Mama started that, and my throat got better. It got to the place it didn't hurt at all. But even so, I was having trouble swallowing. The fact was my tonsils had gotten so large that they almost met in the middle. So, they took me back to Dr. Bailey. He looked at my throat and said, "Well, his tonsils will have to be removed." My mother asked where she should take me. The doctor replied, "Oh, I can remove them myself. Bring him up here next Friday morning." The next Friday morning he took me into his office and had me lean back in a chair and open my mouth. He then got out his syringe. I asked, "What are you going to do now, Doctor?"

He said, "I'm going to inject you with some cocaine, so you won't hurt, and I'll take your tonsils out." Sure enough, after a needle prick, I didn't feel any more pain. His instrument consisted of a knife in the form of a ring with a fork attached to the contraption so that when he placed the ring over my tonsil and pushed a lever, the fork would go through the tonsil and the ring would cut it off.

Suddenly, there was a gush of blood. Now, get this! He had me gargle with some hot water to stop the bleeding. I don't know how I lived through that surgery. He took out one tonsil that day. I think he got a little panicky because I was bleeding. He told me to come back the next Friday, and he'd remove the other tonsil. I went back, and he repeated the previous procedure. Aside from a little sore throat that followed, everything was all right. The only reason I didn't bleed to death was because the good Lord wasn't ready for me yet. I get cold sweats now when I recall how my tonsils were removed.

Later, after I had finished my medical studies, I went back home for a visit with my folks and saw this same doctor. He was very old and feeble. I walked up to him and asked, "Dr. Bailey, do you remember me?"

He said, "Well, let's see."

I prompted, "Do you remember that little skinny fellow whose tonsils you took out?"

"Oh, you're that little skinny fellow! You're still skinny! I was afraid you were going to die on me that time. I think about that, and it scares the heck out of me. You know one thing?"

"What, Dr. Bailey?"

"That was the first set of tonsils I ever removed. And that was the last."

I really did feel panicky then.

***

When I was in about the fourth grade, I had said so much about being sick, feeling weak, and having headaches, that one day my parents called Dr. Sherrod in to take a look at me. Dr. Sherrod put on his glasses and called for a glass of water to stick his thermometer in. After rolling it around in the water, he stuck it into my mouth. I don't know where it had been before that, but anyway, that's the way he did things. He took the thermometer out and gazed at it for a while. Then he asked my parents to go out of the room with him. After about ten minutes they returned without Dr. Sherrod, who had gone back to his office.

My mother said, "If you don't want to go to school, that's all right. You go when you feel like it."

I went back to school and finished through the fifth grade. I decided then that I would tell them I felt so bad all the time that I didn't think I wanted to go to school any longer. You know what they said? "Well, okay, that's all right. If you don't want to go, you don't have to." They let me out of it right then and there. Boy, was I having myself a ball! As a result of their decision, I didn't enroll in the sixth grade that September.

It was along about this time that some building was going on in town. A brick mason needed a place to stay, so he came around to the Quigless Boarding House. The man was Mr. Milton Brooks from Paducah, Kentucky—a real Kentucky gentleman. His main occupation was bricklayer, but he also did cement finishing on floors and walkways. He loved to talk, and he also loved his bourbon.

He was a tough hombre and would talk all about the fights he had been in. Once, he said, he had killed a man in self-defense during a fight. The man was Black, so the law didn't bother pressing charges against Mr. Brooks.

Once, he installed a sidewalk in front of a business. The cement had been poured late in the afternoon, and he couldn't finish it until the cement had set. Around ten o'clock that night, I held a lantern for him while he put the finishing touches on the sidewalk, finishing the job around two o'clock in the morning.

After he had been with us about two days, he noticed me hanging around. He asked, "Mrs. Quigless, why is that boy not in school?"

Mama answered, "He stays sick all the time, so we just thought it better to let him stay out until he felt like going again."

He replied, "Mrs. Quigless, that boy is not sick. He just doesn't like going to school." My mother reflected, "That sure is the truth."

Mr. Brooks suggested, "Let me take this boy in hand." So, from that day on, we got to be good buddies. He loved to talk, and I loved to listen. He liked fishing, and I loved to go fishing. It got to the place that every afternoon, after he finished work, we would go to the creek and put the line in and fish until dark. The whole time he would be talking. He asked me, "Son, I think you're a pretty good little fellow. What's wrong that you don't want to go to school?"

I said, "I just don't like school."

"Why don't you like school?" he pressed.

"You sit there all day long and hear the same thing over and over," I answered.

He reasoned, "Son, that's the way it is. You've got to do that in order to get some place. What would you like to be when you grow up?"

"I'd like to be a doctor. That's the only thing I want to do."

He said, "Son, you can't be a doctor unless you go to school." His son was a doctor and had finished medicine at Old Leonard Medical School. He talked about how his son had gotten through school, how hard he had to work, and how successful he was. He said, "My son finished medicine and is a big doctor out in Oklahoma. You could do the same thing."

I queried, "You think so, Mr. Brooks?"

He said, "Yes!" Then he started talking about his granddaughter. He said, "Now, I tell you, son, you're a nice little boy, and I'd like for you to meet my granddaughter sometime."

That man worried me talking about his granddaughter. She was this, that, and the other. She could play violin and piano; she could do this; she could do that; she could do everything. I got tired of listening to him.

On Saturdays he'd send to Vicksburg and get a quart of bourbon and sip it all weekend. He liked me so well that he said, "Son, I'm going to get you something that you can drink. You can't drink no liquor, but I'm going to get you something so we can drink together." He got me a quart of Crème de Menthe, which I thought was the best stuff I had ever tasted in my life.

Bricklayers and carpenters all liked their liquor, so they'd all get together to do their drinking. On Fridays they would order a keg of beer and put it in the ice house overnight. They'd also buy a box of crackers, along with a round of cheese and a case of salmon. Saturdays they would drink beer while eating salmon and cheese with the crackers. One day, Mr. Brooks told my mother that he thought he knew something that would make me fat. "All he needs to do is drink beer every day or at least on the weekends with us."

Mama exclaimed, "Oh Lord, drinking beer at his age?"

"Now it won't hurt him, but it'll make him fat." The next weekend when he got ready to go for his beer drinking spree, he said, "Come on boy, let's go and get some beer!" We entered the place, and everybody looked at me.

"What the hell are you doing, bringing that boy in here? What will people say about him drinking beer?"

"That's all right. Let him drink some beer."

They responded, "You can't do that!"

He told them, "Damn it to hell! I'm in on this beer keg, and he is going to drink it if he wants to."

There was another man there—Mr. Lindsey, a barber. He had a son about my age called "Brother," whom I used to whip all the time. Mr. Lindsey said, "If he can drink beer, then I'll bring

Brother in and let him get some too." So, the next weekend, he brought Brother and gave him some beer. Brother didn't like the stuff because it was bitter. The old man tried to make him drink it, but he wouldn't.

I drank beer every Saturday for about three months, and it didn't put a pound on me.

During the spring when the weather became warm, our fishing trips began again. Mr. Brooks would get home about five o'clock, we would eat dinner, then light out for a fishing hole. We would fish until it got so dark, we couldn't see the cork bobble up and down.

I shall never forget the first trout I ever caught. We went to Lake Karnak, a beautiful lake of about six acres surrounded by Cypress trees of all sizes. Some had been blown over by the wind. With the roots being on shore and the trunks in the water, it was easy to walk out nearly forty feet from the shoreline. I walked out on one almost to the very end and dropped my hook in with a wiggling worm on it. Something grabbed it and started carrying it away. I yanked it as hard as I could, and the fish was hooked. I was very excited but still managed to get the fish onto the log where I was standing. Mr. Brooks took a look and said, "Good boy! You caught a trout that time, and what a fine one it is too!"

I was tickled pink, but I made a big mistake when I took the fish off the hook. I was holding the trout in my hand while trying to put it on a stringer with the other two fish I had caught. However, the trout gave one good flip and was gone back into the water. I went right into the water after it. I couldn't swim, but it so happened that the water was only about three feet deep. Mr. Brooks jumped in and pulled me out by my britches. He gave me a good lecture on water safety, how to handle fish, and how to keep cool and not become too excited.

Along about the middle of August that year, I began tiring of the fishing trips. So, during the day when Mr. Brooks was at work, I'd wander all over town. I would wander to the garage and watch Mr. Fitzmore work on automobiles. I would go up by the pressing shop and watch Gus Lefure clean and press clothes. All the time I was getting more and more bored. Then I began running around with a little gang of what could be called juvenile delinquents. There were about seven or eight of us who spent days on end picking up scrap iron anywhere we could find it, though mostly around the blacksmith shop. We would sell it to Mr. Charlie Waterman who never asked any questions. We would sometimes run errands for anyone who asked. However, when pickings became slim so far as the scrap iron and errands were concerned, some of the gang decided to steal any little thing that could be sold on the corner. There was even talk of breaking into houses whenever it was known that the occupants would be away. That's when I quit the gang. I became a loner, and the gang went on its merry way. Within the next two years, three members of the gang were sent to reform school for stealing.

After I quit running with the gang, I began amusing myself by walking around town looking in on anything that caught my interest. There was a small, one-room frame building near my mother's boarding house that was Arthur Watson's barbershop, who was more familiarly known as "Bo." Each day I'd hang around his shop and listen to the talk. There were two barber chairs in the shop. Sometimes, especially on Saturdays, another barber would come in to work with Bo. There were twelve chairs for the customers.

Bo would place small towels under the chins of his customers on which he could wipe his razor as he shaved them. I offered to keep his towels washed, and he paid me fifty cents a dozen. At that time, I also considered myself efficient at shining shoes. There was a shoeshine stand in the shop, and Bo Watson suggested that I use it in exchange for keeping the shop clean. I agreed.

Two or three afternoons each week, especially during the winter, a few guys would get together in the warm barbershop and sing. There was Gus Lefure, Sid Belk, Wesley Williams, Joe Welbert, Rufus Thomas, and one or two others whose names I can't recall. It was an informal group, and anyone who thought he could sing was welcomed to chime in. If they did not sing well enough, we would just boot them out the door and keep on singing. They would sing spirituals, popular songs, and songs that different members of the group composed. I joined the group. My voice had not changed at that time, so I sang first tenor. We'd start with "Sweet Adeline," go into "In the Evening by the Moonlight," and go from there to spirituals and "soulfuls." The singing experience helped me later in life.

My cousin, Fred King, was a shoemaker. He had a nice place where I liked to go to hear tall tales being told. Cousin Fred came from the country, went to Alcorn College to learn shoemaking, and came back to Port Gibson to set up his shoe repair shop. He did very well. He even worked up to a huge Singer sewing machine that sewed soles on shoes—without a motor. It was run by heavy foot power but was still a great contraption to me.

I really enjoyed watching that strong needle carry the heavy thread in and out of the shoe soles, attaching them firmly to the sides of the shoes. I liked it so well that I decided that I would probably become a shoemaker.

Along about that time, the largest and most important drugstore in the town was totally destroyed by fire. Jabbo, the Black man who assisted Mr. Joseph, the pharmacist, struck a match close to the turpentine barrel. The match head flew over into the sawdust that was spread around the turpentine barrel to catch the drippings.

A huge blaze developed immediately, and the turpentine barrel was engulfed in flames. Jabbo ran out just in time to avoid being caught in the explosion when the turpentine barrel erupted. The fire raced through the entire drugstore in about ten minutes. By the time the fire department arrived, the blaze was completely out-of-control. It burned about four hours. That really gave me something to watch!

The reconstruction of the drugstore was done mostly by Blacks. I watched the workmen clear out the burned fixtures and the carpenters come in and do their jobs. A Black plasterer was brought up from Natchez to finish the inside of the building. Tile men came in and laid the floor. Across the front of the floor was the pharmacist's name "J.G. Joseph," spelled out in the tile. When they started putting in the fixtures, I was always around to see what was going on. When they unpacked the showcases, it was noticed that the interiors needed cleaning. Since I was the smallest thing around there, Mr. J.G. Joseph took one look at me and said, "Kid, get in there and clean those showcases, and I'll give you some change."

I cleaned the showcases to his satisfaction, and he paid me thirty-five cents for doing so. I spent about half a day on that job, then he decided that there were other little things that needed to be done, so he started calling on me. "Quig, do this. Quig, do that," he said. I had found a place where I was wanted and needed. I was very happy with that. When the time to reopen the drugstore drew near, Mr. Joseph looked around and said, "Well, we're going to need a delivery boy. Would you like that job, Quig?"

"Yes sir, that is the very thing I would like to do," I answered. I loved the idea. I'd be at the drugstore where I could eat all the ice cream I wanted, drink all the Coca Cola I wanted, and not have to work too hard at that. The time finally came for the reopening, and Mr. Joseph chose the people he would need to operate it. First, there was himself, the owner and registered pharmacist. Then there was a white man by the name of Neal Hacket, but we all called him Mr. Happy Hacket.

Also, there was Abram Graves, whom we called Jabbo. He acted as the chief janitor, stockman, and the fellow who made that good store-bought ice cream. My job, of course, was that of delivery boy. I enjoyed sitting in the pharmacy watching Mr. Joseph filling prescriptions. He gave me the job of washing and sterilizing bottles so they could be reused for prescriptions he filled. Later he gave me the job of filling one-ounce and two-ounce size bottles with turpentine, castor oil, and spirits of nitre (a strong-smelling substance that the country folks used for bellyaches and fever).

Jabbo started calling on me to help him freeze the ice cream. The ice cream room was in the rear of the drugstore. Jabbo was a master at fixing the milk, cream, and flavoring with some gelatin to give the ice cream smoothness. I liked that part of my work because after the ice cream was frozen and transferred to the big ten-gallon cans at the soda fountain, there would always be enough for me to fill up on before beginning the task of cleaning up the ice cream freezer and flushing out the room. I kept the job at the drugstore for three years.

However, there was a department store further down the block where a delivery boy was needed. Mr. Joseph was paying me four dollars per week, but Mr. Krauss at the D. Bock Department Store offered to pay me six dollars per week. I couldn't turn the offer down. While sitting around Bo Watson's Barbershop, I mentioned the fact that I was going to change jobs. John Odom, one of my old gang buddies, asked me to recommend him for the job at the drugstore.

I told him I would recommend him under one condition: if I ever wanted to get my old job back, I could come and take it from him. He agreed. I told Mr. Joseph that I had a good boy for him and introduced him to John. Would you believe it? John Odom worked at that drugstore from 1915 until his retirement in 1970.

I started work at the D. Bock Department Store, which was also a very interesting job. The owner, Mr. David Bock, was a Jew who had immigrated from Poland and traveled throughout this portion of the South as an itinerant peddler with a pack on his back. He sold cloth, lace, and anything else that women needed to make clothes for the family.

Mr. Bock made enough money to open a small store in Port Gibson. He instinctively knew what poor people wanted and needed. He furnished the merchandise at an attractive price, which caused his business to grow to such a degree that his store was ultimately enlarged, taking on the impressive name of D. Bock's Department Store. He went on to establish a wholesale business in Vicksburg. After opening the store in Port Gibson, he sent back to Poland for Felix, his younger brother. Felix Bock became the bookkeeper and cashier at the store.

Mr. Sid Krauss, a member of a family of merchants with a store in Fayette, Mississippi, was Mr. Bock's partner. As I understand it, Mr. Krauss was able to amass enough money to invest in the department store with Mr. Bock. Later, when the Depression hit hard, he was able to take over the store and push out all the Bocks. It ended up as S. Krauss's Department Store.

Mr. Johnny Watkins, the son of a butcher in Port Gibson, was the chief salesman at the department store. In addition, there was a younger fellow who worked there named Hix Anderson, the son of an immigrant from Sweden.

I brought up the rear as porter and delivery boy. I liked the job at the store. It made me feel important. It made me feel good to know that I had certain duties to perform and that I carried out my duties to the satisfaction of the owners. I was in that job about three years. However, I became more and more dissatisfied with my lot in life and questioned, within myself, the wisdom of deciding to quit school.

One day, Mr. Watkins said there had been another porter who had worked at the store for sixteen years before quitting to go north. I was getting paid six dollars a week, so I asked Mr. Watkins how much he'd paid this fellow, George, who had preceded me. He said, "Well, he worked here for many years, so he was being paid fifteen dollars a week."

That sounded bad to me. I couldn't see myself working in a store for fifteen years and only being paid that much. During the Christmas holidays, other young boys my age were employed to help out. However, all of them were in school and were talking better than me. They could also read faster. I was soon beginning to envy those fellows.

In the meantime, Mr. Brooks had decided to bring his wife from Kentucky and buy a home in Port Gibson. Mom Brooks, as I called her, was a very impressive little lady. We took to each other right away. Mom Brooks tried to get me fat too. She fed the heck out of me. I could eat at home and then go to Mom Brooks's house and eat some more. But to no avail—I never gained a pound!

I saw Mr. Brooks one day, and he said, "Well, Milton, my grand-daughter, Mattie, is coming to spend the summer with us. I know you are going to like her."

One day, while I was arranging a display in one of the store's three show windows, I looked up to see Mr. Brooks looking in. He was with the cutest little brown-skinned girl I had ever seen in my life. I almost fell out of that show window getting out to speak to them. Mattie was a little short, but she had two long plaits of black hair that hung just about to her waist. She had a soothing voice without that Mississippi drawl to which I was so accustomed.

Mr. Brooks said, "Well, what do you think about my granddaughter?"

I couldn't do anything but just stand there and stammer. I believe I said that I would be down for supper that day. I wanted to get acquainted with Mattie right away, and that I did. Mattie and her mother had come down to visit her grandparents. Mattie was a junior in high school, and here I was having only finished the fifth grade. That didn't set well with me either.

Come Sunday morning, I went to church, and Mattie was there. She played a solo on her violin. I had gone nuts over that pretty little girl by that time. In no time flat, we were going steady with the smiling approval of Mattie's mother. Mattie's father was the General Secretary of the A.M.E. Church and traveled all over the United States. When he came to Port Gibson to visit his family, I met this tall, dignified gentleman who apparently approved of me also. I was on Cloud Nine by that time. After church, and after eating dinner, I would turn up at the Brooks' home to take Mattie out. We would go off on our Sunday afternoon walk. In that day and time, we had no disco, TV, or radio. But, boy, was it fun to take those long walks around town, returning home at just about dusk. And, if nobody was looking, I would steal a kiss just before we got to the Brooks' house.

It just so happened that Mr. Tom Johnson, a very successful Black farmer who owned a three-hundred-acre farm about five miles from Port Gibson, had a son just about my age. But, unlike me, Tommy had continued to go to school. He met Mattie and took a shine to her, just as I had. He began paying a little bit too much attention to Mattie for my comfort. To make matters worse, Mr. Johnson had a big, long Studebaker car.

One Sunday, I went around to Mattie's to take her out on our regular Sunday afternoon walk, and she had just left with Tommy in that big, long Studebaker. Boy, was I upset! That guy had started making moves on my territory. I resented his intrusion just as much as Mattie seemed to enjoy the current turn of events. After he started riding her around in his Studebaker on Sunday afternoons, I could be found sitting on the corner turning green with envy whenever they passed by.

All my buddies sensed the situation and tried to give me some consolation. They tried to figure out a way to get back at Tommy without having to be put in jail. I would still go around to the Brooks' house at intervals, but it seemed as though I had been toned down from making any headway. As the summer drew to a close, time came for Mattie to go back to Kentucky, and back to school. She let it be known to everyone, including me, that Tommy Johnson and the Studebaker were just passing fancies. In the end, I was the guy who walked with her to the railroad station where she was to board the train.

Backtracking just a little, I went to the graduation exercises in the spring when the boys and girls that I had been going to school with were graduating. All of a sudden, I realized that I was just about to miss the boat, even though the school only went through the ninth grade. As a rule, Port Gibson graduates who went on to Alcorn College were put in a senior high school class there. They could work their way up through the twelfth grade and then be admitted into college.

But there I was, left in Port Gibson, having finished only the fifth grade. I had also met Mattie and knew that I wanted to see more of that beautiful young lady at a later date, but I couldn't see myself getting anywhere with her or in the world. I could see myself being pushed aside by someone like Tommy Johnson who had continued with school. I saw myself having to be satisfied with a job that paid as little as fifteen dollars a week for the rest of my life.

I went home and had a talk with my parents. "Mama, just why was it that you didn't make me go to school like you made Thelma? Why didn't you lay the switch on me and make me go?" Though she tried to evade my questions, I insisted on knowing.

Mama reminded me of the time I was "sick," when they had called the doctor in to see me. She reminded me that the doctor had called them aside and spoken to them for a little while. She explained the doctor had examined me and had told them that, in all probability, I would not live to get grown. He thought the best thing they could do for me was let me have all the fun I wanted, and if I didn't want to go to school, not to make me.

You could have knocked me over with a feather because first of all, I had not been sick at all, and secondly, I did not anticipate dying before I had a chance to make my way in this world.

CHAPTER 4

SCHOOL DAYS

There was one smart boy who had been in my class: Henry Johnson. Although he had only finished the ninth grade, Henry had taken the entrance examination at Alcorn College, and his intelligence was such that he was admitted to the freshman class. I envied him because he was going on ahead of me. When Henry came back to Port Gibson at the end of his first year, I began talking to him. I explained my problem and told him that I wanted to go back to school and wanted him to help me. I did not intend to go back to the sixth grade with all those little, snotty-nosed kids.

I had been down to Alcorn on many occasions and talked to several of the students there. I asked them what classes they were in. Several of them told me that they were in the sixth grade! I asked one of the fellows why he was in the sixth grade and not in college. "Well, I had finished the fourth grade and dropped out of school to work on the farm. After I got grown, I decided that I wanted to go back to school and become a teacher," he answered.

He went to Alcorn and was given an entrance examination. It was found that he was intelligent and able to learn, which meant that he would have to start in the sixth grade, the lowest grade taught at Alcorn. He pointed out a senior at Alcorn at that time. That senior had been at Alcorn for eleven years. During that time, he had advanced from sixth grade to his final year as a senior.

In other words, if a person would come to Alcorn, even as an illiterate, they would put him in the sixth grade and keep him there until he could go into the seventh grade, eighth, ninth, etc.

When I talked to Henry, he asked me what I had been reading. I told him that I had read everything from the *Saturday Evening Post* to Shakespeare and Greek mythology. With that background, he thought that if I could be admitted to the eighth grade, I could go on from there. So, we planned for him to tutor me so I could take the ninth-grade examination. We both knew that I would flunk the exam, but the admitting teacher might put me in the eighth grade, and I could work my way from there.

My mama would make five gallons of ice cream, and Papa would sell it on Saturdays to people from the country. There would always be some left, so I made a bargain with Henry that I would give him all the ice cream he could eat on Saturdays if he would tutor me. That was fine with him.

I had to review arithmetic to get ready for the eighth grade, which would go into algebra. This was all foreign to me, but I caught on anyway. I remember when we were talking about the circumference of a circle, and Henry said something about "pi equals" this, that, and the other, and I wondered why in the world he had called it pi. "That's what you call it. That's a Greek word," he told me. "Oh, yeah," was my response.

Henry taught very well. We talked about all the parts of speech, definitions for the parts of speech, and he gave examples of how to use them in sentences. When he had started with me, I hadn't known a preposition from a proposition, but during that summer I worked very hard. In mid-July of that year, I went to work in the department store and found Mr. Krauss to be a very kindly man. Several times we talked, and he said, "Boy, you should go back to school. You have a lot in you that could come out if you just had some education." He was delighted when I told him that I had decided to go back to school in the fall. In fact, everybody in the store was delighted.

The next thing I did was scrawl a letter to Mattie to tell her that I was going back to school. I got a three-page letter back from her saying she was delighted also. Yes, I was ready to go now.

I wrote for an application for admission to Alcorn, and it came back in due time instructing me to go to Alcorn College. I felt very big that day.

I got down to Alcorn and went to the teacher in charge of admissions and told him I had come to be admitted to the ninth grade. He asked, "Did you bring your records from school?" I said the principal was out of town and had not gotten back in time for me to get my transcript, but that I would be very glad to take the examination anyway. That was one of the biggest lies I ever told. Anyway, he put the examination up on the board. The passing mark was 70, and I think I made about 52, which I thought was great. He said, "Well, my young man, I'm sorry, but I can't let you go into the ninth grade, because you failed the examination, which was very fair."

Henry and I had planned for this. He'd said, "Look, Quig, if you will just raise a little racket in there and insist on going into the ninth grade, I'll be outside, and when I hear you raise your voice, I'll come in. We'll go out and talk this thing over. Then you go back in and say that you'll go to the eighth grade."

Sure enough, that's what happened. I said very loudly to the instructor, "I know that I am supposed to be in the ninth grade!"

On cue, in stepped Henry Johnson. Henry said, "Wait, Professor, let me talk to this fellow. I think I can make him understand what is going on." We went out behind the building and danced a jig. Everything was turning out just fine.

I came back with a downcast look on my face and said, "Okay, I'll take the eighth grade, but I really should be in the ninth!"

The teacher started in, but Henry jumped up and said, "Don't worry, Professor. It'll be all right. I'll take care of him." It was all right too. I was admitted to the eighth grade, and the next day, when class was organized, I had such a big mouth that they made me the class president. Now here I was, president of the eighth-grade class, and I was so dumb that I hardly knew a noun from a hound.

***

The colored people—as they were called then—in Port Gibson seemed to have average intelligence, maybe even a little above average. Somehow, they learned to appreciate good music and had a brass band composed of Black musicians. The band director was George Comfort. My daddy played in the band, and all the members were a close-knit group of men. One day, one of the band members left his trombone at our home, so I asked if I could play it. Daddy told me to go ahead and try and see what I could do with it. I began picking out tunes. My sister, Ruth, would come in and play the piano, and soon we made our own duo. The next thing I knew, I was picking out entire pieces that were popular during that time.

In addition to the brass band, there was a group of men who played stringed instruments. The string band was composed of two violins, three guitars, two mandolins, and a bass viola. They played for dances, parties, and any other type of gathering. I asked them to let me sit in with them and play my trombone. I was playing by ear and was doing it pretty well. Subsequently, they included me in the group, and I made anywhere from two to five dollars playing for a dance or other function.

It just so happened that Mr. Comfort was chosen by the President of Alcorn College to direct the college band. In addition to that job, he was what we called "supervisor of food services." There were about five hundred students at Alcorn College, and at mealtime anywhere from fifteen to twenty minutes were wasted getting the students in and out of the dining hall for their meals. Mr. Comfort (my father made me call him Uncle George) found a way to get these students in and out of there in a hurry.

He developed a small orchestra which started playing a stirring march as the bell rang for a particular meal. The students, both men and women, would march in, march to their assigned tables, and be waiting for the blessing to be sung in just about two minutes. Uncle George Comfort had charge of the dining hall orchestra as well as the college band, and it so happened that the trombone player in the group had graduated that spring.

When I came around with my trombone, Uncle George gave me the job of playing with the group. We received our board as payment for our services of playing at mealtime. Therefore, I was assured of my board from the very first day I got to Alcorn. Tuition was very cheap, about twenty-five dollars a year, because it was a state-supported school.

At Alcorn, an emphasis was put on trades. Studies offered at high schools and colleges were also part of the curriculum. There were about three hundred to four hundred students enrolled in Alcorn during the time I was there. Most of the students came from other schools throughout Mississippi. Many came from rural areas and had never been to school before. Some were men and women who had developed the urge to do more with their lives than work in cotton fields.

I was working in the department store when I left to go to Alcorn, so I could get clothes at a reduced rate. I had two or three good suits, hats, shoes, and plenty of socks. When I was ready to leave, I tried separating my socks from those of my brother Johnny. We couldn't separate them to our satisfaction, so I decided to take all the white socks and leave him all the colored ones. I ordered a handsome seersucker suit from a famous New Orleans department store. Now, I think I probably looked pretty silly in it.

My first day at Alcorn was very interesting. Each room was heated by a large fireplace. Some of the students earned their tuition and board by remaining at school during the summer to cut firewood for heating the buildings throughout the winter. When I went to school, I was advised by Henry and the other students who had been there awhile not to take a room in the modern buildings with steam heat, but to try arranging to stay in one of the older buildings where there were fireplaces. Why? Because we could supplement our diet of grits, gravy, corned beef hash, and navy beans with such delicacies as rabbits, squirrels, fish, and from time to time a "misplaced" chicken, which we could cook in our dormitories after all the lights were out and the shades were drawn. Although cooking in the dormitory rooms was strictly forbidden, the monitors would never turn anyone in for cooking as long as they were allowed some of whatever was being cooked.

I was assigned to a room with Henry Johnson, his brother, and one other student. When I got to the room, I found a dresser, a fireplace, and four beds with new, empty mattress covers lying on each one. "Where is the mattress?" I asked.

Henry replied, "Come on, you'll see." We took the mattress covers to the barn and filled them with fresh-mown hay until the mattresses were well-stuffed.

"Why do you put so much hay in the mattresses?" I asked.

They answered, "After a month, it will be padded down and will be a nice, comfortable place to sleep."

Oh boy! That first night it was all I could do to keep from rolling out of bed because of that overstuffed mattress. The next morning, I was awakened by the chapel bells at six a.m. I had half an hour to get out of bed, get dressed, and get down to the dining hall to join the rest of the students. That was a stirring experience for me. At last, I had another chance to get more education and realize my dream of becoming a doctor.

On the first day of school, we were given our books, and lessons were assigned. Now, here I was in the eighth grade, having finished only the fifth, with five or six books and classes beginning the next day. I had no idea how I should study, but I was kept in line by Henry. When I went to class, I found that I wasn't too bad off when it came to reciting the lessons. However, in view of the fact that I had missed the sixth and seventh grades, I found it necessary to read up on the lessons for the next day with Henry's help. It was tough on me for about six months, but after that, I caught on pretty well. I found myself being able to keep up with the other kids in the class. As a matter of fact, I was able to stay ahead of a lot of them because I had done a good deal of reading in those years that I had been out of school. I did so well in history that the teacher, who was also dean of the college, allowed me to conduct the class while he sat over in the corner and attended his duties as dean.

Now as to math (it was arithmetic in those days) and grammar, I had to study hard to make up for the years I had missed.

However, near the end of my first year at Alcorn, I found myself competing with the other kids who were considered to be the best students in the class.

A rivalry developed between me and Emma Weathers. Having had a much better background, Emma was much smarter than me. But, in discussion classes, such as history, I somehow always managed to get higher marks. She was a better student than I was, and from then until I left Alcorn, I felt guilty because I believed some of the teachers gave me better marks because I was a boy, and she was a girl.

I really loved life at Alcorn. I was a new person and eager to learn. The types of classes available for men were painting, carpentry, blacksmithing, or shoemaking. The women had elementary education, nursing, or domestic science. English and grammar were taught, along with mathematics, up through geometry, elementary physics, Latin, French, and chemistry. The white folks said that all the Black men needed to know about chemistry was how to read fertilizer bags. We had good teachers in all the subjects. If a student wanted to get ahead in education in all branches, they could do it. It just depended on their eagerness.

I enrolled in the shoemaking class, but Lord knows, I soon learned that I did not want to be a shoemaker. Reverend Craig, the instructor, was a master shoemaker and would come by every now and then to give me instructions. One day, he stopped by my bench and saw me fooling around, doing nothing, and said, "Son, let me tell you one thing. You don't want to be a shoemaker, and you never will be a shoemaker. You are just wasting your time and mine fooling around here in this shoe shop. Tell you what, you clean up the shop, and I'll give you marks until the end of the year. Then, I want you to change your trade, you hear?"

"Thank you, Reverend Craig! You told the truth. I don't want to be a shoemaker," I answered.

I started paying more attention to my music at that time. We had chapel services every morning, Monday through Friday. The chapel bell would ring for fifteen minutes. After that, all the students at the school—and I do mean ALL—had to be in their assigned places in the chapel for the beginning of the service.

The president of Alcorn at that time was Dr. Levi B. Rowan. He was born and raised in Claiborne County, the county in which the college was located. He had been taught in a one-room schoolhouse by a missionary and had gone to Colgate University where he received his PhD in education. He was a man well prepared for the job.

The teacher in charge of music, Mrs. Ruth Rowan Saunders, was Dr. Rowan's daughter. Mrs. Saunders had received her master's degree in music from Fisk University in Nashville. When I walked into the chapel, I saw a petite lady seated at the Steinway grand piano playing some of the most beautiful music I had ever heard. Mrs. Saunders was usually playing one of Chopin's nocturnes, or sometimes she would play her own arrangement of "Oh Lord Our Help in Ages Past," or "Deep River." I could always be moved by her renditions of the works of the masters. I have records of Chopin's music played by Arturo Rubenstein.

However, when I listen to those works of the old masters, I do not think of Arturo Rubenstein. I think of Mrs. Ruth Rowan Saunders.

As I stated before, some of my earliest memories revolve around "loud singing" in the A.M.E. Church in Port Gibson. The singing that I heard there always fascinated me. Now at Alcorn College, listening to Chopin's nocturnes and preludes and to anthems being sung by a well-coached choir, I wanted to join the choir. When I went back at the beginning of the second year, the first thing I did was try out for the choir. My voice had begun to change, so I tried out as a baritone and was accepted. Mrs. Saunders worked very hard with us. She was able to take students from the backwoods, pick out the best voices, and develop them into serious singers with an appreciation for classical music. We learned to appreciate works of Handel, Bach, Beethoven, and other masters. Every year we presented operettas such as Gilbert and Sullivan's *H.M.S. Pinafore* and *Madame Butterfly*. I worked very hard at my music as well as with my studies.

I tried out and received a place in the choir's octet. At the beginning of my third year at Alcorn, I tried out and received a place in the senior chorus as well. Among three teachers who came to teach at Alcorn from Morehouse College in Atlanta, Georgia, was Mr. Joe Brooks, who taught Latin and English. He had been a member of the quartet and male chorus at Morehouse College. When he came, he brought all his know-how. He took over direction of the octet, chorus, and male quartet. I was not a member of the male quartet, but I was allowed to sit in and sing with them. One day, when the baritone singer had a sore throat, I was right there to take his place. You know what? That student never got a chance to sing with the male quartet again.

I had always been very skinny, and when I got to Alcorn, I knew that I would need some protection. I looked around for the biggest guy I could find. E.T. Hawkins came from out in the country to Alcorn and was in my class. This guy weighed about two hundred pounds and had the biggest feet I had ever seen in my life. He had a deep bass voice but no singing training whatsoever. Even so, I knew that Hawkins was basically better than the guy who was then singing bass in the quartet. So, I said to Hawkins, "With your voice, one of these days, I'm going to get you into the quartet. If the bass singer gets sick for any reason, you will be able to step in and take his place. Once you get that, you will be able to do better than he is doing."

I copied all the songs that we practiced and would go about half a mile from campus and practice the bass parts with Hawkins. I told him, "Now you just hang in there and be there when we practice, and your chance will come along sooner or later." Well, it did come along. When the bass singer became ill, I suggested to Mr. Brooks that he try Hawkins in his place. Hawkins had a better voice, and it was no trouble for him to take over the bass spot in the quartet.

Mr. Brooks taught us to sing "Invictus," which became my theme song. I could never forget the first verse: "Out of the night that covers me, black as the pit from pole to pole, I thank whatever gods that may be, for my unconquerable soul."

There was another teacher by the name of Mr. Busby, who came to us from Bordentown, New Jersey. Officially, he taught elementary agriculture. All the male students at Alcorn had to take agricultural courses. Mr. Busby talked more about current events than he did about cotton and fertilizers. He would look around the classroom and say things like, "Now we have a room full of boys and girls, men and women, coming up. Some of you are going to drop out when you finish high school. About one tenth of you are going on to finish college. Of that number, about five percent will be teachers, and the remaining five percent are going to do something more than teach."

He continued, "I can look around right now and pick out the five percent of you who are going to college and on from there to bigger fields." I thought that he was looking at me all the time, and I was drinking it all in.

I was dead set on becoming a doctor. My family didn't have any money, so I had to figure out a way to get the necessary training. The college physician was a young man who had finished Meharry Medical College. One day, I cut my hand and had to go to him for treatment. Dr. Bond was the first Black doctor I had talked to since talking with Dr. Sherrod when I was eight or nine years old. I questioned that man to death. He became interested in me and asked, "What do you want to do? Do you want to be a doctor?"

I said, "I know that I can be a doctor, and that's what I want to be. But I have several things going against me."

He prompted, "Such as?"

I told him about missing four years of school, that my people did not have the money to send me, and I didn't see how in the world I could make it through medical school. We sat down on the steps, and the first thing Dr. Bond asked was, "What about your brothers and sisters?"

I told him that both my sisters were in Chicago, one working as a maid and the other as a cook. My oldest brother, Charlie, was also in Chicago, and he worked at a hotel near the stockyards. He said, "Hell, you don't need anything else if you've got all those folks there. All you need to do is go to Chicago. There are three colleges there where you can get a pre-medical course. You can go on down to Meharry and study medicine, and let your brothers and sisters help you out. Won't they?"

I said, "I'm sure they would."

"Well, you need to get ready now. The first thing I want you to do is go to see Joe Brooks. Tell him your story. He will get you ready, and I'll do what I can as well. The best thing for you to do is finish your third year of high school, go to Chicago, catch up on your classes, and finish high school there. You can then transfer to Crane Junior College and get your pre-med work." It sounded like a lot of work, but he said there was nothing to it if I made up my mind and did it.

I said, "Wait a minute here. When I get to Chicago, I've got to help myself. I will need a job of some kind."

"All you have to do is get a job as a Pullman porter. You can work during the summer and make enough money to pay your tuition and board at Meharry. The board and tuition are cheap. You can make it, that is if you have the guts to go ahead." That sunk in, and I went to see Joe Brooks.

He said, "Boy, I've been studying your papers. You write okay, but you can't spell worth a damn. Your sentences are all right, and you put everything in order, but you just can't spell. What's wrong?"

I told him, "I was never in the sixth and seventh grades."

He asked, "How in the world did you get into the eighth grade?" I told him my whole story. "Okay, I'll tell you what we can do. I need to know what else you need to learn. I want you to write something every night and bring it to me. Write about anything that crosses your mind. I can check it and see just what you need in the way of English and everything else."

I had some old journals that I found before leaving Port Gibson. They had a lot of unused pages—great big, long pages—that I cut out and brought to Alcorn with me to use as scratch paper. I pulled out one of those old sheets and began writing everything I could think of. I wrote about hunting with Charlie. I wrote about things that happened in Port Gibson. I wrote about things that happened in school.

I took what I had written to him, and he commented, "That's fine. Where did you get this paper?"

"I brought it from Port Gibson," I answered.

He said, "Okay, I want you to fill both sides of this paper every night and bring it to me." I did just that for about one month. He studied everything I had written and finally said, "I see what you need, and I am going to give you extra work to do, and darn it, you are going to have to do it."

I replied, "Yes, I'll do it."

"Now get on that French so you can catch up with your class and stay with that math. I'm going to do grammar, Latin, and English with you. Then you'll be ready. Don't worry about it. I know you will be able to get your relatives in Chicago to help you and give you a place to live." The man encouraged me to no end saying, "You have got to go, and I am going to see that you do."

The next thing I did was write to my brother Charlie in Chicago that I needed some help. I told him that I wanted to go to school, and I wanted to come to Chicago to do it. His reply was, "Yes, I'll give you a ticket, and you can come this summer." He thought I would be able to get a job and find out how I liked Chicago.

My sister Ruth was working for Dr. Lownesberry, the chief surgeon of the Chicago, Milwaukee, and St. Paul Railroad. She told him about me and asked, "Dr. Lownesberry, do you think he can get a job here?"

"Oh yes, he can get a job, and I'll see that he does." Dr. Lownesberry told my sister that when he was studying medicine at Northwestern University, he worked on the Chicago police force. He had done all right for himself and was sure that if I had the stamina, I would be able to do all right for myself.

My brother, Charlie, gave me the ticket, and I went to Chicago. I found one or two odd jobs around Chicago that summer. Charlie didn't push me; he just went right along with me because he wanted me to see whether I would like it well enough to come up and work my butt off. I told him that I thought so, and he said, "I'll help you so long as you help yourself. But the day you stop working yourself, I'm going to put your butt out. Do you understand?"

"Oh yes, I understand!"

"Okay then," he said. By the end of that summer, I went back to Alcorn with my mind made up.

CHAPTER 5

MINSTREL SHOW

The Alcorn College band was tops, and I considered myself to be a pretty good trombone player. I played first trombone in the band and felt that I was equal to, but no better than, any trombone player in any college band. However, the time was not long in coming when I found out that I was not quite so hot.

The first trumpet player in our band was named DeWitt Buckingham, but we called him "Buck." He was short in stature and a darned good trumpet player with quite a bit of experience. He had been playing his trumpet since he was about ten years old and made a little extra change during the summer by playing with a minstrel band. It just so happened that the minstrel show had its headquarters in Port Gibson. The idea came to me to get with the minstrel band that summer so I could make some money and buy some extra clothes for the coming school year in Chicago. That would give me some traveling experience as well. I asked Buck about my chances of being hired to play with the band during the coming summer. He queried, "You do know that the home base is at Port Gibson? Do you know Mr. Walcott?"

I did. The Honorable Fred S. Walcott, Esquire, owner of the Rabbit's Foot Minstrels, was a short man who was duly decked-out, no matter how hot the weather, in a high black silk hat, a wing-type, high white collar with a wide bowtie, a colorful vest, Prince Albert-type black coat, striped pants, colorful spats and black patent leather shoes. He would step into the circle formed by the

band and give a five-minute-long, entertaining spiel to entice people in whatever town his minstrel troupe was performing to come
to the show. He would then doff his hat, bow gracefully, and stride
from the center of the circle. The band would strike up a march,
and the parade would return to the railcar from which it came.

Mr. Walcott knew his business for sure. In fact, he became the
owner of Huntington's Mighty Minstrels in addition to the Rabbit's
Foot Minstrels. He liked my hometown of Port Gibson so much
that he made it his headquarters and bought a plantation with an
imposing antebellum mansion. When he first came to Port Gibson,
I was a very skinny, twelve-year-old lad who had quit school.

During the winter, Mr. Walcott began assembling his cast in
preparation for his show for the next season. It was then that I
came to know the performers. My mother's boarding house was
the nearest thing to a hotel the Blacks had in those days. My
mother only took in married show couples such as Mr. and Mrs.
Brown, the bandmaster and his wife, who had the stage name of
"Sweet Georgia Brown." Mrs. Brown had a wonderful voice.

Later, when traveling Black theatrical groups, such as the Smart
Set group based in New York City, began including our little town
of Port Gibson in their stops, I was thrown into contact with such
stars as Tut Whitley. I found all the stars whom I met to be very
intelligent people. I did not have contact with the single men and
women who made up the remainder of the troupe. They were, for
the most part, uninhibited, prone to fights, drunkenness, and various misdemeanors. They were responsible for the bad reputation
with which minstrel performers were labeled.

On one of my weekend trips to Port Gibson, I approached
Mr. Walcott and asked him to take me on at the beginning of
next season's tour. I explained to him that I was a student at

Alcorn, had been playing trombone for about five years, and was considered a very good first trombone by my music teacher. I told him I was acquainted with Buck, one of his minstrels. He said he would think about it and talk to Buck about me. The very next weekend, I got Buck to come to Port Gibson and talk with Mr. Walcott about me. He convinced him I would probably be a good addition to the band. Though Mr. Walcott already had two trombone players, he said he would hire me for fifteen dollars a week. Buck, a veteran in show business, received twenty-five dollars a week. That was perfectly all right with me; this pay was much better than the six dollars a week I earned working at D. Bock's Department Store.

Buck notified Mr. Walcott of the date we would leave school, and Mr. Walcott said he would send him our tickets. Buck received our train tickets along about the first of May. The day after our final examination at Alcorn, we caught the train in Port Gibson to meet the minstrel show in Greensboro, North Carolina. Though I had been to Chicago, I considered a trip to Greensboro to be the greatest event ever to happen in my life. The train carried us east through the Mississippi and Alabama cotton plantations, through the foothills of Georgia, around and through the tree-covered foothills and mountains of South Carolina and North Carolina, and finally to Greensboro, taking about eighteen hours. Of course, we had to ride the "Jim Crow" car—a half-section of a passenger car attached close to the engine just behind the whites' baggage car. During most of the trip the car was crowded, but I was too busy looking out the window to notice, and time passed swiftly. We had no lunch with us on the trip to Greensboro. However, when the train stopped along the route, we were able to find a "colored" restaurant where we could get any type of food, from sandwiches to full meals of soul food, including collard greens, ham hocks, black-eyed peas, and corn bread.

At that time, I did not own a trombone, but my music teacher at Alcorn let me borrow one from school. It was in first-class condition, silver-plated with a gold-plated bell. I was excited about being on the trip and looked forward to joining the minstrel band to become a full-fledged trombone player. My real education was about to begin.

We arrived in Greensboro around eleven-thirty p.m. The first thing we had to do was find a place to spend the night. There was no such thing as a hotel for colored people. They, along with other transients and travelers, had to be content with rooming houses. Most rooming houses had thin mattresses, and the springs stuck in your sides, if there were any springs at all. In addition, bedbugs chewed on you from the time the lights went out until daylight.

Nevertheless, that was where we had to sleep that night. We were directed to a rooming house about two blocks from the railroad station. We knocked, and a young lady came to the door. She asked, "What can we do for you?"

Buck spoke out, "We would like to rent a room for the night."

"Okay, come on in. What are you doing in Greensboro?"

"We came here to join the minstrel show."

"Minstrel show!" the lady exclaimed in a loud voice with a look of disdain on her face. "Mama," she called. Her mother came out in her robe and nightgown.

"What's the matter, daughter?"

"These two guys want a room, but they are going to join the minstrel show tomorrow. We don't want them in here, do we, Mama?"

Her mother said, "I don't guess they can find any place else to stay. We can give them the back room down at the end of the hall."

"Mama, are we going to let them stay here?"

"That's all right. They need someplace to stay, and we can't put them out. They're just going to be here tonight. They will be going out tomorrow morning."

After having come from Port Gibson where I had always been regarded as a harmless and nice young boy, I now found myself in a situation where I was looked upon as something to be disdained and kicked out. I was beginning to get a little leery about how we would get along, but Buck was very reassuring. He said, "Ah Quig, don't pay them any mind. After all, you know we're better than they are. Just don't let on that you know it."

We had arrived in Greensboro a day ahead of the minstrel show. However, we knew one person there, a young man by the name of Joseph Smith, who was an accomplished musician. He could play all the wind and string instruments and had been allowed to direct the band and orchestra at Alcorn. He had taken the position of music director at Bennett College in Greensboro. We also knew one of the teachers at North Carolina A&T College, Professor Garrett, who taught in the Agricultural Department. The next morning, we asked the landlady, who was much more civil than her daughter, to let us leave our bags and band instruments in the boarding house until we could find another place to stay. And in the meantime, we went to Bennett College and got in contact with Joe.

At that time, Bennett was a co-educational institution founded and maintained by the American Missionary Association, providing educational facilities all over the South for training Black youths. Bennett College was not very large and was about to be converted to an all-girl college. The orchestra Joe conducted was supposed to play for the graduation exercises. However, the orchestra had no trombone, and the trumpet player was not so well trained. So, Joe was very glad to see us and asked us to join the college orchestra to play for graduation.

When the graduates and other students began assembling for the exercises, who do you think was in the fourth row? That same young lady who had been so nasty to us the night before! She ran over to us, full of apologies. She said, "If I had only known that you were friends of Mr. Smith, I never would have acted so ugly last night." We accepted her apologies.

Because we were already familiar with the music that Joe had arranged, I believe we added somewhat to the occasion, much to the satisfaction of the entire audience.

A dance was held in the gymnasium of A&T College that same afternoon, and we went. The music was performed by the college's jazz band. We enjoyed ourselves, doing the one-step, two-step, and waltzes. Neither of us was so bad looking so we had no trouble finding dance partners. However, something else happened at the dance which led me to realize that minstrel life wasn't so hot. I was dancing with a cute young lady who was really cutting the rug. She asked me where I was from, and I told her that I was from Alcorn College. She thought that to be very interesting. We talked a little longer, and she queried, "What are you doing in Greensboro?"

"We are joining the minstrel show tomorrow."

She replied, "Oh, excuse me, I have a headache." She sat down and spoke to the young lady sitting next to her. In ten shakes of a lamb's tail, I found out that all the girls had headaches.

I pulled Buck aside and said, "Look here, Buck, what's the matter with us? All of a sudden nobody wants to dance with us."

He asked, "What did you tell them?"

"I told the girl where we were from, and she wanted to know what we were doing here, so I told her we were joining the minstrel show."

"You damn fool!" he said. "Don't ever tell anybody that you're a member of the minstrel show. Don't you know that people don't like minstrel folk? They think all of us are nasty, lousy cutthroats and thieves. We better go on home. We're not going to get any more dances this afternoon." That was bad, but he said, "Don't worry, you know who you are. You know what you are, and you don't have to take their word for it."

"I've had it, and I'm ready to go back to Mississippi right away," I replied. At least the landlady's daughter knew we were friends of Joe Smith. Word had gotten around that we were top-flight musicians, and we had no trouble remaining in the boarding house for another night.

The next morning, the minstrel show arrived. They had a car attached to one of the local trains. This car was switched to a siding, and we went to meet it. Mr. Walcott came out saying, "Okay, come on fellows. The parade is at twelve o'clock, and we've got to get ready to go on." He then looked at me and said, "Well, here you are, boy. Let's see what you can do." I smiled and thanked him. I was in high cotton. I was grinning from ear to ear.

All the other members were seasoned musicians. They greeted me warmly and offered to help. Mark Veal, the band leader, took me under his wing at once. He was a dignified-looking gentleman weighing about one hundred eighty pounds. He had mixed gray-and-black hair and a deep rumbling voice. When he played the clarinet, you could hear him filling in whenever he felt help was needed to emphasize certain parts of the music.

The lady who took care of the wardrobe measured my skinny frame and cut the costume down to fit me. It was a nice costume—light, sky-blue satin, modeled after a French Army uniform, complete with silk hat. It had gold braid covering the front of the jacket. There were bright, gold stripes down both sides of the trousers. Our caps were patterned after the type of headpiece worn by the military. They were decorated with gold braid, too. I must confess that I thought I looked very good in that uniform.

Then another real letdown came along. We ate breakfast and were about ready to line up for the parade. The trombones were to be in the first row. They passed out the music, and I found that I was familiar with some of the marches. I said, "Oh, this is going to be duck soup to me. I've got it made."

Then Mr. Veal, the band leader, came out with a stack of music and said, "Well, boys, I just got this music out of the post office, and we're going to play these marches this time. All of them are new, and I know you don't know any of them, but you guys can cut it."

I looked at the new music. I was puzzled, confused, scared, angry—every damn thing. I had never seen that stuff before. I turned around and said, "Mr. Veal, when are we going to practice?"

He laughed and said, "Son, what did you say?"

"I said, when are we going to practice?"

He replied, "Son, we don't practice. We do our stuff, and you'll have to catch it on the fly. Come on, don't worry about it."

Well, I was scared as hell because I was accustomed to practicing new music until it was perfected. The others were seasoned musicians and took to the music like ducks to water. I was shaking all over when we lined up for the parade. We walked down the street, and I had a real wake-up call because I realized that I really was not a trombonist. I was just a scared amateur about to drown in a sea of professionals. The drum major waved his baton, brought it down, and that started the parade. The drums started, but they were not throbbing nearly as loud as my heart was at that moment.

We started the first piece. I think I hit about every third, fourth, or fifth note. Nobody seemed to be paying any attention to it, however. The weather was hot, the sun was shining brightly, and I was really sweating. After a while, I was catching on a little better and could play three out of every four notes. I was so intent on keeping up with the music that I didn't see the young drum major twirl his baton to the right, indicating the route the parade would take around the corner. I marched straight ahead, still playing like hell. It came to me that the music was getting faint. I looked around and saw the band going in another direction. I turned and ran to catch up with the others. People were laughing. The band members did not tease me about it, but I was really embarrassed. Lord, I was so ready to go back to Mississippi that very day.

But Buck said, "Look here, you know you can't go back now. You had a ticket out here, but you don't have one back to Mississippi."

Well, brother, I started studying that music like hell. I studied all afternoon, and when the time came for the pre-show concert under the tent, I had a little more confidence. We played four or five songs, and everything we played was fast. Following this, everyone was invited into the tent to see the show. The grand opening followed. The orchestra would go into a fast number, and the curtain would be drawn back, revealing the entire show troupe. At either end of the stage there would be comedians in blackface, who we called "end men." Next would be the "side men and women." There would be two or three couples on both sides of the stage. The bandmaster would be seated in an elevated chair just a little above the other members of the band. After a spirited song, Mr. Walcott would step forward and greet the audience.

At this juncture, the star, or stars as the case might be, would come to center-stage and either sing or do a comic performance.

The opening would be concluded with another song. There would always be a round of applause when the curtain was drawn. Other acts would follow. There were bicycle acts, knife-throwing acts, comedy, dancing, and singing. During the show, the orchestra would play the songs for the performers. There was music going the whole time. The show usually lasted between one-and-a-half to two hours. The grand finale was like the opening act, with everyone on stage. After some songs there would be dancing and someone like "Sweet Georgia Brown" with a beautiful voice would sing the final song, and the curtain would drop.

I made it through the show somehow. But after the show was over, another great disappointment was in store for me. The railroad car the minstrel show was traveling in was half Pullman car and half baggage car. The tent and all the paraphernalia were stored in the baggage compartment. There were eight upper berths and eight lower berths in the other half of the car. That was all the space provided for thirty-six members of the minstrel troupe. The troupe slept two to a berth, which left four of us with no berths on the car.

I was the last person hired, so I was paired with the contortionist named Barrel. We had to go out in the afternoons and find a sleeping place in whatever town we were in. After the show, we would go to the lodging place and spend the night. We would have to be up in the morning in time to catch the train when it moved on to another town.

Barrel found our lodging for one night. It was one of those typical lodging houses, lit by kerosene lamps with dirty sheets infested with bedbugs. That was the most miserable night I ever spent. The next morning, we had to catch the train. The show car was so crowded that the four of us who could not find sleeping space in the car had to stand in the aisle from one town to the other. Everyone else in the car would be sleeping late.

They fed us breakfast about nine o'clock in the morning. As a rule, there was plenty to eat. Most of the time it would be grits and sausage, occasionally ham and eggs, and the usual coffee and biscuits. It would be enough to fill you up anyway. We had two meals each day. The other meal was served around four o'clock in the afternoon. This would consist of soul food and some type of pudding dessert. Sometimes there would be lemonade.

After breakfast I set out with Barrel to find another lodging place for that night. This was always a problem since minstrel players were depicted as the scum of the earth. We passed down a street and saw a sign, "Room for Rent." Barrel went up and knocked, and a lady came to the door. Barrel asked, "Do you have a room for rent?"

"Yes, we have one."

"How much is it?" he continued.

"A dollar a night."

"Can we have it?"

"Yes, come on in and take a look at it," she answered. We did, and it looked halfway decent. The lady asked, "What are you doing in Salisbury, North Carolina?"

"We're here with the minstrel show."

The lady retorted, "Minstrel show? Get out of my house! I don't allow no minstrel niggers in my house! Bastards! Filthy, stinking, low-down, thieving niggers! GET OUT!" She even said she was going to beat us up.

I was becoming more and more disenchanted with the idea of spending the summer being chased out of one chinch-ridden boardinghouse after another, standing up between towns, trying to learn all that foreign music, and being scorned by everybody in the street who thought we were a bunch of no-good minstrel niggers.

The next night's show was in the little town of Albemarle, North Carolina. All the white folks lived on one side of the railroad, and the Blacks lived on the other. We looked all over the "colored section" for a place to stay and finally came to a rundown two-story house where the proprietor said we could sleep that night. After we performed our show, we found our way back across the tracks and up the hill to the lodging house.

When we got there, we found a great commotion going on. A guy called "Boll Weevil" had caught some boy running around with his girlfriend. He promised to go home, get his shotgun, bring it back, and "blow the hell out of the damn place." Now I had never been exposed to anything like that, but everybody was laughing about it. "It's going to be something. You just wait around here. When old Boll Weevil gets back, he is going to raise some hell."

"Barrel, let's go to bed," I countered.

So, we did. But I didn't sleep that night, even though Boll Weevil never did come back to raise all that hell. I was curled up in a knot of fear until broad daylight, waiting for him to come back. We had to get up at 6 a.m. to catch the train that left at 6:30. I got going so fast that I didn't have a chance to wash up, but I found out that most of the guys on the car didn't do much bathing either. I now could understand some of the reasons why minstrel performers traveling from town to town were looked upon with such disfavor.

It was about a two-and-a-half-hour ride to the next town where we were to do another show. I soon found myself fast asleep standing up. When we arrived, I got off the train, found myself a nice shady tree, and took a short nap. Buck woke me to eat breakfast, and the day was just like the last. We performed in High Point,

North Carolina, that night. Before the parade, I found the telegraph office and wired Mama to send me fifty dollars so I could go back home.

Buck said, "Well, Quig, don't leave now. When you get your money, just keep it, and stick around until the man fires you; then leave. I wouldn't just quit and leave or walk off. Make him fire you."

That sounded pretty good to me. Anyway, we were getting farther and farther from Mississippi all the time. I went back to the telegraph office about 4 p.m., and my fifty dollars was there. I took the money, put it inside my sock, and kept that sock on until we got to Danville, Virginia, where Mr. Walcott asked Buck to inform me that I was fired. I was so glad to be fired that I didn't know what to do. That was just one of the two times I was ever fired in my life.

I did not report for the parade. I went straight to the railroad station and waited for the Southern Railroad train to take me back to Meridian, Mississippi, where I could take an Illinois Central to Vicksburg, and the Y&MV to Port Gibson. I got back to Port Gibson a very despondent young man, but I was glad to be there. The first thing I did was take a bath. I was in the tub one solid hour before I felt clean. And then there was the food. I thought I would never get filled up on that wonderful home-cooked food. Because I was also so despondent, my parents offered me a lot of consolation and helped build up my self-confidence again. It was so great to be home!

CHAPTER 6

ALCORN & THE RAILS

I t took about two months until I was my old self again.
The following spring, I was in a group that played for a festival in Natchez, Mississippi. One afternoon we were all sitting around kidding each other, as guys in school will do. This fellow, who was not a particularly good friend of mine, turned to me and said, "Quig, tell us what happened on that trip." I thought everybody had forgotten it. I had almost forgotten it myself. But when I was asked about it, I became depressed again.

That was when my good friend Hawkins pulled me aside and said, "Now look here, Quig, you can't let something like that get you down. You know that guy doesn't like you, so tell him to go to hell and forget it." With support from people like Hawkins, Henry Johnson, and other classmates, I overcame my depression, and by the end of the year, which was my last year at Alcorn, I felt like my old self again.

During that spring the time came for the trustees' visit. All the trustees were white, of course. Most of them were also members of the legislature. In order to get a halfway decent appropriation for the school, we had to take great pains not to antagonize those "good white folks." Mrs. Saunders had to prepare three or four old spirituals for us to sing for the trustees. We also rehearsed the "Hallelujah Chorus" from The Messiah by Handel.

When we sang our spirituals and the "Hallelujah Chorus," one of the good trustees was so carried away that he applauded wildly. He spoke up saying, "That was the best spiritual I ever heard.

Keep up the good work." Dr. Rowan rolled his eyes at us, and we had to keep straight faces. A number of appropriations for the year were at stake. But when they drove off in their cars toward Jackson, Mississippi, we laughed for fifteen minutes or more. And the appropriations came through nicely that year.

I began feeling homesick when I finished my third year of high school at Alcorn. Looking around, feeling the balmy breezes, I remembered vividly one warm day in December. Then I thought about Chicago. I had read in the newspaper that they were having a blizzard. Now it was up to me to determine my way. Should I stay here in this idealistic environment, finish college, and become a backwoods teacher? Should I go on to Chicago with the cold wind and buckle down to some hard studying?

Misgivings ran through my mind about moving on to Chicago. One Friday night, the quartet I was in was to sing for a program presented in the chapel. What did Joe Brooks pick for us to sing that night? "Invictus!"

That night when I lay in bed, the words of that song came to me again. "Out of the night that covers me/Black as the pit from pole to pole/I thank whatever gods may be/For my unconquerable soul."

I slept well all night long. I was ready to go to Chicago.

My brother Charlie and both of my sisters, Virgie and Ruth, lived there, so I had no trouble with living arrangements. But I had to get work somewhere.

Dr. Bond, the school physician at Alcorn who suggested that I study medicine in Chicago, had also told me to get a job as a Pullman porter. When I told Dr. Bond that my sister was working for the chief surgeon of the Milwaukee Railroad, Dr. Lownesberry, he remembered that the Milwaukee Railroad operated its own sleeping cars and frequently hired students to take care of the increased summer tourist travel. He said, "Now, boy, you really have a break."

Dr. Bond advised me to get in touch with my sister and have her talk to Dr. Lownesberry. She told him that I wanted to study medicine and would need help from my senior year in high school through medical school. Ruth said that the doctor smiled, leaned back in his easy chair, and started talking. He told her of his lean days in medical school and how he was employed as a part-time policeman in Chicago to pay his tuition. He told Ruth that he would be glad to help me. So, there I was, set up in Chicago the first of June 1925.

The transition from a small town to a big city had some effect on me. It took me some time to get accustomed to the hustle and bustle of the big city. First of all, down in Mississippi, if you had a slight cold or headache, you stayed home until you got better, and when you returned to work, you would find your job waiting there for you. However, in Chicago I was told very early that if you failed to show up for your job for two days, you would go back to find that the job had been taken over by someone else.

Then I had to get accustomed to the transportation system. I had to learn to use streetcars and the elevated system. The first week or so that I was in Chicago, I walked a lot to become acquainted with my neighborhood and try to determine north, south, east, and west. I soon learned how to get to Union Station, where I had a job, to Wendell Phillips High School, which was within walking distance, and then to my sister's apartment where I lived when I first arrived.

My brother, Charlie, laid down the law with me. He would look out for my living quarters as long as I kept a job and tried to help myself. My first paycheck from the railroad enabled me to repay him for the money I borrowed to buy books and the porter's uniform I had to have before starting the job. I tried to pay my way as I went; I didn't want to be a burden to Charlie. However, after taking care of my transportation expenses, buying books, and paying for meals whenever I couldn't eat at my sister's apartment, I didn't have too much money left for baseball games or shows. Furthermore, I was too busy trying to keep up with my schoolwork. I made it a point to sign up for the classes I needed with the strictest teachers. I knew that when I went to medical school, I had to be able to absorb a lot of information in the shortest possible time in order to keep up with my classes.

On Sunday afternoons, as a rule, I was able to attend local theaters on the South Side. There was one on South State Street known as the Vendome Theater that I liked to visit because they had a live orchestra that played a lot of popular and classical music. I took pains to save a little change so that I could attend elaborate productions staged during the holidays downtown at such theaters as The Chicago and shows such as the Ziegfeld Follies offered at the Auditorium Theater on Michigan Avenue. I was able to see and hear such stars as Bert Williams, Eddie Cantor, and Al Jolsen. Although I did not like to think that some of them performed in blackface, I liked the material they presented.

On the day after arriving in Chicago, I went down to the Central Station to Dr.

Lownesberry's office. I was ushered into his office. He took one long look at me — this skinny kid from Mississippi.

"Dr. Lownesberry," I began, "I'm Ruth's brother. I'm the one she has been telling you about who wanted to come to Chicago to get a job and study medicine."

"Okay, come in, son." He called his secretary and dictated a letter to the superintendent of the sleeping car division, asking him to give me a job. "Take this down there, and you'll be put to work right away. Don't worry about your size. I wasn't any bigger than you, and I was a policeman. I know darn well that you can take care of yourself on a sleeping car. Don't forget to come back, and let me know how you're getting along, hear?"

That was it.

I took the letter to the superintendent of the sleeping car division. He took one look at me and said, "Huh! Okay, if Dr. Lownesberry says to give you a chance, I will. But it's going to be up to you."

"Thank you, sir."

He sent me to the "sign-out man." He was responsible for assigning porters to sleeping cars. He said, "Well, we can use some good college boys, but first you have to go out and be trained. Now you come down here at six o'clock this afternoon, catch one of the trains that is backing down to the railroad yard, and report to Sam Donnell, the porter on the Olympian, car number nine."

"Thank you, sir."

I went down and met the porter.

"Okay, kid, come on in, and we'll see what we can do. You're a little light, but you ought to be able to make it."

He instructed me on taking down the berths in the sleeping cars, making the beds, hanging the curtains between each bed, and making the beds in the compartments and drawing rooms. During the night, all you would see was a corridor with green curtains on either side, extending from the ceiling to the floor with each berth's number in white letters. There were from twelve to sixteen sections in each car. Twelve sections were in the open portion of the car, and there would be what was called a drawing room and one or two compartments at one end of the car.

Now the Olympian, "The Flagship of the Milwaukee Fleet," ran from Chicago to Seattle, Washington. The most modern cars were assigned to that particular train. It was easy to unlock the berths so they would drop down slowly from near the ceiling. The mattresses were firm and tended to slide from the upper berth to the lower berth easily. The sheets were folded so that a bed could be made up in less than one minute.

On my second night, I was assigned to another porter who instructed me on "making down the car," as we called it, and "setting it up" for passengers to go to bed. He also instructed me on preparing the washrooms, taking care of the dirty linens, and everything else related to it. I was assigned to a porter named McGuire on the third and final night of my training. All these fellows were old, experienced porters who talked a lot and explained things that I should and should not do as a sleeping car porter.

McGuire was most interesting. He took a lot of time with me. We sat for about two hours until it was almost time for the trains to be backing up into the station to receive passengers. We had to work real fast, and he showed me just how fast the job could be done once you had the hang of it. About that time, a more elderly porter came through the car and spoke to McGuire.

"What are you doing with that little skinny kid? He can't do nothing. He ain't never going to be no sleeping car porter."

McGuire responded, "Don't bother him. He'll be all right."

"He's too damn skinny. He'll get tuberculosis before he gets to Butte, Montana."

He made me feel bad until McGuire said, "Don't pay that ornery old bastard no mind. You're all right. You're ready to go now."

McGuire gave me a note to give the sign-out man which read: "This boy is ready to be assigned a run." Man was I happy then.

They issued me a set of keys, and I got a second-hand cap from one of the porters and a second-hand coat from another. A pair of pants was all that I had to buy. Then I got my shoe-shining kit. My brother loaned me his old handbag, so I marched triumphantly to sign up for my first trip out of Chicago. All the new porters and youngsters were assigned to a train that ran up into the lake country of Wisconsin. Mostly fishermen went up there, along with some of the more affluent Chicagoans who had cottages there.

My run left Chicago on Saturday afternoon and arrived at Star Lake, Wisconsin, on Sunday morning. It was hot in Chicago in June, but it sure was cold when we got to Star Lake. I was enthralled by the beautiful countryside and the many lakes with surfaces that were as smooth as glass. That area is muskellunge country. Muskellunge is a game fish that puts up a hell of a fight, and serious fishermen go up to see how many muskies they can land. When I got there, the only thing I could think about was going fishing. Instead of sleeping all day, I fished all day, and believe it or not, I caught a musky using a worm for bait. I was so proud of that fish that I had to bring it back to Chicago. On the way back, I filled my cooler half-full of ice and half-full of muskellunge. That was the best part of my story. Now here comes the worst.

I was trained on the most modern equipment. The berths had to be unlocked from the sides of the car, pulled down in place, and made fast, so they would not spring back up and lock the passengers inside. In a sleeping car, two seats faced each other from one end of the car to the other. These two seats had cushions that could be pulled into the center space between them, and a back cushion pulled down to make a base for the bed. An innerspring mattress, stored in the upper berth, would be pulled down and placed on top of these drawn-out seats. The bed would be made up with top and bottom sheets, a blanket spread over the top sheet, and another sheet placed over the blanket so that only sheets were left showing. Next, a rod would be pulled out from the side of the car and fastened in position so curtains could be attached to the rod, affording privacy to the upper and lower berths. Everything worked well with the new equipment. The berths could be made down in two minutes or less, depending upon your dexterity.

However, on weekend specials and fishing trains, old wooden sleeping cars were used that creaked and groaned whenever the train rounded a curve. The springs that assisted me on the new steel cars were all worn out on these wooden cars, and if you didn't jump back when the berth was unlocked from the side of the car, it would knock your brains out. Some of the locks which held the upper berths to the sides of the car were worn so badly that it took super-human strength to unlock them. I only had a few passengers going up to Star Lake, so I was able to take my time working with the old car. It took me two hours to get six passengers to bed. On the return trip, passengers crowded in. All the berths were filled on both sides. I started making the berths at 8:30 p.m. that night and didn't get the last passenger to bed until 1:30 a.m. the next morning.

Even so, they were very patient and considerate.

One passenger asked, "Porter, how many trips have you made?"

I answered, "This is my first trip."

"Well, take your time. Everything's all right," he replied.

I had to get the passengers up at 7 a.m. for their arrival in Chicago at 8 a.m. Some of them wanted to get up at 6:30 a.m. and have breakfast before getting off the train. Getting them up and out was great confusion. I was told that as soon as the passengers got out of the upper and lower berths, I was to make them up so they would have a place to sit. By the time we got to Chicago, I only had four berths made up, so the people were having to stand in the aisle. I was so tired that I could hardly move. I was sore and aching all over. One passenger reassured me, "Well, young man, I know you'll be better next time." They tipped me twenty-five cents, fifty cents, and a dollar.

"Thank you, thank you, thank you, sir."

All the passengers left the train at Union Station in Chicago. I tried to get all the dirty linen off the berths and into bags, put mattresses in the upper berths, and then close them. Boy, oh boy! I just didn't have strength enough to do it. The passengers left the train, and it was one hour before the train was backed down to the railroad yard. During that time, I think I may have put away three more berths. When we got to the railroad yard, the crew came in to clean for the next trip out that night. When they came into the car I was in, I had sat down and was just about to cry. The fact of the matter is that I did cry a little bit. I felt that I had lost my chance because I was too weak to properly put away the cars.

"What's the matter, son?"

"Well, I don't know. I just can't make it. I can't push these berths up."

"Okay, we'll get them up for you. You go home and get some sleep."

Man, I was truly disgusted. I got my fish out of the cooler, wrapped it in several layers of newspaper, and put it in my handbag along with my uniform. Then I went back to the sign-out office. I decided the job was a little too much for me, and I couldn't make it.

When I got to the sign-out office, I put my keys on the desk. Old Man Gray, who assigned cars to the porters, looked up and said, "Boy, you don't have to say a word. I know you're disgusted and want to turn in those keys, but I'm not going to accept them. I'll tell you what I want you to do. Go home, get in the bed, and rest for two or three days. The first of the week, we have a special train going to Ann Arbor, Michigan, carrying the last of the Civil War veterans for their final reunion. Most of them can't walk or will be walking with sticks, and some are in wheelchairs. You'll be in Ann Arbor for three days. You won't have to make down the car, but you can use that time practicing. Drill yourself real well. Another thing, you're going to have better cars on the trip to Ann Arbor. They'll be steel cars, and the berths will be easier to make up and down. I will see what I can do about keeping you off these old wooden sleeping cars from now on. Does that sound all right to you, son?"

"Yes, sir, that sounds all right."

"Okay, let's hop to it now. I'm not going to keep these keys. You're just going to have to do your job. That's all."

I went on the Ann Arbor trip with the Civil War veterans. They were northerners—Yankees. After making the berths down for them to sleep the first night, I was advised to leave them down because they would be resting during the day as well. When they came in and out of the car, they related stories of the things that had happened during the war. They would laugh about how they beat the hell out of the Rebels. They were glad to tell these stories, and I was glad to listen. Down in Mississippi, I had heard the Rebel stories, and here I was now hearing the Yankee stories. I was all ears. Many of them were too disabled to leave the car to attend the festivities.

Mr. Gray had been right about the steel cars. They were easier to make down, and the cars were enclosed and comfortable. They moved along at high speed, and all you could hear was a clicking as the wheels passed over the rail joists. I had three days to get acquainted with the job, and by the time we got back to Chicago I had enough confidence to go to Mr. Gray and tell him, "Mr. Gray, I believe I can make it now."

He said, "That-a-boy! That's the spirit."

I found myself assigned to overnight runs out of Chicago, mainly to Sioux City, Iowa; Kansas City, Missouri; and Omaha, Nebraska. The runs were very good for indoctrination. However, the overnight runs directed to the Midwest were not very rewarding financially. The usual overnight tip was from twenty-five cents to fifty cents. Every now and then passengers in the drawing rooms and compartments would come across with a crisp one-dollar bill. All in all, I was learning the game, counting up those half dollars and quarters, and every two weeks I received a check for $32.50.

On the days I was not assigned to a car for a run out of town, I was eager to grab the job as standby porter. Trains carrying sleeping cars had to leave the station on schedule. Those cars had to be covered at all times, so whenever a porter was unable to report for duty because of an emergency or because he had a hangover from a big weekend, there had to be a porter present to take the car out. There were always two porters assigned to standby duty.

Because I very often took standby duty, I became acquainted with all the porters manning the top trains, such as the Pioneer Limited to St. Paul/Minneapolis, the Olympian to Seattle/ Tacoma, and the Columbian to Seattle/Tacoma. Almost every afternoon or night when I went down to check on the cars and see that the porters were present, some of the regular porters would ask me to go and pick up a paper for them or get chewing gum or a pack of cigarettes.

When I did, I usually got tipped fifty cents or a dollar from the man who had asked me to get whatever he needed. I let it be known that I was a student planning on staying in Chicago. This helped my tips along. Some of the porters, having been on the same runs for a long time, had become well-acquainted with some of the passengers. They had earned their trust and respect to such a degree that the passengers entrusted their children to the care of these porters.

Whenever I managed to get a trip to Marquette, Michigan or Omaha, the passengers would come on board asking, "Where is Dave White?" or "Where is John Smith tonight?" I explained where they were, and the passengers would tell me to be sure to tell those porters they missed seeing them. If any of the porters or their families were ill, the passengers always asked that their well wishes or sympathies be conveyed. I made it a point to call the regular porters and convey these messages. In return for these little niceties, the old fellows would look for me to take their runs in the event they couldn't make them. In other words, I tried to make myself useful. I was well-satisfied with conditions as I found them.

As Labor Day approached and the time came for students to be laid off so they could go back to their respective schools, I began worrying about getting a part-time job to hold while attending school. As far as I knew, all the porters hated to be assigned to standby duty, but I thought this would be a good spot for me if I could persuade the man in the office to allow me to become a permanent standby porter. I talked to the other porters, asking if anybody ever held a job as a regular standby porter. They had never heard of that arrangement.

Finally, Labor Day rolled around, and on the second day of September, which was also payday, the sign-out man announced loudly, "Now all of you students, I think you have done a good job this year, and this is your final payday. You go back to school, and please contact us when you get out next spring to see if we have an opening for you. If possible, we will hire you back next summer. Goodbye and good luck." I sat back in the corner until the last porter had received his check and left. Mr. Gray looked around and said, "Quig, why are you sitting back there? What are you waiting on anyway?"

I said, "Mr. Gray, I've got a little proposition to make. I was just thinking that it might be possible for me to stay on and work as standby porter to take some of the weekend runs."

"Oh no, we don't have anything like that."

"But you need me around here."

He replied, "Son, this railroad has been in operation for fifty years without you. So, why in hell do you think we need you?"

"Oh, there are a lot of things I could do around here. When Number One train to Minneapolis/St. Paul backed in to be loaded, the dining car didn't have any napkins aboard. I had to run around, get some off a train coming in, rush them over to Number One, and sign the requisition showing that I had transferred them."

Mr. Gray said, "Is that right? I didn't hear anything about that around here."

"Yeah, I know you didn't. The steward didn't want me to tell anybody, and you know the waiters didn't want me to say anything. But that is just one example of what I have done. Another time the train backed up, and the porter was half-drunk and had not set up his car. He wasn't too tipsy to go out but just needed some help. I set up his car in about twenty minutes."

"Why didn't you tell us about it? We would have grounded him."

"Yeah, I know you would have. If they had grounded him, I would have had to go out on that run, and I didn't want to go that night. And furthermore, a lot of these old men around here would like to stay home some on the weekends, and I could take their runs out."

"Naw, that wouldn't work. Give me your keys."

"Wait a minute. I'll tell you what we can do, Mr. Gray. Let me stay around here this month. I'll keep the keys and see if I can make a job for myself. Just put me on permanent standby duty during the week and allow me to take a run out on Friday. I could get back on the car on Sunday and be ready to go to school on Monday."

"No, I don't believe that would work. Give me the keys."

"No, I just won't give you the keys. You don't have to pay me. Don't put me back on the payroll. Just go ahead and let me do my number around here. I think I could do something that would make you fellows ready to keep me forever. Okay, sign me up for regular station duty."

"No, I'm not going to sign you up. Just give me the keys."

"Well, I'm just going to hang around here anyway."

Sure enough, when the trains backed in to be loaded to go in their different directions, I would go down and inspect every sleeping and dining car and ask, "Do you need anything? Can I help you out in any way?"

I found a lot of little things to be done. One night a car was backed down, and there wasn't any toilet tissue on the sleeping car. I hustled over to the next two or three cars and got a few rolls of tissue and took them to the porter. I didn't say a word about it until the train was gone half an hour. Then I went to the office and said, "Mr. Gray, you know one thing? There wasn't any toilet tissue on car number eighteen on train number one."

"Well, what the hell happened?"

"I don't know what happened."

"Did you do anything?" he asked.

I answered, "Oh, yes. I got three rolls and put them on the car. That will be enough until they get to Minneapolis tomorrow."

The next night, the Olympian backed into the station for loading, and the steward was about to have a fit because nobody had brought the crescent rolls down for the next morning's breakfast. I scooted over to the Fred Harvey Restaurant, which furnished the rolls, and took them to the dining car just as the train pulled out. I waited half an hour, went to the sign-out man, and said, "You know something? They didn't have any crescent rolls on the Olympian. You know they were listed as a specialty for breakfast."

"What the hell happened?"

I said, "The guy was drunk and didn't bring them over from the diner, but I took them over just before the train pulled out."

In the meantime, I enrolled at Wendell Phillips High School on the South Side of Chicago. At the end of the first two weeks, I had my books and was studying assignments for the next day when the porters came in to get their checks. The sign-out man called each one by name, and they came up and got their checks. I was sitting back in a corner, struggling over the assignments, when I heard somebody call my name.

"Quigless, where are you? Quigless, come here."

"What do you want?"

"Come, get your damn check. Now you are assigned to standby duty for Monday through Thursday, and damn it to hell, you be here on time and in your uniform at three o'clock in the afternoon."

"Yes, sir! Oh, by the way, Mr. Gray, would it be possible for me to work standby from Monday through Wednesday and let me have Thursday off, so I can catch up on my schoolwork?"

"Well, if that's the way you want it. What about Friday?"

"I'll be back Friday, and ready for an assignment on the road. Somebody is going to want to miss out on the weekend."

"Okay, we'll see how it goes."

Boy, I was off and running then!

CHAPTER 7

WENDELL PHILLIPS HIGH

There were about ten high schools in Chicago and the surrounding area. Wendell Phillips High School was an old, dilapidated school situated in the middle of South Side, an area of Chicago heavily populated by Blacks. I don't recall how many years it had been in operation when I got there in the fall of 1925. It was within walking distance, about six blocks from my sister's apartment where I was living at the time. It was easy for me to walk to school in the mornings, then leave school and take the streetcar or elevated train to Union Station where I worked. Most of the time I used the elevated train because it got me to Union Station faster.

At that time, all the high school students, except maybe four or five, were Black. Our principal and about two-thirds of the teachers were white, and all but about four of them were elderly. My English teacher, Mrs. Arbell, and one of my math teachers were Black. Most of the white teachers were somewhat senile and plagued with arthritis, much like Mrs. Arbell, who walked with a limp. She was the best and the toughest English teacher at the school. I found the teachers, both Black and white, to be proficient, intelligent, and dedicated to their profession. They tried to give the students as much training and education as they could.

I enrolled in the senior class with the understanding that my records would be transferred from Alcorn. Whether or not I would be able to graduate would depend on the results of my records, along with the progress I made at Wendell Phillips. While checking on the requirements for graduation, I noted that two years of high school music, two years of freehand drawing, and four years of physical education were required.

The only way to get four years of physical education was to be a member of ROTC. That suited me nicely since the band was under the auspices of the ROTC, and I could join the band. I figured I wouldn't have any trouble with high school music since I was a member of the band. I was right. But freehand drawing was something else. It was required before I could finish high school. What could I do about that? I intended to be there for one year, so I tried to figure out how to get around that roadblock. I enrolled in the third semester of freehand drawing. The teacher was a serious artist and seemed interested in her students. She did what she could to try and help them with their work. She spent a lot of time at my desk, thank goodness. She said, "You are about the worst student we have here. I don't see how you got into this class."

One day I told her, "Mrs. Aires, I don't want you to kick me out of this class, but I want to tell you something. I must get out of high school this year. I have to confess to you that I have never had freehand drawing."

She looked hard at me for a minute and then said, "I think you have a lot of nerve enrolling in a third semester of freehand drawing."

I said, "This freehand drawing is the only thing that's going to keep me from graduating."

She answered, "I'll take a few extra pains with you and see what we can do about it."

We were taught the fundamentals of background development. Mrs. Aires brought pictures for us to copy. I remember one with a girl dressed like Whistler's Mother. We sketched her in a costume. My sketch was judged the best in the class. I did not think it was the best and was somewhat embarrassed to have mine chosen. Mrs. Aires spent a lot of time at my desk every day correcting my work and suggesting steps I could take to improve my grades. In addition to that, she was putting 80's and 90's on my papers. Some of the others near me were getting 30's and 40's, and whenever anyone spoke about it, I would change the subject. The lady was definitely in my corner.

The band and ROTC were the best things that happened to me at that time. We had a school orchestra directed and conducted by Mrs. Mildred Bryant Jones. I was familiar with many scores that she taught, and in a short time, she had me helping the other students. Every now and then though, she would fly off and raise hell with all of us about our deportment—the way we looked, talked, acted, and dressed.

We had orchestra practice from one to two o'clock on Tuesday and Friday afternoons. I had to be down at Union Station at three o'clock on Fridays, so I would smuggle my old beat-up handbag into the orchestra room and throw it over in the pile with the cases holding the orchestra instruments. Mrs. Jones was a stickler for discipline. One day we were practicing the "William Tell Overture," and she got mad at two or three boys. She stopped us right in the middle of the score and started raving at us about everything in the world she could think of.

Finally, she got around to the way we piled up the instrument cases. "And one more thing," she raved. "I want to tell whoever it is that brings that old, ragged suitcase in here to get it out and keep it out. I don't want to ever see it in this room again." Mrs. Jones was the only person in there who didn't know who that old, ragged suitcase belonged to. Some of the kids snickered, and some laughed out loud, all except me. I got hot under the collar.

After she dismissed the orchestra, I remained in the room until everybody had left, then went up to her desk and told her, "Mrs. Jones, I'm sorry about the old suitcase. It belongs to me. You see, when I leave here, I have to go down to Union Station, put on the uniform in that suitcase, and work as a sleeping car porter. Most of the time I don't get back home until Sunday morning. I love to play in your orchestra, and I think you are a very fine teacher. I am sorry, but I think I will just have to withdraw from the orchestra."

She looked up at me, turned and looked out the window, looked back at me, then looked out the window again. "Quigless, I am so sorry. I didn't know that you were having to do all that in order to play with us. I'll tell you what. You bring that suitcase in here and put it anywhere you want, and I'll never say another word about it. And furthermore," she said, "please accept my apologies."

"Oh yes, I accept. Thank you, Mrs. Jones." The lady had tears in her eyes.

Being in the ROTC band automatically made me a member of ROTC, but I still had to get a uniform. I got a secondhand one, and both the jacket and pants were too large. The uniform had wrap leggings—the same type issued in World War I. My legs were so skinny that I wore two thick pairs of wool socks underneath so I would look half-way presentable. The band instructor, Major N. Clark Smith, was a Black retired U.S. Army major and a believer in strict military discipline. All band transfer students were assigned the rank of Private.

After two weeks of practice, Major Smith called me over and said, "You know something about that trombone, don't you?" I told him I had played a little before going there. "Where are you from?" I told him where I was from and where I had played. "Well now, I am commissioning you First Lieutenant." He announced this to the rest of the band. After two months, he called me over in front of the band and said, "You've done so well as First Lieutenant that we're going to skip the rank of Colonel and give you the rank of Major and put you in charge of the brass section of the band. Good luck, young man." I saluted, and he walked off. Ha, ha!

Now, what did the officer in charge of the brass section do? He kept the guys in line, bawled them out for fouling up the music, and told them to act like men, not boys. Cole was the smallest fellow in the band and played a tuba. I later learned that his brother was Nat King Cole. He had a sousaphone wrapped all around him, and you could hardly see him for the instrument. He was a mouthy little rascal, too. I was always bawling him out about talking in line, but he handled that tuba very well.

I believe it was early in January 1926 that Soldier Field in Chicago was finished and dedicated before the first football game there. We practiced about two weeks before the dedication ceremonies. Each high school band in Chicago had to play one number and then march to an area of the stadium reserved for the bands. The mass band then played one number under the direction of the Army bandmaster. I felt we were honored to have been selected as part of the mass band for the dedication ceremony. Following our number, the West Point cadets marched around the stadium and did fancy drills. Next, the Annapolis midshipmen marched around the stadium and did fancy drills. The weather was rough, cold, and snowy during the entire ceremony. I looked around at those assembled at the end of the field on which we were located and noticed that some of the soldiers had lost their shoes. They had walked right out of them and kept on marching, never missing a beat.

That was the first big college football game I ever witnessed. For the life of me, I couldn't understand why those guys would get out there in that mud, snow, and cold and beat each other up without complaints. If that game had been played in Mississippi, it would have been postponed until all the snow was gone. We were really glad to get away from that stadium on that January day.

As a part of our English class work at Wendell Phillips, we had a short course in public speaking. While at Alcorn College, although I was in high school classes, I was thrown together with college students especially in choir and other vocal organizations. We made many public appearances, and during that time, I became immune to stage fright. In the public speaking section of English, we made presentations in front of a very critical audience composed of teachers and our classmates. Most of my classmates at Wendell Phillips suffered from stage fright, some to the extent that they stammered when standing in front of an audience. However, I had lost all my fear of audiences, and my presentation was satisfactory to the teachers in charge.

So, when the time came for characters to be chosen for the annual senior play, they chose me as one of the students to read the script. The play was a comedy entitled, "Captain Applejack."

The person playing the lead character had to be able to become dramatic in some places and portray a very comical individual in others. In reading the script, I felt I could portray Captain Applejack very well. However, in looking at the costume, I noted that they depicted a character wearing boots that came half-way to the knees. He also wore pants that came half-way down his thighs, leaving his knees exposed. The costume of another character named Borolsky, on the other hand, had the knees covered. I was so sensitive about my skinny knees that I decided against playing Captain Applejack because of the costume. But my teachers, Mrs. Prescott and Mrs. Cuthburt, strongly insisted that I take the role of

Captain Applejack. And just as strongly, I refused. Time after time they asked me why I didn't want to portray Captain Applejack, but I evaded their questions by telling them that I thought I could portray the villain Borolsky better than Captain Applejack. Both teachers finally accepted my wishes. However, after rehearsals began, they continued asking why I refused the lead role.

About five weeks into rehearsal and three days before the play was to be presented, I finally confessed that I refused the role because my skinny knees would have been exposed. Mrs. Cuthburt responded, "Why in the world didn't you tell us that in the beginning? You didn't have to wear that costume. You could have worn another one if you were too sensitive about your skinny knees. Why, oh why, did you have to turn down the lead role?"

The play was presented on two nights in order to have more students involved. My group presented the play the first night. In my portrayal of the villain, I received tremendous applause, which was very surprising to me. My teachers were all the more dismayed, because they thought my portrayal of Captain Applejack would have been far more effective than the student who had received the part. They immediately began trying to get me to try out for parts in other plays that were being produced in Chicago with the idea of involving Black youths in the theatre. However, I reminded my dear teachers that my mind was set on becoming a physician, and nothing could change that.

Early in March, I was called before the credentials committee to assess my credits and decide whether I would be able to graduate that spring. I was interviewed by Mrs. Burof, who reviewed my credentials from Alcorn and noticed that I had transferred and had done well in my senior year at Wendell Phillips. She asked about my background, knowing that I was from Mississippi. She was from Sioux Falls, South Dakota. I informed her that I had been there at least fifteen times the previous year as a sleeping car porter. Trying to get on her good side, I tried to point out all the good things I could about Sioux Falls. I said that I was elated to be in that part of the Midwest where history had been made many years ago. That pleased her very much.

In checking over my credits, she noted that I had no grades for high school music and freehand drawing from Alcorn. She said, "Now, what are we going to do about this high school music?"

"Mrs. Burof, I came to Wendell Phillips as a Private and was promoted to Major in the ROTC Band. In addition to that, while at Alcorn, I was a member of the college choir, quartet, octet, sextet, and chorus. I think that should take care of the music part, don't you?"

"Oh yes, yes. That's all right. I'll just mark it out here. Now, what about this freehand drawing? You are supposed to have four semesters of freehand drawing, and you only have two here."

I was already way ahead of her there. "Mrs. Burof, we had free-hand drawing in Mississippi." That was a lie. "However, it was not considered a required course for graduation. Please check the marks I received in the two courses here." She noted that at the end of the first month, I had averaged a "D." At the end of the third month, I averaged an "A". Now, how could I have received those marks from a very strict art teacher if I had not been exposed to freehand drawing before coming to Wendell Phillips?

Mrs. Burof said, "Well, I guess you're right there, so I will clear you for graduation. Good luck, young man."

"Thank you, Mrs. Burof."

Everything seemed to be working out well for me. I had gone to Wendell Phillips to get myself totally ready to go to Crane, which was to prepare me for medical school. I wasn't going to let anything get in the way of this plan.

High school graduation day finally came. My brother, Charlie, who was not given to expressions of emotion, smiled at me as I walked down the aisle. He was so elated with my having finished Wendell Phillips that he got me high on Scotch and soda that night.

CHAPTER 8

BACK ON THE RAILROAD

My second summer with the Milwaukee Railroad began. They were forming a crew to man one of the tourist trains that regularly left Chicago on two-week tours. Tourists would travel to such places as Yellowstone Park, Seattle, Alaska, Vancouver, and the Canadian Rockies.

On my first trip to Vancouver, also my first time ever out of the United States, I experienced all kinds of feelings. I can't explain it, but I felt more protected as a U.S. citizen in Canada. I always felt like the underdog in the States because I always felt like I was being looked down on.

I somehow felt prouder to be an American while being in Canada. Although I was on Canadian soil at the time, I felt freer than I had anywhere in the United States.

We had a layover in Vancouver from Friday afternoon until Monday morning. The first thing we did after arriving was get a full meal, followed by a trip to a beer parlor. The parlors resembled old-time saloons in the United States. They had counters with seats, a brass foot rail, tables, and chairs, and all the fixtures of polished mahogany were kept in good condition by waiters who continuously polished and cleaned them. At each parlor, there was a stack of sandwiches, cheese, and crackers for the patrons to munch on while they imbibed their brew.

Since prohibition was the law in the United States, I, along with the rest of the crew, could not wait to begin guzzling that good, strong Canadian beer. I would be more or less stoned by the time we left the beer parlors.

Some of the porters had told me about Stanley Park, a big, beautiful park. I was anxious to see that wonderful place, so we took a taxi there. I don't remember much about the place because of my state of drunkenness. However, I do remember that never in my life had I seen trees so tall. The trees resembled columns of a great cathedral. The ground was covered by brown carpet, made of dried needle-like leaves from the tall redwood trees.

We came upon a clearing in which a bandstand, in the shape of a huge clam shell, had been constructed. A band was giving a concert, and we stopped right there. The band played "God Save the King" as their last selection. As they played, everybody, except three or four of the porters, rose and put their hands over their hearts. I rose along with the other people. They asked me, "What the hell are you standing up for?"

"Man, you better stand up too!"

"They aren't playing 'My Country 'Tis of Thee;' they're playing 'God Save the Queen,' and that's the Canadian national anthem."

Another fellow said, "Hell, I don't stand up for nothing but the 'Star Spangled Banner!'"

I answered, "If you don't stand up here and now, one of those policemen is going to pop you across the head and put you in jail." He immediately stood up.

About 10 a.m. on Monday, the passengers boarded the train again for a trip through the Canadian Rockies and back to the United States. The route took us along the Frazier River with its clear blue water cascading toward the sea. I could watch that river all day, especially when we got to the rocky area known as Hell's Gate, a small waterfall in the region. As we went along, we could see

American Indians poised along the riverbank with what we called gigs, spearing salmon as they swam upriver to spawn. At that time the American fishermen were allotted certain days and hours when they could fish for salmon. However, the Indians were free to fish for salmon at any time. They stood poised along the banks, and as the salmon swam by, they speared them with gigs, dressed them, hung them up under a canopy of tree boughs and smoked them, just as we would smoke other types of meat in the South.

Shortly, the tracks left the Frazier River, and the climb would begin toward the Rockies. After dark, some of the passengers retired to the recreation car to dance or play cards. Some asked that their berths be made down so they could go to bed early.

A stop would be made at 4 a.m., at a station near Mount Revelstowe. At that time, if one looked to the south, he could see the peaks of the rugged, multi-colored mountains shining in the rising sun, along with snow-white glaciers in the spaces between the mountain peaks that seemed to descend into the pre-dawn darkness that still enveloped the valley. After my first trip over the Canadian Rockies, I always told my passengers about this early morning view and that I would awaken them in time to enjoy it if they wanted me to, and most of my passengers would. After the train had left the station, I would direct them to the club car where they could obtain hot coffee and doughnuts. Invariably, my passengers would insist that I come back to the club car and enjoy the hot coffee and doughnuts with them.

Our first scheduled stop was at Lake Louise, which was advertised as "Lovely Lake Louise." The passengers could leave the train and board buses for a trip to Chateau Lake Louise, an alpine-type hotel situated at one end of the crystal-clear lake. The passengers could take a swim in pools fed by hot springs, which bubbled out of the ground all over the region. Later, they would return to the train and take off for Banff, Alberta.

All the areas around Banff were considered a national park, so another bus trip was scheduled for that resort. After the passengers departed on the buses, we would tidy up our cars and make the beds down because we knew that the passengers would be ready to go to bed as soon as they got back from their day-long trip. We would then take in the resort areas and stop and rest for lunch at noon. On one such trip, we stopped at a restaurant and were greeted warmly by a waitress who said she knew they had something special for lunch that day that we were going to enjoy. We tried to find out what it was, but she would not tell us. At the end of our lunch, she brought out this baked concoction covered with a sweet sauce. She inquired, "What do you think of it?"

I asked, "What is it?"

"Cornbread."

"Cornbread! Lady, where I come from cornbread is not served with sweet sauce. It's covered with collard greens and black-eyed peas."

The waitress had never heard of collard greens or black-eyed peas. Soul food was not being imported to Canada in those days. I took time to explain the types of foods we ate in the southern United States.

Because Banff was a national park, animals such as moose and deer could be seen roaming around the area. The deer were quite tame and enjoyed being petted and served cakes, candy, or anything that was offered. One day we saw a pair of bear cubs. I started feeding them peanuts, and the old mama bear saw us, grunted, and started in our direction. We were not there when she got to the cubs.

Usually after lunch, we would retire to the King Edward Beer Parlor, imbibe more of that good old cold Canadian beer, and get half high again. Then we would go back to our stations and welcome the passengers. We spent the next day traveling through the central plains where nothing could be seen except wheat fields. The next morning, we arrived at Moose Jaw, Saskatchewan, and transferred to the Sioux-Saint Marie Railroad, better known as the Soo Line, which carried us into St. Paul, Minnesota, and on to Chicago, arriving on Saturday, fourteen days later.

On my third summer as a porter, I found the tourist trips to be more stable and lucrative than the other overnight runs out of Chicago, so I asked to be put on one of them for the season. I was put on a crew with a conductor named Andy Johnson. Andy had been employed by the railroad for about twenty years and had been a brakeman. The brakeman couples the cars together on a freight train. He had been involved in a wreck in which he lost three fingers of his left hand. Instead of retiring, Andy then trained to be a conductor. He was not too bright and required help in doing his reports and filling out requisitions.

One day, I found him sitting at a table, scratching his head, and trying to figure out just what he should do next. I started helping him and soon found myself in a mess. Andy began depending on me to do a lot of things that he could have done himself. One day he said, "Quig, as long as you are with this railroad, I want you to run with me." I remembered that I had been in tough spots once or twice and had to depend on other people to help me, so I agreed to help him the best I could. That was the beginning of a strong friendship between us.

Each crew of sleeping car porters was under the supervision and direction of the sleeping car conductor. At intervals, an inspector would board the train somewhere along the route, after it left the terminal and before arriving at its destination, to check on the service given by the conductor, dining car stewards and waiters, and the porters. None of the members of the dining car or sleeping car crews were supposed to know where that inspector was or when he was going to board the train. However, during the day, the porters had a system whereby they could indicate by sign language the general location of the inspector. They could communicate from one train to another as they met and passed along the route.

Now, if this inspector boarded your train and found the washrooms not in order, the linen closets dirty or in disarray, dusty windowsills, or unclean corridors and the like, the porter would be reported to the superintendent and called in for a hearing. If the offense was severe enough, the porter would be laid off for up to two or three weeks, and in the most severe cases, he would be discharged.

The most feared of all inspectors was the hard-nosed, wiry, cussing Mr. Copenall. I was warned early in the game to be on the lookout for him. Most of the older porters were definitely afraid of him. I noted that whenever he boarded a train, they became overly polite, bowing and scraping, and obviously nervous. I didn't see any need to become nervous as long as my work had been done properly. I passed this word along to the other porters, and they would say, "Oh no, you just don't know that man. He's going to find something to beef about no matter how careful you are doing your work." I just couldn't see it that way.

However, when he inspected my car, I would go along with him, and if he caught anything out of line, he would tell me what to do to straighten it out. I would thank him, and he would go along to the next car.

Whenever he checked the other porters' cars, they would end up sweating and exhaling great sighs of relief after he left. I asked one of the older men just why they were so nervous. "I don't want to be grounded for a week or ten days and lose the pay and tips I could make," he said.

More than one porter expressed hope that Copenall would not be in their car that night. If he slept in their car, they couldn't take a snooze in the aisle, because he might get out of bed to check on them and find them asleep. All the porters on duty were supposed to be alert and ready to answer any bell whenever a passenger required their service during the night.

One of the regular duties of the porters was to shine the passengers' shoes, which were usually left beneath the lower berth when the passengers retired. Copenall was around sixty years of age. He loved smoking a great long meerschaum pipe, so he frequently sat in the smoking compartment with the porters late at night while they shined shoes and did other chores. On one trip, he brought along his two young sons. One was about eight and the other about ten. The boys were very energetic and loved talking to everyone who would listen. The other porters seemed to be afraid of the boys. However, I was glad to talk with them.

After the passengers retired, Copenall came to the smoking compartment and sat while I shined shoes. Copenall and I got into a conversation that lasted about two hours. After a while he said, "Well, I guess I had better find some place to sleep." I told him that I would be glad to have him sleep on my car. He answered, "Huh, nobody else seems to be glad to have me around."

"As long as I do my work, I don't see any reason why I should be afraid of you."

"That's right, young man. That's the right idea."

One night en route to Seattle/Tacoma, he boarded our train at a little town in North Dakota. After inspecting the cars, he came into my smoking compartment while I was shining shoes and said, "Well, Quigless, I'm going to bed. Get me up at five o'clock in the morning."

"Yes, sir."

I took great pains to wake him at exactly 5 a.m. We were approaching the entrance to Yellowstone Park at Gallatin Gateway. He went into the washroom and called out, "Quigless, go on up to the dining car and get your breakfast now so that you won't have to wait until eleven before you have a chance to eat." I went ahead to the dining car and found the dining car crew just as busy as could be.

I was confronted by the steward in charge, and he asked, "What are you doing up here this time of morning?"

I replied, "Mr. Copenall told me to come up here and get my breakfast so I wouldn't have to wait so late before I ate."

"Mr. Copenall don't run this damn dining car. I run it, and you just get the hell on back there and wait until it's time for you to come and eat." About that time, he started stammering, and his eyes widened. I turned around and Mr. Copenall was right behind me.

"Just what's going on here?" he inquired.

The steward answered, "Oh, I was just questioning Quigless here about coming up at this time of morning and was just getting ready to serve him."

One of the waiters got busy setting up the table. He brought me a menu and asked, "Well, little brother, what would you like for breakfast?"

I asked for a tall glass of orange juice to be followed by a slice of country ham, two eggs over light, toast, and coffee.

Copenall commented, "You ordered a nice breakfast." He took a seat at my table and said to the waiter, "Repeat that order for me, please."

The waiter said, "Yes, sir."

Just as he turned to go back into the kitchen, he rolled his eyes at me. I looked out the window.

I did not know it at the time, but I had incurred the wrath of the sleeping car porters by reporting incidents of shortages I found on the cars being backed into the station to take on passengers. Because I reported that I had taken care of these shortages, some of the porters were called in and reprimanded for not having properly supplied the car. I didn't know it, but I was making enemies for myself. I made enemies among the porters, the stewards, and the dining car waiters. In my mind, I just did my job and saw to it that the cars were properly equipped and stocked.

Meanwhile, the superintendent got a message that an extra sleeping car was needed in three days at the Seattle terminal. That meant a sleeping car would have to be sent out from Chicago for passengers. In other words, it was supposed to be what we called a "deadhead" trip, and a porter had to be on board to guard against vandalism. I was eager to get to Seattle anyway, so I volunteered for the trip. The empty sleeping car was attached to the train just behind the engine with the baggage and mail cars between it and the rest of the train.

We were two days out of Chicago, and I went back to the dining car for dinner. The first person I saw was one of those porters who had been called on the carpet because he hadn't properly supplied his car for the passengers. When I had to re-stock his car, I reported him. So, he was mad at me. As I came through the dining car door, he said, "Oh, there you are. You're the guy

I want to see. What the hell are you doing reporting me to the superintendent?"

"I didn't report you," I emphasized. "But I had to report the fact that I had not found any towels on your car and had to transfer some from another car so you wouldn't be short the next morning when the passengers wanted to wash up."

"Naw, that won't do. I'm going to get your tail before we get to Seattle."

I got my dinner but was afraid of that big guy. It so happened that by the time I finished my dinner, the train had already stopped. I tore out of that dining car, got to my car, and locked myself in. I did not come out of the car until we got to Seattle. I went around from one end of the line to the other, explaining that I was doing a job and hadn't reported anybody out of malice. I explained to the porters that if I had not discovered the shortages, they might have been fired or at least grounded one or two weeks. That quieted the waiters and even the porter, who was trying to get me to apologize.

On another deadhead trip to Seattle, the conductor decided that the train was a little too long to make it over the Rocky Mountains on scheduled time. My car was cut off the train at Mobridge, South Dakota, where I had to layover for three days waiting for another one to take me on to Seattle. Mobridge was a division point. The train engines changed there—one train crew would be dropped off and another taken on.

The town had one street, which began at the railroad station, and five or six stores were located on either side of the street. There were about thirty-five houses just past the stores, and beyond that point, the road stretched out into the horizon. There was a restaurant in the little station for the convenience of passengers transferring from one train to another. All they served were bacon and eggs, ham and eggs, toast, canned juice, hamburgers, and coffee.

I was there for three days, and the first day I ate bacon and eggs for breakfast, ham and eggs for dinner, and bacon and eggs for supper. The next day I ate the same, except for dinner when I had two hamburgers served on stale buns. They had a special of what they called custard pies, but I'm not sure what they really were. They looked like cooked starch with sugar in it. I knew that a special train was arriving the next morning, so I stationed myself about where I thought the dining car would be when the train stopped. When the train came to a halt, I boarded it and went through the dining car into the kitchen where I saw a chef I knew.

"What's up?" he asked.

"I'm about to starve to death around here. All I've had to eat for two days is bacon and eggs, ham and eggs, pie, stale hamburgers, and coffee. Give me some food! I must have some food!"

While they were serving breakfast, an order of ham and eggs was about to go out, and he said, "Here, eat this ham and eggs."

"No! I'd rather finish starving than eat more ham and eggs. That's all I've been eating for two days."

He put a roast duckling that had been left over from the night before in a small tablecloth. He also put on two pounds of cheese, three or four cans of fruit, a loaf of bread, and three cans of sardines. Then he tied it up into a bundle, shoved it to me, and said, "Get the hell out of here." I was just backing off the car through the kitchen door, when all of a sudden, he looked like he had been shot. Then he jumped back in the car through the door.

I looked around, and who should be standing there but Inspector Copenall. I was galvanized. Copenall looked around and then back down the track in the direction from which the train had come. He was giving me a chance to run. I ran like hell through the station to a point where I couldn't be seen and sat there, praying and puffing. I just knew my railroad career had ended right there, and I felt so sorry that I had involved their best chef.

But I never heard a word about that episode. I thank the good Lord for looking after me, and for such people as Mr. Copenall. That man saved my life. If he hadn't looked down the track in the other direction, I probably would not be here today, writing my story.

CHAPTER 9

IN THE PACIFIC NORTHWEST

On two or three occasions, I walked around the town of Tacoma, Washington after finishing my work. I found Washington far different from any of the other parts of the United States I had been. The Pacific Ocean appears blue, whereas the Atlantic Ocean appears green. There were few Black people in Tacoma.

Timber and fishing were the main industries. I saw many fishermen, but I saw more lumberjacks on the streets. They were tall, sturdy, bearded, tobacco-chewing men. They all wore hob-nailed boots and cussed like hell. I remember July 4, 1927, when I was in Spokane, Washington with another porter named David Daniels, who was a student at Fisk University. "They're having a great celebration in town," he told me. All we could hear was what we thought was fireworks exploding.

We finished our chores and set out to take a sightseeing walk around the city. When we got about four blocks from the railroad station, we turned onto a side street. What we had thought were fireworks exploding were drunken lumberjacks shooting their pistols. We stopped in a nearby restaurant for lunch, and it didn't seem too safe in there either, as a tall lumberjack with a two-week beard on his face was stone drunk and singing to a waitress, who was ignoring him. When he saw us, he turned around and said, "Hello there, boys. How're you doing?"

We were scared but said, "Oh, we're fine."

"You like it around here? You came on the train, didn't you?"

"Yes, we came on the train."

"You like it out here?"

"Oh, we like it fine."

"I like it, too. You know something else? I like you boys, but I don't like damn coons."

I looked at Dave, and Dave looked at me.

The man said, "I don't mean you boys. I mean those damn Indian coons. I saw one outside and knocked his damn head off and heaved him into the trash can out back."

We didn't enjoy that lunch very much. As we hastily left the restaurant, we looked down the alley, and sure enough, we saw half of a man's body and legs sticking out of the garbage can. We went and pulled the fellow out. His face was beat up and bruised, and he seemed hardly alive. We washed his face, and he said he would be all right, so we left him there. We felt sorry for the Indian, but there wasn't anything else we could do. We probably would have gotten in trouble by trying to help him. We went back to the train. Goodbye, Spokane!

Back in Seattle, we wandered along the waterfront and saw sailors of all nationalities who were unable to speak any English. They talked and gestured, but we didn't know what they were saying. We passed a restaurant that had a sign in the window: "Oysters – 45 cents – 1/2 dozen." That was interesting to me. Where I came from, you could get two dozen oysters for forty-five cents. We went in and asked the man at the counter what kind of oysters he had for forty-five cents a half dozen. He said the oysters were plants. "I bet you couldn't eat half a dozen."

I knew good and well that I could eat a half dozen of any kind of oysters. Low and behold, he brought out a large platter with what appeared to be six boneless filets of breaded fish. However, when I cut into the things, I saw that they really were oysters. He explained to me that "plants" were oysters kept in beds or enclosures where they were fed cotton seed or soybean meal. That caused them to grow very large in a short period of time. I really could not eat six of those oysters because they were so large.

I liked Tacoma much better than Seattle. All in all, the people in Tacoma were more friendly. Tacoma reminded me of a Midwestern town, except there were many hills. With about thirty-five thousand residents, the town had about three or four boulevards crisscrossing with cherry trees in the center of the two-way streets. When ripe, the cherries were free to pick and eat. Little Japanese boys ran around picking all the cherries you could eat and charging twenty-five cents for them.

As I walked around town, I noticed that there seemed to be a lot of animosity toward the Japanese residents in Tacoma. I was talking to a young white boy who was about my age and brought up the subject. I asked him, "Why is everyone so prejudiced toward the Japanese?"

He said, "You don't understand. These Gooks got over here and started taking all the jobs. Unless a white boy is willing to work as a lumberjack or on one of these ships leaving port, there ain't much else to do. The easy or minor jobs are taken over by Japanese, and we're left without any work to do."

I asked him what type of work they were taking over, and he said, "Oh, everything—housework, gardening, farming."

I asked if he would be satisfied doing that type of work.

"No, not necessarily. However, I would like to have the choice of taking it or not taking it."

The Japanese residents didn't seem to pay any attention to the sneers of the whites. True, they were working as gardeners and street maintenance workers, and many operated stores and restaurants. I saw buses passing by with the rising sun painted on the sides, loaded with children going to a school with Japanese hieroglyphics and characters on their entrances. A young Japanese man told me that the children were sent to their own schools because of the treatment they were subjected to in the public schools. I saw picketers walking in front of Japanese stores and restaurants.

One day I decided to buy lunch in a Japanese restaurant. The place was crowded with Japanese and white Americans. There was one vacant seat at the end of the counter and sitting next to it was what appeared to be a Japanese farmer. He wore a wide straw hat, overalls, and rough shoes. Instead of taking a seat next to him, I felt a surge of anger pass over me. I said to myself, "Just why in hell should I sit by this guy and eat my meal?" I turned around and walked out of the restaurant.

Suddenly, I realized that I was exhibiting the same prejudice toward this man that I had been subjected to all my life. Here I was being kicked around by all the whites in the world, not because of anything I had done, but because of prejudices instilled in whites toward Blacks. I felt ashamed of myself. I turned around, walked back into the restaurant, and sat down to eat my meal.

That incident had a humbling effect on me, and at the same time allowed me to look into the minds of prejudiced individuals. For the first time I felt that these unreasonable and uncalled for resentments toward my fellowman were brought on by misconceptions as to the equality of individuals regardless of race, creed, or color. Not only were the Japanese looked down upon, but other ethnic groups were made to suffer embarrassment and humiliation because of prejudice. In talking to the young white fellow, I learned further that Chinese individuals were subjected to the same type of prejudice as the Japanese. Filipinos were also looked down on, but most prejudices were directed toward the American Indians.

I asked the young fellow, "What do you think about colored people?"

"Oh, colored people don't give us any trouble. First of all, there aren't many of them out this way, and since they are mostly connected with railroads, they give us no competition as far as taking our jobs." So much for prejudice. So much for *blind* prejudice.

CHAPTER 10

CRANE JUNIOR COLLEGE

The next stop on my overall plan was my matriculation at Crane Junior College. Crane was one of several junior colleges situated in and around Chicago. It was located on the West Side, right off Jackson Boulevard, and established as part of the Chicago Public School System, where high school graduates of limited means could continue their education and prepare themselves for various professions, such as law, chemistry, pharmacy, medicine, and some mechanical trades. There were probably around three thousand students there at that time, but not many of them were Black. I was attracted to Crane because it was a city school and as part of the public school system, it did not charge tuition. In order for me to carry out my plans to get through medical school, it was necessary for me to find a school where I could get the proper training for little or no money. I had to have advanced organic chemistry, advanced biology (including zoology), and a foreign language.

The very first thing I did after enrolling at Crane was to contact some of the students who had been there at least one year ahead of me. I wanted to know who the toughest teachers were on the faculty because I was not at Crane just to be able to go to college. I was there to get properly prepared to study medicine. High school physics was not taught at Alcorn, and I had not been able to incorporate it in my program at Wendell Phillips. As a result, I found it necessary to take a whole year of high school physics in one semester. I sought out the toughest, strictest teacher in physics and was advised that I should enroll in Mrs. Zoe Ferguson's class. For chemistry I was directed to Mr. Faucett; for freshman English I was advised that Mrs. Bourne was the most exacting teacher; and I understood that Mrs. Knight was the best teacher in biology.

Because I had done so well in French at Alcorn and Wendell Phillips, I decided to try another foreign language, German. Now that's where I messed up. You see, proficiency in one foreign language was required as a prerequisite to medical school. One not only had to know the foreign language but had to be able to read and understand scientific subjects in that particular language. After enrolling, I went to Room 301, looked through the glass door, and saw the teacher and the students. I opened the door, and all I could hear was "Gooten Morgan." I didn't know what in the hell they were talking about. I was looking around, not knowing what to think. I started backing out of the room, when the teacher asked me, "What course are you looking for?"

"German I."

"This is German I."

"No, lady. Everybody in here is already speaking German, and this was supposed to be a beginner's class."

"It is, but these students are German Jews. They hear German at home and are taking it because it's easier than taking another foreign language."

Well, there I was, and I didn't even hear good English all day. However, I was determined not to give up on anything that I started, so I made up my mind to go ahead and take German. I would like to say here that with a schedule made up of English, high school physics, chemistry, and biology, I spent an hour and a half at night studying German and another hour and a half on the rest of my studies. Believe me, it was a dog.

I liked physics and found Mrs. Ferguson to be a very good and interesting teacher. She didn't hurry over everything, and I rarely had to ask for explanations. As for Mr. Faucett, on our first day in his class, he said, "This is the first course in college chemistry. If you expect to pass my course, you will have to put up with my insistence on following directions. Further down the road, you will take examinations and be required to identify an unknown substance. It will be necessary for you to follow a prescribed set of directions. If you are not able to follow these directions, you will not be able to identify the substances and will not pass my course."

"You will be seated alphabetically," he continued. "When I give a test, those with a last name beginning with an 'A' will turn your paper over and pass it to the next seatmate whose last name begins with 'B'. He will turn his test paper over and pass it to 'C', and so on, until the end of the row. Beginning on the second row, you will follow the same procedure. After the last paper has been turned over, I will be able to collect them, and when I get to my study, I will find them in alphabetical order. If I find a paper that is not in alphabetical order, I will throw it out, and it will not be graded. Those are my simple instructions. Now, as to the quality of your work. Don't expect me to take anything for granted. You are going to give me what I ask for or you will fail that particular test. And, to make it worse, you will fail my course."

Mr. Faucett was true to his word. For the first month or so there were very few passing marks. But, to this day, I feel the system he gave us has been one of the most important factors in my life.

Mrs. Bourne, the freshman English instructor, was teaching us English composition, and she gave out subjects on which we were required to write a theme. When the class met, Mrs. Bourne picked out two themes—the one she considered the best, and the one she considered the worst. She then gave us a lecture indicating the points that she wanted stressed in our next assignment.

When class met for the second time, she picked out two papers and stated, "I have picked one each from the two themes—one I consider to be the best, and one I consider the worst. I shall not call the students' names but will use these papers to emphasize my criticisms and suggestions. The theme I considered the best is best in one respect, but it is the worst I have ever seen in another. The subject matter is excellent. However, the spelling is atrocious!"

She began reading my theme! After reading it she said, "Now the subject matter warrants an A. The sentence structure is good and carries forth the thought very well. The spelling on the other hand warrants an F, so I'll split the difference and give the writer a C, and I am insistent"—she raised her voice—"that this person find someone to check his theme before turning it in to me!"

My mind traveled back to Mississippi and to the fact that I had skipped the sixth and seventh grades. Because I had continued to read everything I came across, I developed a feeling, even before getting the training in grammar in high school English at Alcorn, that would allow me to combine words into phrases and then put the phrases into sentences that would make sense. Even so, my spelling continued to suffer, and, unlike high school English, I did not have time to go over all those words and look up their spelling. It so happened that one of the other porters was a student at the University of Chicago, majoring in English. I latched onto him and asked him to check my themes before I turned them in. From that time on, the teacher continued reading my themes as the best and graded my papers with A's throughout the remainder of the course.

I distinctly remember the Crane orchestra. The director, Mr. Jones, was from England and had a heavy accent. He was a very demanding director. Some of the students were professional musicians who enrolled in Crane to obtain college credits. You had to be on your toes to play with those guys. There were only three Blacks in the orchestra—a girl who played organ and piano, Irby Gage on clarinet, and me on trombone. We all got along very well, and, as far as I can remember, none of us ever got reprimanded by Mr. Jones.

Mrs. Knight, my first biology teacher, was an interesting teacher, and I have not found her equal yet. Her lectures were so complete that there weren't any questions to ask afterward. All the way through medical school, I found that I was able to correlate some of the basic principles that she laid down with the subjects at hand.

As a person, however, I found her to be quite different. First of all, she was married to an Englishman, and, to hear her talk, if you weren't an Englishman, you were next to nothing. I remember her discussing some findings that were discovered by a biologist from India. One of the other teachers felt that the findings were amazing, but Mrs. Knight said, "Now, look here. You have to take these statements by the Indian with a grain of salt. Those people from India are so filled with romanticism that you have to dissect their findings to the 'nth' degree before you can accept them." I call that lousy.

We entered her classroom one day, and she looked around and stated, "There are thirty-five of you in here now. Out of the thirty-five, two and a half of you are going to finish medical school." She may not have been talking about me, but she looked straight at me when she said that. I said to myself, "Damn, you don't know what you're talking about, lady." I was glad to finish her course and go on to zoology, which was taught by Mrs. Aline Cullinson.

Mrs. Cullinson took great pains with us and as much time as necessary to explain anything that was unclear to us. She had two laboratory assistants, one of whom was Black. Kirsey was a young fellow from Chicago who had finished Crane and gone on to study medicine at the University of Illinois Medical School. Kirsey specialized and took his boards in obstetrics and practiced for many years in the Chicago area. Our first year in zoology began with the study of the lower forms of life, from the amoebae up to, and including, the frog. The second semester began with the study of vertebrates, from dogs and fish through mammals.

Periodically, we were given oral examinations. Either the teacher or the lab assistants would bust us out on the points that we were supposed to have studied. I did not realize it then, but they were preparing us for the oral examinations we would get in medical school. When we got to the cat, each of us was given one to dissect. I never thought of them as animals, only specimens. I knew I had to understand them before I could get into the study of human anatomy. I never thought of a cadaver as being human, only as a specimen that I had to dissect in order to learn the construction of the human body. The cats had been prepared by embalming. The arteries had been injected with a red jelly-like substance and the veins with a blue jelly-like substance, so they could be easily identified. We carried out the dissections during two-hour laboratory periods, three times each week.

It was the early 1920's, and gangsters were ruling Chicago. Every day or so we would pick up the paper to see that a gang fight had erupted, and two or three gangsters had been killed.

Crane was situated on Jackson Boulevard. There was a cemetery out on the boulevard beyond the school. The laboratory was on the fourth floor of the school, and it was nothing to look out the window every two or three days and see a large funeral procession going by with an ornate hearse and five to twelve Lincoln touring cars filled with floral pieces headed toward the cemetery. Somebody would say, "Uh-oh, another gangster."

I had gotten a little behind in my dissection, so Mrs. Cullinson allowed me to take my cat specimen home with me so I could catch up the work. I wrapped the cat, whom I had named Felix, in oil cloth and several layers of newspaper, so it wouldn't smell on the elevated train. During that time, my brother, Charlie, and I were rooming with a cousin from Mississippi on East 52nd Street. Cousin Annie was a nice lady but superstitious. When I got home, I put the cat under the bed and ate my dinner. She came through, and her very sensitive nose picked up the odor of formaldehyde. She looked around and sniffed until she found the package under the bed. "Come here at once!" she yelled.

"Okay, Cousin Annie. What's the trouble?"

"What's that thing that smells so bad in there?"

I answered, "The cat that I brought home to dissect. I have been working on it in the laboratory at school."

"You mean to tell me that you have a dead cat in this house?"

"He won't bother you. You won't get an infection from him. He is preserved with formaldehyde."

"Yeah, I smell that terrible stuff. I'm going to tell you something right now. You're welcome to stay here, but that cat has got to go. Get that thing out of my house...NOW!"

"Okay, Cousin Annie. I'll do just that."

"Now! You just get that thing away from here!"

"Cousin Annie, I'll get it. I'll take the cat back to the laboratory and do my extra work there."

Soon after that we were to make a detailed study of the cat's skull. The skull was much easier for me to smuggle into the house. One Thursday, when I was off work, I jumped into the bed, got the cat's skull, and started memorizing the foramina, that is, the holes in the cat's skull. Each hole, or foramen, had a name, which I memorized along with the names of the nerves that went through those holes. As I was studying, I got a phone call. I dropped the skull on the bed and went to answer the telephone. In the meantime, my brother, Charlie, came home. He pulled off his clothes, put on his pajamas, and jumped into bed, landing smack dab on the upturned cat's skull. The cat's teeth sank right into Charlie's buttocks. He yelled, jumped out of bed, and threw back the covers to find the skull.

"What the hell you got in here?" he demanded.

"Oh, that's nothing but the cat's skull we are studying about."

"That damn thing bit me on the butt. Don't you ever bring it back."

"Okay, okay," I answered.

Every morning I awoke at 6:30 a.m., fixed my breakfast, and caught the elevated train by 8 a.m. My classes went until 3 p.m., then I would catch the elevated train to Union Station, where I would quickly change into my porter's uniform and either check on the outgoing trains or hustle down through the railroad yard to prepare a sleeping car for an overnight to Kansas City, Ohio, or Minneapolis. Though I felt my life was boring at times, I never thought of giving up.

Sometimes I had trouble getting up in the mornings. I hated getting up to the jangle of an alarm clock. I bought a record by

Paul Whiteman with the title, "When the Red, Red Robin Comes Bob, Bob, Bobbin' Along", and whenever the alarm clock started, I would turn on the Victrola. That song made getting up very easy for me, especially the part that went, "Wake up, wake up, you sleepyhead; Get up, get up, get out of bed." I'd jump out of bed and start fixing breakfast. I just about wore that record out in the two and a half years I was at Crane College.

Every now and then I would get depressed, thinking about how long it was going to take me to reach my goal. Everybody else was having fun, going to the Big League baseball games, to girlie shows downtown two or three times each week, on trips to dances, and so much more! I sat home and missed it all. I would begin thinking about all the good times I was missing, then I'd just try to push it out of my mind and think about how well I was going to do when I got to be a doctor.

I was reading the *Chicago Tribune* one Sunday when I came across an article describing a picture entitled, "The Song of the Lark" that was on exhibition at the Chicago Art Institute. In describing the picture, the writer described a girl in a field with a scythe in her hand, looking up at the lark winging its way through the sky while it sang. The way the writer described the picture served to excite my curiosity. That afternoon, I went to the Art Institute to see the picture. When I saw it, I was even more impressed than I had been when I read the description of it. The painting was huge and perfect, down to the most minute detail with the background highlighting the figure of the girl. I sat on a bench in front of the picture and went over every detail.

The thought came to me, "This peasant girl has nothing to look forward to. She is going to follow the flight of the lark and listen to its cheerful song. But when it disappears into the distance, she will be left standing there in the field with her scythe in her hand and must start harvesting the grain with nothing to look forward to, except the end of a dismal day and the beginning of another."

I looked forward to the time when all this working, hard study, and being denied the pleasures that so many of my friends were enjoying would end, and I would be able to do what I had always wanted to do—practice medicine. I left the Art Institute in much better spirits than when I arrived. I think that was the last time I became deeply depressed.

While I was at Crane, my sister, Virgie, who worked on the Far West Side of Chicago, decided to move to the West Side so it wouldn't take so long to get to work from where she lived on the South Side. At that time, Blacks were moving to the West Side in large numbers. Virgie rented an apartment just off Division Street. Because she was alone, she asked me to move in with her. I did so but hated leaving the South Side of Chicago where all my friends were.

The apartment was at the rear of a building and three flights up. I could look over Division Street from the back porch and see the backs of other apartments with washing hanging on the porches, kids playing in the alleys, and hucksters traveling through the alleys hawking their wares. It was about that same time that Dean O'Banion, a noted Chicago gangster, was gunned down in his florist shop on Division Street. I didn't see the gangland slaying from where I stood on my back porch, but I could look over into O'Banion's florist shop from there. I didn't like that very much. I told Virgie, "I don't like the West Side. I prefer the South Side."

She answered, "Oh, don't worry about that. They're not after you. They're after their own kind."

One Sunday morning about 10:40 a.m., I was on my way home after traveling from Minneapolis to Chicago. I was walking down one side of the street, and a drunk was on the opposite side. Suddenly, about eight or ten boys, not a one of them over twelve years of age, surrounded the drunk, pinned him down, rifled through his pockets, and then scattered like a bunch of frightened sparrows. I told my sister again, "Look here, I want to go back to the South Side. I can't take this any longer."

"But they're not after you."

"How about that drunk out there? They threw him down and robbed him in less time than it took me to tell you about it. They might do the same to me next time."

She still insisted that everything was all right, but I was suspicious of everyone I met on the street. Then, all of a sudden, it came to a head. I picked up the morning paper, and there it was staring me in the face: the St. Valentine's Day massacre. When all the shooting had died down, the police found several gangsters perforated by machine gunfire. A mechanic was also found. The only thing that was left alive in that garage was a dog. Apparently, according to the newspaper account, they had been lined up against the wall and executed by machine guns.

I thought if they would do that to the mechanic, the same fate might await me if I happened to be too near them at some point. I thought that if I removed myself from the area, my chances of living a while longer might greatly improve.

I turned to my sister and said, "Some gangsters got ripped off; that's fine. But what about that mechanic? If that dog could talk, he probably would have been dead too." That afternoon I got my few belongings together and told my sister, "You can stay here if you want to, but I'm going to Ruth's place on the South Side if she'll take me in." Virgie also returned to the South Side about two weeks later.

At the end of my second year at Crane, I graduated with my Associate in Arts degree and had enough credits to be admitted to medical school. I decided to take bacteriology, advanced physics, and advanced zoology to become a laboratory assistant in zoology. In liberal arts, I decided to take Old English literature. That was a mistake.

I was reading Chaucer, memorizing Old English terms I would never use, and reciting stuff in Old English brogue that I could never master. I stuck it out until we got to "Beowulf." That was my undoing! In order to understand what I was reading, I had to spend a lot of time looking up definitions of the Old English terms being used in the story. I quickly decided that I didn't need that much culture and didn't want to waste my time learning it when I very probably would never use it. I knew all my energy had to be aimed toward getting the pre-medical education I needed. I just said, "To heck with 'Beowulf ' and Old English literature." I checked out of school, went down to the railroad station, and signed up as a regular porter for the remainder of the school year.

I am indeed grateful to the teachers at Crane for the pains they took with me. I consider them all very fair-minded, and they thought of me as just another student, not as a Black student. However, there were some incidents at Crane which caused me to leave the school with mixed feelings. First, there was a man teaching a medical subject called histology. I was putting my whole soul into my work, and whenever I asked questions, he snapped at me. I didn't pay him any mind and at times just laughed at him. It was quite evident that he was a racist.

We were given bits of tissue to be stained and made into microscope slides for part of our lab work. He gave me a section of fetal pigskin tissue, and I was to make slides of the material to be passed into the department in order to get credit for the course. I followed his directions explicitly. I avoided the teacher and called on one of the assistants for help. I finished my slides and was proud of them because they surpassed those of my classmates. I passed them to the teacher. He took one look under the microscope and said they didn't reveal what he wanted because the hair follicles had not developed. He insisted it be done over, not because of technical error, but because the development stage he wanted to demonstrate wasn't shown. I didn't argue with him; there was only a week left in the term. I took the slides to Dr. Lawrence, head of the department, and was given a coveted A. Thankfully, when this racist protested, he was put in his place by Dr. Lawrence.

Second, there was a white girl who had classes along with me. My locker was on the fourth floor hall where I had three of my classes. We had to lug our books from our locker to the classrooms. Because her locker was on the first floor, it was rather difficult for her to race down to the first floor with her books and back up to the fourth to class without being late. One day she came to me and said, "Quigless, is it too much trouble for me to put my books in your locker? I have to go up and down to classes. I'd appreciate your letting me put them in your locker, so I won't have to make so many trips to the first floor."

"Yes, it's all right with me," I said.

So, she placed her books in my locker. One day one of her white male friends passed by, looked at her, and said, "What the hell are you doing, putting your books in there?"

"What's wrong with you?" she asked. "I put my books in his locker because it's more convenient."

"Well, I don't like it a damn bit!" he said.

This fellow wasn't any bigger than me, so without caring who was passing by, I said, "Well, what the hell are you going to do about it?" He turned red in the face and went on about his business.

And there was a third incident at Crane. I was approaching the school with one of my white classmates when we were met by about eighteen white boys. One of them looked straight up in the air and said, "Ooh, look at the jiggaboo."

Knowing that he was referring to me, I started for him, but my friend said, "Wait a minute! Don't get into that. I know he hurt your feelings, but if you get tangled up with that gang, you're going to get your bones broken." I thought about it and decided that he was right. I ignored them. I decided the advantage of being at Crane would far outweigh the difficulties, and I shrugged it off.

The worst slap in the face I got from Crane was concerning class pictures. The students in all the class pictures I had seen heretofore were in alphabetical order whether they were Black or white. My class picture was delayed a whole year. I was furious when I finally did get it. All the Blacks were on the first row at the top of the picture. There was about one inch between that row and the second, so that the first row could easily be cut off if anyone wanted to do it. There wasn't anything I could say about it, but I decided that there wasn't any need for me to go back to Crane for anything.

CHAPTER 11

MEHARRY MEDICAL SCHOOL

I applied for admission to four medical schools: University of Minnesota, University of Illinois, Northwestern, and Meharry. Northwestern turned me down when they saw my picture. I had strong feelings about going to the University of Minnesota Medical School. However, during one of my weekend runs to Minneapolis, I went down the street to where I could get four hotcakes, a slice of ham, and all the coffee I could drink for thirty-five cents. As I walked along to the restaurant, there wasn't any wind, but I felt a stinging sensation about my ears. I got to the restaurant, got my order, and started eating. About that time, a man came in delivering supplies to the restaurant, and one of the workers asked him, "How cold is it out there now?"

The delivery man replied, "Twenty-seven below. It was thirty below when I got up this morning."

Well, I started getting cold right there in the restaurant and nearly froze to death on my way back to the station. I decided that the University of Minnesota was out. O-U-T!

During the time that I worked as a sleeping car porter in Chicago, I had been in contact with many medical and dental students attending Meharry Medical College in Nashville. I listened at length to the descriptions and accounts of their medical studies there. I came to know the different teachers, their mannerisms, their good points, and their bad points. I decided that Meharry Medical College must not have been such a bad place.

With that in mind, several other medical students and I boarded a train headed for Nashville. I met another incoming freshman by the name of Seabrooks. He had not had the benefit of pre-med courses. However, he had finished college with a Bachelor of Science degree from one of the schools in the Nashville vicinity. He had been exposed to some chemistry and physics, and a smattering of biology.

Because he had been around Nashville for four years, his assistance was invaluable to me when it came time to find a place to reside. Seabrooks knew one of the neighborhood merchants who lived near Meharry. The man had a large, rambling house, and all his children were grown and gone. We made a beeline for the house and asked him and his wife to take us in as roomers. They showed us a large room, which seemed comfortable. The bed seemed all right, the mattresses firm and not lumpy. We felt that because the merchant operated a small grocery and market, we would, at the very least, be assured of having ample meals. The merchant also sold coal as a sideline during the winter; thus, we were assured of being warm as well. Seabrooks found two more of his friends who were looking for a place to stay, and the room accommodated the four of us without any crowding. The rate for the rent and board was twenty-five dollars per month. Try finding that in this day and age. The next morning, we had a good breakfast and were at Meharry by 8 a.m. for our first assignments.

So, there I was at Meharry Medical College. Why was it named Meharry? Fifteen or twenty years prior to the founding of Meharry, there were five Irish brothers named Meharry operating a farm in southern Indiana. At that time there was no such thing as refrigeration, so one of the most important commodities in a farming area was salt. One of the Meharry brothers took their horse-drawn wagon to the nearby town to get their year's supply of salt, which would enable them to preserve the meats and kindred farm products used during winter months.

On his way back, he encountered a great storm. As he drove along, his team got mired in the muddy road, and all he could think about was that the salt he was carrying home would be ruined. He looked around and saw a log cabin nearby. A former slave came to the door, saw that the man was in distress, and went out to help him. He hitched two other horses to the wagon and pulled it from the mire and under a shelter, thereby saving the salt and asking for no compensation in return. The Meharry brother was so impressed with the willingness of the freed slave to help him that he vowed that someday, in some way, he would do something to help the formerly enslaved people.

During this same period there was a young officer named George Whipple Hubbard, who witnessed the pitiful state of the recently freed slaves. After receiving his medical degree from Vanderbilt University, he offered his services to the Methodist Episcopal Church. He developed a medical department at Central Tennessee College, which was under the auspices of the Methodist Church, to train Negroes for the practice of medicine. Here is where the Meharry brothers come in. When the Methodist Church sent out a call for funds to establish a school, the five Meharry brothers gave fifteen thousand dollars to the church. When Dr. Hubbard heard of the Meharrys' gift, he suggested that the school be named Meharry Medical College in grateful appreciation for the first donation toward the establishment of the school.

Meharry opened in 1876 as a medical department of Central Tennessee College with Dr. George Whipple Hubbard as dean and faculty. The name was changed to Meharry Medical College of Walden University in 1900. Then with the decline of Walden University, it obtained a separate corporate existence on October 13, 1915.

When I enrolled at Meharry in 1929, the many faculty members at that time were learned and dedicated physicians. Dr. D. Victor Romans was also one of the founders of the National Medical Association, which exists today as a forum for the dissemination of medical information to Black physicians and surgeons as well as a mouthpiece for the Black medical profession in all matters— scientific, political, and otherwise.

We also had two white teachers from Vanderbilt, both of whom were in the Department of Medicine. That was the only relationship Meharry had with Vanderbilt.

I was concerned with learning all I could. My teachers not only taught from the textbooks, but they also related personal experiences. I was pretty well prepared for whatever I might run into when I got there. When I started Meharry, I was making about one thousand dollars per summer. Tuition was four hundred fifty dollars per year, and board was ten to fifteen dollars per month, so that left me very little money to live on. At the beginning of my third year at Meharry, I returned to Nashville with just over one hundred dollars in my pocket. That shows how bad times were. We were a few years into the Great Depression by then, and it was beating the hell out of us.

But prior to all that, on a bright September morning in 1929, before the stock market crash could wreak havoc on the U.S. economy, the incoming Meharry class of 1933 assembled in a small lecture room on the second floor of the administration building. I recognized one member of the incoming class—Don

Watkins. He had been one of my classmates at Alcorn. I was surprised to see him because he had been studying agriculture with plans to return to Sunflower County, Mississippi, to help the farmers. There were three or four fellows from Morehouse College in Atlanta, two from California, two cousins and two sisters from Texas, four fellows from North Carolina, and one student from Kenneth Square, Pennsylvania, who later became my buddy.

The remainder of the class was from various colleges. We made the rounds of the different classrooms and were given a list of books and supplies we needed to get before reporting to class the next day. The three subjects that we would study the first semester were physiology, physiological chemistry, and anatomy. I was forewarned that physiology would be the easiest subject and physiological chemistry the most difficult. Anatomy would be the most exciting to some and the most devastating to others.

At the beginning of my freshman year, I had enough money to buy the books required for the entire year. I might add that this was the only year I was able to do so. Following my freshman year, money began getting tight and stayed that way until I left Meharry. Physiology was my first class. The teacher was strictly a textbook man.

Physiological chemistry, now called biochemistry, was my next class. The teacher had a doctorate in chemistry and was a brilliant chemist. However, he did not fit very well as a teacher. He would put a formula on the board with his right hand, erase it with his left, while at the same time rapidly give an explanation. He also discouraged any interruption. In addition to these roadblocks, he demanded complete notes. He'd say, "And I mean complete notes, because my examinations will be taken strictly from my notes." As a result, we had to figure out a way that we could attend classes and come up with completed notes in time for weekly quizzes. So, four of us got together and decided that one of us would copy the beginning of a formula before he erased it, the next man would copy the last, the third would write out the beginning of the teacher's explanation, while the fourth would write out the end of it. Then we'd put all four parts together after we had eaten dinner.

The afternoons from 1 until 5 p.m. were given over to anatomy, which was taught by Dr. V. G. Tolbert, a Meharry graduate. He had done postgraduate work at the University of Pennsylvania and was a very colorful character. His first lecture was an outline of the subject matter of his course, and he made it plain to all that we would have to know anatomy before we would be allowed to go to our sophomore year. "If you don't learn it," he said at the beginning of the year, "you can just make plans to go back home and plow." The upperclassmen had told us Dr. Tolbert's bark was worse than his bite. If it became evident that any student was having trouble, he would help him if he thought the student was making an honest effort. Dr. Tolbert could weed out those students who needed more help and determine which students would be most likely to fail.

I could tell that there would be a lot of casualties in the freshman class. From the very first day, Don Watkins, my classmate from Alcorn, was as much out of place as a catfish would be on Main Street. He managed to hang on, however, until one day, Dr. Tolbert walked into the amphitheater and said, "Now, ladies and gentlemen, the time has come for me to introduce you to the cadaver—that is, the human body—that you will dissect during the remainder of this course." That was the day we began the study of anatomy in earnest.

There was a big difference between the study of anatomy in 1929 and the study of anatomy today. When a student begins a course in anatomy today, the cadaver is prepared for him. That is, the cadaver has been suitably embalmed and carefully wrapped in plastic so that evaporation will not occur. In 1929, the cadavers were embalmed and preserved in a solution containing salt and formaldehyde. It was the duty of the students to clean up their specimen, shave it, if necessary, apply a thick coat of Vaseline to make the skin supple, and place it on the dissecting table.

We were placed in groups of four for each cadaver. A large vat contained the bodies which had been embalmed. I grabbed a hook and started pulling a cadaver out of the vat, coming up with a leg. Dr. Tolbert yelled at Watson, who was standing beside me, "Grab that leg, and get him out of there!" Watkins then grabbed the leg but fainted when he attempted to pull it out.

Dr. Tolbert laughed and revived him by throwing water on him. Watkins got up off the floor and walked out, never coming back. When we got back to our boarding place, I was told that Watkins caught the train back to Mississippi. I heard later that he became an agriculture teacher there.

My anatomy group included Orvil Walls of Pennsylvania, Reuben Foster of Beaumont, Texas, and a fellow named Simmon of Louisville, Kentucky, who replaced Watkins. I was glad to have Walls on my team because I weighed around one hundred ten pounds, and he was about two hundred pounds. It was an advantage having the biggest fellow in the class as your buddy. I might add that my friendship with Walls continued as long as we were classmates.

Human anatomy was very interesting to me as I had been prepared for the subject through various courses in zoology at Crane. My roommate, Seabrooks, had trouble keeping up with us. The daily assignments were too much for him. One day, Dr. Tolbert started quizzing Seabrooks, and he went all to pieces. He couldn't utter a word. Dr. Tolbert noticed his nervousness and went to another table. When Seabrooks regained his voice, he told me, "Quig, I'm going to tell you something right now: I'm quitting today."

"Oh, Seabrooks, you can make it all right. Of course, you get nervous every time Dr. Tolbert comes close to you, but you can make it. Suppose we study about an hour longer every night?"

Seabrooks answered, "No. I'm leaving tomorrow morning on that train to Chicago, and I'm going to stay there for the rest of my life." I couldn't do anything to dissuade him. After all, I could see that he wouldn't be able to keep up with the class.

With Seabrooks gone, I was left alone at my rooming place. I decided to move into a fraternity house so I could have three roommates who were also classmates.

As to social aspects of Meharry, there wasn't any campus life. Most of us were in that town to study medicine, and that was foremost on our minds. In the fall, we did take time out to go to football games between Fisk University and other schools. We also saw games between the Black campus of Tennessee State and other schools. Other forms of recreation were the Friday night dances at the Black Masonic Temple in downtown Nashville. No outsiders came to those dances because most of the time, if they came, they came for trouble. Whenever they started anything, they were promptly thrown out by the members of the Masonic Temple.

At the end of my freshman year, I returned to Chicago and to my job as a sleeping car porter. The year was 1930, and the Depression was getting much worse. However, I made enough money to return to medical school. I moved into the fraternity house with my classmates, Reuben Foster, Orvil Walls, and Joe Jones. Joe was from Rocky Mount, North Carolina, and was a brilliant student.

After getting our room in the fraternity house, the next order of business was finding a boarding place. There were several small restaurants scattered around that catered to medical students. The board was cheap, anywhere from fifteen to eighteen dollars per month, which included breakfast and dinner. Breakfast usually consisted of one or two eggs with some bacon, grits, coffee, and biscuits or toast. Dinner was served between 5 and 6 p.m. and consisted of vegetables, meat, bread, and iced tea or coffee. We usually treated ourselves to a hamburger and Coke for lunch. I knew that my money wouldn't last throughout the entire year, so I contacted my younger sister who was still teaching in Mississippi. She agreed to advance my board money whenever my funds were exhausted. My funds lasted until January, at which time I wrote to her, and she readily sent the money to pay my board.

My sister was married, and they had a young son. She and her husband were both working—he was the principal of the school where she taught. His salary was eighty dollars a month, and hers was sixty-five dollars each month. Because they were in a country school, it was easy for them to obtain food with very little money. As a result, she could see her way clear to send me eighteen dollars a month to pay my board. She sent me the money for two months. But along about April, I got a letter from her husband stating that she could no longer send me money because they needed all they were getting paid for their own expenses. I had nowhere else to turn and was frantically trying to get my relatives in Chicago to help me out.

The Depression was very bad at that time. I was two weeks late paying my board, and the lady who ran the boarding place informed me that she would give me three days to get the money together. After three days, the lady called me aside and told me that I would have to find some other place to eat because she couldn't afford to carry me any longer. Every morning and every afternoon I ran to the post office, only to find no mail. Then the day came when I was told not to come back for breakfast. The next morning, we got up, and Walls said, "Come on, Quig, let's go to breakfast."

I lied, "I'm not hungry today. You go ahead, and I'll see you later." I was hungry as hell. Lunchtime came, and Walls said, "Let's go get a hamburger and coffee, old boy."

"I'm not hungry. Go on and get yourself something to eat."

When dinnertime came, Walls said, "Quig, let's go to dinner."

"Nah, I'm still not hungry."

"You're telling me a damn lie. What the hell is up?"

"I'll tell you, Walls. My board money didn't come through, and the lady says I can't eat there anymore until I can pay my bill."

Walls started cussing. "Why in hell didn't you tell me that before now?" "Because I knew you didn't have too much money."

"But damn it to hell, we can't let you starve around here." So, Walls, Foster, and Joe Jones pitched in and paid my board bill. The next morning, I ate two breakfasts, and the next evening I ate two dinners.

Everything went on smoothly for a while after that. They paid my bill again the next month. The good lady became more insistent that everyone pay his bills. One morning, we went out for breakfast to find the restaurant closed. We got worried and went to her home. She wasn't there. She had left town with everyone's money.

A white couple owned Neal's Hamburger Stand about three blocks from the school. Often, we would study until midnight and then retire to Neal's stand after to get a cup of coffee and a hamburger. After the lady absconded with our board money, we all went over to Neal's to talk over our plight. Walls said, "Well, fellows, here we are. We gave her all our money and don't have any left. We'll have to find some way to eat until the end of the school term." He turned to the owner of the hamburger stand and said, "Mr. Neal, if you heard us talking, I'm sure you understand the position we are in. Would it be possible for you to let us board with you until the end of the school term, and let us send the money back to you during the summer? You can be assured that you'll get your money, because Dr. Mullowney would not allow us to re-enter school if you were to go to him and tell him how you had helped us, and we had refused to pay as promised. You know, Mr. Neal, that a lot of Meharry students patronize your hamburger stand, and it shouldn't be too much of a hardship to carry us along. Would you do us that favor?"

Neal went back into his living quarters and talked it over with his wife. Finally, he came out and said, "Well, fellas, I think I can carry you through." We had our first meal of hamburgers, apple turnovers, and coffee right then. From that time until the end of the school term, we were assured of a place where we could eat enough to keep body and soul together.

With all the studying we had to do, there was little time left for social activities. However, there were four all-Black Greek-letter fraternities represented at Meharry—Alpha Phi Alpha, Kappa Alpha Psi, Omega Psi Phi, and Phi Beta Sigma. Each of the four fraternities had a basketball team, and a healthy rivalry had developed among them. Saturday nights, a basketball game would be held between two of the four fraternities at the Masonic Temple's gymnasium, followed by a dance. The rivalry was friendly at all times, and the basketball games and dances gave us a chance to relax from the intense strain connected to long hours of study.

The Meharry upperclassmen formed a combo and performed the music for the dances. The combo included a couple of trumpets, a clarinet, one or two banjos, a bass fiddle, and drums. The leader of the combo and three other members were slated to graduate at the end of the school year. The combo continued with me on trombone, R. W. "Bobo" Miller from Arkansas on drums and banjo, and Julius C. "Juicy" Hines, from Edenton, North Carolina, on clarinet. Another classmate, Frank Avent, played the trumpet, and Ned Stanfield was the pianist. For playing a gig, we each were paid five dollars. With the prospective continuation of the dances, I found a way to pay for my board.

In addition to the basketball games and dances, we occasionally picked up another gig on Friday nights, playing at the country clubs in small surrounding towns such as Columbia, Tennessee. Each of us earned $7.50 for those engagements. I remember one cold Friday night we were returning from Columbia when the ignition system of the car caught fire. There we were, out in the country, with no one around who could put out the fire. We felt doomed to spend the night in the freezing cold. However, the driver yanked up the hood and yelled, "All out! Piss on this fire and put it out!" At our astonished looks, he said, "That's the only thing we have to put it out with. Piss on it!" We managed to put the fire out—but try to imagine the odor that floated up from that hot engine. After about fifteen minutes, the ignition system dried out enough that we were able to start the car and get on into Nashville.

There were two or three radio stations in Nashville at that time. One of them was not doing very well financially. They were glad to pick up any combo or person who thought they could sing or play to round out their programs. One day they approached me and invited us to appear on their program, provided we would not charge them anything. We were glad to have any exposure we could and agreed to play. I shall never forget that program because that was the time I sang the song "Three Little Words." Some of the fellows listening at the frat house said we did pretty well. However, I wonder just how well we did because shortly after that program, the station filed for bankruptcy and moved away from Nashville.

We usually played for the dinner and dance every Friday night, and it was the usual custom for Dr. Rolf to give a short physiology test on Saturday mornings. I usually didn't have a chance to study for the test before we went over to Columbia, so I took my notes and textbook along with me. Because I knew the music we played each week, it was not necessary for me to put the music up on the stand. Instead, I put my notebook up there and studied while we were playing.

One Friday night during intermission, Juicy Hines, the clarinet player, looked over and asked, "Quig, what in hell are you doing with that notebook here? You know you're not going to absorb anything tonight. You'll be as bad off tomorrow morning as we will."

I replied, "While you turkeys are over there twiddling your thumbs, what about a little quiz? Let me bust you out a little, so you'll be ready for tomorrow morning's test."

"Naw, man, go on. We're not ready for that stuff."

"Well, at least you could listen while I read over these notes, so you can have something under your belt."

"Oh, forget it!"

"Okay. Remember, I warned you, and you got the chance to read my notes."

The next morning, we got to the classroom on time, and Dr. Rolf came in, put his questions on the board, and believe it or not, covered the same subjects I had reviewed the night before. I began writing the answers and chuckling. Dr. Rolf came up and said, "Quigless, what are you laughing about?"

I replied, "Doctor, you're asking the same questions I went over last night while we were playing down in Columbia. Now I want you to compare my answers with those of Bro' Avent, Juicy Hines, and Bobo Miller." I looked around at them, and they were sweating like hell. Dr. Rolf posted the grades the following Monday. He had given us ten questions, and our marks were recorded from one to ten. I had been given the coveted ten. Bro' Avent had a two, Juicy Hines had three, and Bobo Miller had zero. That was so amusing to me, but not very funny to my friends.

About this time, I was experiencing severe financial difficulties again. My money was out; I was eating from day to day and wondering how I would travel from Nashville to Chicago for next summer's work. On one particular Saturday morning, my nerves were all to pieces. I could hardly sit still.

I went to Dr. Rolf's physiology class as usual. He put the questions on the board, and I tried to write. My hands were shaking, and I felt like I was smothering. My heart was beating so fast and furious that I could feel a throbbing sensation in my temple. I tried concentrating on the questions, but I couldn't. I began to shake all over. Dr. Rolf approached, looked at me, and inquired, "Quigless, what seems to be the trouble?"

"Doctor, I am just as nervous as I can be. I just need to get myself together. If I could just get out into the air a few minutes, I think I would be able to make it all right. Would you allow me to take a few minutes to get myself together?"

"I'm sorry, Mr. Quigless, but if you leave the room, you'll have to leave your paper and will not be allowed to finish it when you come back."

He was concerned I'd try to look up an answer while I was out of his sight.

"Doctor, I don't need to look up anything. I would just like to get up, walk around, and get my nerves quieted so I can finish this examination."

He replied, "I'm sorry, Mr. Quigless, I can't allow that."

"Doctor, I guess I will just have to sit here and write you 80 percent, or what I think would amount to that and walk out and get myself some air."

He said, "Okay, Mr. Quigless, if you write 80 percent, I'll give you 80 percent." I answered eight of the questions as fast as I could, turned the paper over to him, and walked out of the room. I knew that I could have answered all the questions that he had posted, but I was just wondering if he would be fair-minded enough to give me what I made on that paper. On Monday, the grades were posted, and there was my 80 percent.

Social life was extra drab during my stay at Meharry. Although there were many beautiful girls attending Nashville's Fisk University and Tennessee State College, I could hardly get to first base because I was always in financial difficulty. Other fellows could attend fraternity affairs, parties in the neighborhood, movies, and such, but I had to conserve my nickels and dimes to be sure that I would get by.

I didn't brood over my state of affairs, however. I knew that if I ever got through medical school, I would make up for all those niceties that I had missed. Furthermore, there was always studying to be done, and because many times I had no books of my own, I had to use my roommates' books while they were out having a good time.

Late in my sophomore year, my social fortunes took a slight upturn. During one of the basketball dances, I met a beautiful young lady whose name was Lazinka. I began talking with her during intermissions and found out that she was a teacher in the public school system in Nashville, that she was a divorcee, and that she had a nice little coupe. More importantly, she was very lonely.

Suddenly, life was becoming a little more meaningful to me. I could count on a ride through the countryside on Saturday afternoons with her and occasionally a full dinner on Sundays. After about three or four months, Lazinka suddenly asked, "Why is it that I never see you at any of the dances or parties other than at the basketball games?" I told her simply that I did not have the money to attend such functions, or movies, or even an occasional stop at a hamburger stand or chili parlor. Even after I revealed my financial insolvency, we still spent many weekends together. Occasionally, Lazinka would come up with tickets to dances and parties, and I would be glad to escort her. However, the time approached for final examinations, so the weekly basketball games were terminated.

After the final examinations, I was able to scrape up enough money from my classmates to take a bus back to Chicago. On arrival, I found my ancient suitcase, got my porter's uniform together, and went down to the Milwaukee Railroad sign-out room for an assignment to a sleeping-car run as soon as possible. I did not have to worry about a place to stay while in Chicago because my brother had married and rented a house with an extra room. The officials at the railroad office were apparently glad to see me.

I was greeted with, "Hey, Quig, come in here. I have a run for you leaving this afternoon for Seattle, Washington, on the Columbian." I signed in and, in no time at all, had an assignment for a two-week trip to the coast, carrying a group of tourists from Chicago to Seattle, and from Vancouver through the Canadian Rockies.

I had been in school during the previous nine months with no exercise except a little dancing now and then. I had spent most of my time sitting around classrooms and working in laboratories. The first night, I got all my passengers to bed about 10 p.m., then curled up in the smoking compartment for five or six hours' sleep. Late the next afternoon, my feet began aching a little bit. As the day wore on, my feet ached more and more. By the time we got to South Dakota, my feet were killing me. I got my passengers to bed on the second night, and when everything got quiet, I pulled my shoes off and crept around in severe pain.

My feet got worse. By the time we got to Seattle on the fifth day, I could hardly walk. Luckily for me, we discharged our passengers at Seattle on Friday and had until Monday to rest up while our train was being transferred to Vancouver. By Monday morning when we picked up our passengers again, my feet felt fine.

The rest of the trip was uneventful. I spent the entire summer with the same group of porters and waiters, carrying tourists over the same route. Most of us were students and found it rewarding financially to make the trips pleasant for our passengers. In fact, there was a hospitality car on the train, and some of the fellows in the group organized a small combo. We were able to get away from our duties for an hour or two following dinner and play for the passengers before they retired for the night.

On one of our trips, we left Chicago on August 14. One of the passengers had a birthday the next day, so we gave the passengers a nice celebration. I mentioned the fact that my birthday was the next day, August 16, and thought no more about it. On the night of August 16, the passengers kept me pretty busy in my car until 9:30 p.m. Then one of them asked me to come up to the hospitality car so I could play my trombone with the combo. When I got there, I found that the passengers had gotten together to give me a birthday party. They gave me many presents, candies, and above all, about seventy-five dollars in cash. That gave me a bright idea. From then on, I made it a point to mention to someone in each group of passengers that my birthday was two days away. That gave them two days to get together for the party. I carried on that racket for the remainder of the summer, and when I got back to Meharry, I was able to pay all but one hundred dollars of my tuition for the year. I promised the bursar that I would pay that by the end of the school year.

As I mentioned earlier, the Depression was getting worse every day, and I couldn't depend on any member of my family to help me. I was able to eat regularly because we still had basketball games. However, I was not able to buy a single textbook that year. That did not bother me as long as my classmates had textbooks and let me use them. When time for examinations rolled around, everyone wanted his own textbook, so I would be the quizmaster. I think I got more out of this deal than anyone else.

I found that I could depend on Lazinka for the little extra change that I needed. I told her that I was keeping a record of the money she had loaned me, and she knew that I would pay her back every penny of it. In the meantime, I was becoming increasingly fond of Lazinka. One day I picked up the *Pittsburgh Courier,* a paper that was edited and published by a Black firm. When I got to the society page, I was greeted by the headlines. Mattie,

Mr. Brooks's granddaughter, the only person whom I had ever adored, had gotten married to an Alcorn classmate of mine. He had finished Alcorn and was teaching in Mississippi. Mattie had finished college, majored in home economics, and had begun teaching the course at Alcorn. This is where they had met. I walked around in a daze for about two weeks.

Realizing the futility of this attitude, I soon snapped out of it. I told Lazinka about Mattie, then I got to thinking about the matter. I thought enough of Lazinka to marry her, so I popped the question. However, I let it be known that I would not be of much help to her financially until after I got out of medical school. She said that was all right with her. I hated leaving my classmates, but under the circumstances, I felt that if they tried to carry me along all the time, it would end up jeopardizing their own futures.

I knew that Lazinka had been married before. I had talked with many of her friends in Nashville who had known her from birth. They all assured me that she was a worthy person and that the break-up of her first marriage was due to the man whom she had married and not to her. In spite of all of that, doubts still ran through my mind as to the gravity of the situation in which I would find myself if my dear Lazinka, recognizing the potential afforded to her by marrying an upcoming physician, turned out to be a fortune hunter. Before we married, I made it distinctly understood that I was taking a chance on her and that I would be fair-minded and give her a chance to prove herself. I told her that I had no intentions of marrying a person that I would have to watch, and that I would definitely not put up with any unfaithfulness.

We were married in a quiet ceremony with Walls, Foster, and Joe Jones present. At the end of my junior year, I did not have the money that was due on my tuition. However, I assured the bursar that I would have it before I entered school in the fall. I had to borrow money from Lazinka to get back to Chicago that spring. When I got there, I returned to my job as a sleeping car porter. However, the tourists who made the trip to Canada that summer were not as big spenders as those the year before. I might add that my salary was only seventy-two dollars a month, and we were more dependent on the tips than we were on our small salaries. When the tips were slow in coming in, it left us out in the cold, you might say.

CHAPTER 12

PROHIBITION

My brother Charlie was chief bellhop at one of Chicago's small hotels located near Union Station. The Union was formed by all the meat-packing plants pooling their resources. They built the Stockyard Inn where they entertained the big western ranchers and cattle dealers who brought their cattle to Chicago to be sold to the different packing plants for processing. At that time there was a great rivalry between the meat processors in Chicago and those in Kansas City. The management at the Stockyard Inn went all out to entertain the big cattlemen.

This was during the Prohibition era, and the bellboys made most of their money from the guests by bootlegging whiskey, which they obtained from the racketeers in Chicago. Because some of the ranchers were being blinded and poisoned by bad bootleg whiskey, they started making the bellhops drink some of the liquor first to make sure it was okay. I knew some of the bellhops, and they told me all about the bad liquor they had to sell. They said that if they could get some good Canadian whiskey, they could make some money. They would say, "Why man, we could get twelve dollars a pint for that stuff, especially the Scotch, if you could get it out of Canada."

As I said, tips weren't coming in so well, and it was going to be my senior year in medical school when I got back. I needed all the money I could get. One of them said, "Now, Quig, if you could get a case of liquor over here every trip, we could all make a barrel of money." That sounded good to me!

I knew some of the porters who were bootlegging cigarettes to Canada and whiskey back to Chicago. I told them they would have to get somebody to pick it up at the railroad station because I didn't know how to get it past the policemen. We enlisted one good brother from South Carolina by the name of Odom who said he would be glad to get the whiskey from the station to my brother's house if I would give him one quart of Rock and Rye, made of rye whiskey and rock candy, every time I came back from Canada.

I could get good Scotch in Canada for two dollars a pint. So, I borrowed a pigskin Gladstone bag from a good friend to take to Canada with me, bought a case of Scotch in Vancouver, and hid the pint bottles in bags of soiled linen. The inspectors got on the car and checked it out for contraband before we crossed back into the United States but never thought of opening the bags of soiled linen.

On the way back to Chicago, our last stop was St. Paul, Minneapolis. The passengers had a day-long sightseeing tour there. That was when we took the whiskey out of the bags of soiled linen and packed it in suitcases that we would get rid of in Chicago. When we arrived at the train station in Chicago, my good friend, Odom, stepped up to the car and explained, "My boss, Mr. Jones, said he got off the train in Minneapolis and is going to stay a few days. He told me to come by, pick up his bag, and take it home for him."

"Oh, Mr. Jones. Yes, I remember him. He told me that he would have somebody meet the train and take his bag. Here it is." My friend, Odom, took the bag to my brother's house and stashed the liquor in the basement. He got his quart of Rock and Rye, drank it all in two weeks, and was ready for another trip downtown to the station when our next tour came in.

All the porters were not entirely honest. As you know, there is no honor among thieves. On one trip, a porter opened one of the bags of soiled linen and took six pints of my whiskey out. So, on the next trip I had to find some other place to hide it. Most people were not aware of it, but on sleeping cars (in fact, on all the passenger cars) there was a long tank extending underneath the car in which water was stored for use in lavatories and toilets. This huge tank was insulated to keep the water from freezing during the winter. In order to service it, a trap door was underneath the carpet in the aisle situated about half-way down the length of the car. I found that this was a good place to stash whiskey, especially pint-size bottles. I could put a whole case of it around the water tank.

So, using my new hiding place, everything went along fine until we got up into the Canadian Rockies. When we arrived in Banff, Alberta, for an all-day stop, the passengers got off the train and took a bus tour through the Rockies. They were gone all day, so we had the day off. After finishing our breakfast, we went to the Tap Room of the King George Hotel in the little town of Banff and sipped draft beer for three or four hours. The Tap Room was a typical saloon with a large counter, stools, and a polished brass footrail. There were tables with tops of black glass throughout the room, and all the fixtures were highly polished mahogany. When we had just about gotten stoned, we went back to the train to sleep it off, and then we were ready to receive the passengers when they got back during the afternoon.

On this particular trip, one of the passengers was so car-sick that she could not leave her berth. After being assured that the lady was comfortable, I retired to the hotel with the rest of the gang and proceeded to get high drinking beer. I knew the lady in the car would probably need something, so I went back a little earlier than the other fellows. When I got inside the sleeping car, the only thing I could smell was whiskey!

I got panicky right away. It so happened that it had become chilly, and the heat had been turned on. Those water tanks suspended under the cars were protected from the cold by insulation and steam pipes. When the steam was turned on, the whiskey heated up. When I was hiding the whiskey, I had placed one of the bottles upside down. The heat came on, the whiskey got hot, the stopper popped out, and the insulation was saturated with hot whiskey. The fumes were coming up in the car.

The lady in the berth had not noticed any of this because she was so sick that she didn't know what was going on. After discovering that the place smelled like a distillery, I got two porters to come in with me. "We're going to sweep and clean in here," I told her, "so I'm going to pull these curtains tight around your berth, then you won't be bothered by dust."

We removed the whiskey, took a gallon jug of disinfecting solution, and poured some all over the carpet and down into the insulation. I had no idea where I was going to put the rest of the whiskey. There was a couch in one of the sleeping compartments being occupied by an elderly couple. The man had elected to sleep in the upper berth and his wife in the lower, so no one was using the couch. I stashed the case of liquor under the couch's mattress. When the customs inspector came through the car, he dared not enter their compartment, so I got this case of liquor across the border without any more trouble.

I made four trips to Canada that summer and brought back four cases of Scotch. Each time I was met at the railroad station by the same person, using the same bag. That was dumb because the railroad detectives noticed this fellow coming in, meeting the same train, picking up the same bag, and leaving in a cab. One day they followed him to my brother's house, and when Odom got out of the cab, they came up behind him and asked what he had in the bag. He told them that it was his clothing. They asked, "Do you go down there and get your clothing off a Canadian train every two weeks?"

He said, "Yeah!" They arrested him and took him to the police station. When they opened the bag, they found that it contained a case of Scotch.

They asked Odom, "Whose bag is this?"

"Mine. My uniform is in that bag, too," Odom lied. He weighed about a hundred pounds more than me.

The policemen asked again, "Whose uniform is this?"

"Mine," Odom responded.

The policemen countered, "Is it now? Put the coat on." Odom couldn't do it. They saw the porter's cap and said, "Put that cap on." It rested on the very tip of his head. And so, they charged him with bootlegging.

Odom's wife had been looking out the window and saw the policemen pick him up and take him to the police station. She called me, and I contacted one of the fellows rooming with my brother by the name of Nick. Nick had formerly worked for the police department as a driver of one of the squad cars, and he knew a lot of the policemen. He went to the station, found out what had happened, and got Odom out of jail on bond.

When my brother heard about the deal, he went down to his basement and found three cases of Scotch. He was so mad that he took all the Scotch out and threw it in the alley. Now, just imagine whiskey in an alley in Chicago. It was not there fifteen minutes before scavengers had carted it off. Nick was able to find out who the judge for the case would be. He approached him and gave him seventy dollars. Then he confiscated the whiskey, so the judge was able to dismiss the case for lack of evidence. Now here I was—I had lost two hundred forty dollars' worth of whiskey! In other words, I was just about wiped out. My brother was so mad at me that he wouldn't lend me enough money to go back to medical school.

CHAPTER 13

HARD TIMES GET HARDER

I ended up with a little over one hundred dollars when I got back to Nashville. I already owed the school that much in back tuition. I went to the bursar and explained to him that I had enough to pay the back bill. However, it would take me two or three weeks to get enough to pay my senior year's tuition. The bursar wrote me a receipt for the amount paid and told me that he was sorry, but I could not be admitted my senior year until I had paid at least half of the tuition in advance. I contacted my brother in Louisiana who promised to send me some money in two weeks. No money came. I waited another week, and still no money. I called my brother again, and he said, "I'm sorry, but I was unable to borrow the money."

I went back and talked to the bursar again, but he stood steadfast. I was at the end of my rope. I didn't see how I could make it any further.

I went to the fraternity house, saw my classmates, and told them my trouble. They wanted to pitch in and try to get together enough money to get me in, but I wouldn't stand for it because I knew their financial situation. I decided that I would have to get back to Chicago to my old job and try to make it again the next year. That was a very sad day in my life.

Lazinka's parents were living in Nashville near us. In fact, Lazinka and I stayed with her parents for a while after we were married. When things started getting really tight for me, I asked

Lazinka if she could help me. She said it was all she could do to help her parents; she didn't have the money to help me, but she would try and borrow some money. I told her I didn't want her borrowing money for me, but that if she couldn't help me, I had nowhere else to turn because my family hadn't been able to come through. I would just have to miss my senior year in medical school, pack up, and go back to Chicago to work and save enough money to come back and finish. That is what happened, but first I had to find a job to help me get to Chicago.

The only job I could find in Nashville was dishwashing in the Vanderbilt University Hospital kitchen. When I applied for the job, the lady managing the kitchen told me that they already had someone to wash the dishes. They had made a mistake in the ad, and what they needed was somebody to wash pots. The dishes were washed in a machine, but the pots were scraped and washed by hand. I was to report the next morning at 7 a.m. When I got to the kitchen, I found pots and pans piled nearly to the ceiling. I washed pots all day long, and when I left the kitchen that night at 7 p.m., there were still pots and pans piled to the ceiling.

Payday was eight days away, and I understood that they would not pay except on payday. I had to keep the job for eight days. The detergent ate up my hands, and where the water dripped on my shoes, it almost ate them up, too. At the end of eight days, I was paid off. I don't remember how much it was, but it was more than enough to get me a bus ride back to Chicago. Because I could not be with my graduating class, I would not be able to stand remaining in Nashville any longer, so I prepared to move. Lazinka continued living and teaching in Nashville when I left. We eventually divorced, and I heard that she later married another senior medical student. After he graduated and served his internship, they moved and set up a practice in Virginia.

***

I got my old job back in Chicago. During the winter months, I did not have a regular run. I would get out of town once or twice a week on an overnight run but with the coming of spring, I was able to get on a regular run, and I kept it throughout the following summer. So, I eventually went back to Meharry and joined another graduating class. I missed my former classmates. However, I made a new group of good friends.

I had no trouble academically during my senior year at Meharry. I had enough money to take the first and second parts of the National Board of Medical Examiners, though not enough to take the third part. The basic science was easy for me, and my marks were decent. On the second part of the National Board, I made the highest mark of all the students in the United States taking the exam at that time.

Everyone began thinking about internships following the Christmas holidays of my senior year. In 1934, there were only eight or ten hospitals where a Black medical graduate could apply for internship. The most outstanding hospitals were Harlem Hospital in New York City, Provident Hospital in Chicago, City Hospital No. 2 in St. Louis, the Kansas City Hospital, St. Agnes Hospital in Raleigh, Goodrich Hospital in New Orleans, Good Samaritan Hospital in Charlotte, and a small community hospital in Wilmington. Only three or four of those hospitals paid interns any stipend whatsoever.

Dr. Henry Hampton, Medical Director of City Hospital No. 2 in St. Louis and a Meharry graduate, came to Nashville to recruit interns. At that time interns were given twenty dollars per month with room, board, and uniforms. I applied for an internship and was interviewed by Dr. Hampton. I was a poor specimen at that time—I looked more like a cadaver than a doctor. Dr. Hampton talked with me, and I guess he was impressed by something, but certainly not my appearance.

After being notified that I had been accepted at City Hospital No. 2, my immediate worries all ended. All I had to do was get ready for the Tennessee State Board of Medical Examiners. I buckled down with the other students to study. We were either quizzed by teachers or formed our own quiz groups in fraternity houses. My nerves went to pieces after our final examinations. I had been under so much pressure, especially during the last two years, that I found it impossible to sleep. When I dozed off, I'd have nightmares. I found it necessary to call my good friend, Dr. Sam Freeman, to give me sedatives so I could get some sleep.

We took the Tennessee State Board Examination before graduation. The tests were held in the old Tennessee State Capitol, situated on a high hill in the middle of the city's downtown section. The examination for the State Board was an anticlimax since we had prepared ourselves for whatever we might face next.

CHAPTER 14

GRADUATION & BEYOND

Finally, the great day of graduation dawned on us. The traditional march, "Pomp and Circumstance," was played as we solemnly wound our way from the administration building to the outdoor amphitheater where the commencement address was delivered by Dr. Perry, a veteran surgeon from Kansas City, Missouri.

While accepting that square of parchment from the president of Meharry, I had an overwhelming sense of elation, relief, exuberance, joy, and peace, all at the same time. I will never forget when the organist gave us the signal to be seated after the last doctor had received his degree. I was so busy looking at the coveted piece of parchment that I forgot to sit down. Following commencement, we retired to our various fraternity houses, and most of us, including me, became gloriously drunk on Tennessee moonshine whiskey. The next morning, I awoke with a hangover, but that was the happiest day of my life.

On June 30, 1934, I boarded the L&N train for St. Louis. If I had not been forewarned about the physical condition of City Hospital No. 2, I would have experienced a great letdown. However, the antiquated structure looked like the Taj Mahal to me. City Hospital No. 2 was housed in an abandoned, four-story, rambling structure, the former Barnes Hospital, adjacent to a slightly more modern six-story annex.

City Hospital No. 2 was a municipal hospital used for the treatment of Blacks in St. Louis, while City Hospital No. 1 was where all the white patients were treated.

The surrounding area of No. 2 had been taken over by Blacks ever since the whites had moved out back when the Blacks were migrating to St. Louis in great numbers.

Upon arriving at City Hospital No. 2, we were greeted by the medical director, Dr. Henry Hampton, and turned over to Dr. William H. Sinkler, the senior intern for orientation. He reminded us that although the building was antiquated, we could look forward to a year of hard work. He reminded us that we would be able to derive experience and training in direct proportion to the effort we put into pursuing our goals. There were sixteen junior interns in our class. Four were from Howard Medical College, eight from Meharry, and four from different medical schools from various parts of the United States.

The first ward we visited was male medicine, a huge room with about sixty beds. All types of medical patients were located in that ward. The next ward was the male tuberculosis ward. That's when I got real panicky. The tuberculosis patients were exhibiting every type of behavior possible—vomiting, coughing, screaming, praying. To make matters worse, since it was July 1, the weather was very hot. There was no such thing as air conditioning in those days. However, an attempt was being made to keep the place as cool as possible by droning, oscillating fans. The only thing I could think was that those fans were circulating acid-fast bacteria, the kind of bacteria that causes tuberculosis, and was passing them on to everybody in sight. Remember, I only weighed about one hundred fifteen pounds. While the others were looking around the ward, I eased outside the door and made a short prayer to the

Lord: "God, please help me through this, and I promise I'll leave City Hospital No. 2 as soon as July 1, 1935, rolls around."

Female medicine, female tuberculosis, and OB-GYN were housed in the annex building, which was in better condition. I climbed to the sixth floor of the annex building and developed another case of first-degree panic. Three residents were in bed, suffering from tuberculosis. I said another little prayer right then and there.

Fate was kind to me during those months at City Hospital No. 2. First of all, I was assigned to emergency and admitting services. The hospital was so crowded, and so much was going on, that the interns on emergency and admissions only had eight hours off out of a twenty-four-hour period.

That meant that during those eight hours you only stopped long enough to eat. We were admitting all types of cases—pregnant women in all stages of labor, psychosis patients climbing the walls, crying babies, screaming children, to say nothing of first-aid patients suffering from knife or gunshot wounds, lacerations, and broken bones. In other words, after eight hours of being on emergency and admitting services, you were ready to fall over from exhaustion.

My first shift was from 11 p.m. to 7 a.m. By that time things had calmed down, and after eight hours, I was free to recuperate for sixteen hours. I was next assigned to the 3 to 11 p.m. shift, where the most trauma cases were seen. The 7 a.m. to 3 p.m. shift was relatively quiet with some admissions and a lot of patients coming for dressing changes, laboratory work, and the like.

The interns were housed four to a room, and my roommates were quite interesting. Madison Foster, from Monroe, Louisiana, snored so loudly that we all got into bed and tried to fall asleep before he did. In the event we were unlucky enough to be awake after he fell asleep, we had devised a method of waking him so his snoring would stop, and we could make another determined effort to get to sleep before him.

Another of our roommates suffered from a severe case of hyperhidrosis. In other words, his feet stunk like hell. His shoes had such an offensive odor that the resident mice would come into the room looking for something dead, even when the lights were on. And, oh yes, about the mice. They were so numerous that we paid them no mind. Believe it or not, I've never seen such fat cockroaches in all my life. Our housing was deplorable. I hasten to state, however, that my class was the last to be trained at City Hospital No. 2. When we arrived in St. Louis, the Homer G. Hospital was under construction, and the entire hospital operation moved to a shining new facility the following year.

Autopsies were done by medical interns, divided into groups of two. I was teamed with Dr. Charles S. Finch. When our turn came to perform autopsies, we found it convenient to do them after our morning rounds. At about 11 a.m., we contacted the pathologist, who would advise us either to wait for him to meet us at the morgue or to proceed with the routine. One day, we had two autopsies to perform. We finished the first about 11:50 a.m. and decided to go on with the second. We resolved that we would finish before our noon meal.

We rushed to the dining room about 12:50 p.m. and found that other greedy interns had eaten everything except for some tapioca pudding. I turned to my fellow interns and said, "Why in the hell didn't you save us some food?"

Dr. J. B. Harris laughed heartily. "Too bad about that, fellows. Sorry about your empty stomachs, but you should have been on time." We filled our bellies with tapioca pudding and waited for the evening meal.

About a week later, two autopsies were again scheduled for us. Both patients had died of terminal cancer. One patient had died of carcinoma of the breast, which had been secondarily infected. In the room where her body lay, there was a very pungent cadaveric odor—we could hardly stand the stench. We finished the autopsy about 11:55 a.m. and immediately went to the dining room. You could smell us long before you saw us. We took our seats right at the middle part of the table facing each other. As interns and residents came in, they met with the terrible odor. Everyone backed off and left the dining room. We had the whole place to ourselves. That was our way of getting back at Dr. J. B. Harris — or "The Judge" as we called him.

The number of autopsies came so fast and furious that I would become nauseated whenever the word was spoken. To overcome my feelings of disgust and repulsion, I psyched myself up by saying very loudly, "Autopsy? Good. I love them; bring them on. You can't bring me too many."

The pathologist heard me talking and said, "So you like autopsies, huh?"

I stammered, "Yes, sir. I like them." I did not want to encourage or displease the pathologist, so I pretended.

He said, "Well, Quigless, since you like them so well, I will just call you whenever we have the coroner's cases." My feathers fell. He said further, "Whenever we have a coroner's case, I get paid extra for it. Now if you'll come down here and expose the brain before I get here, that will save me a lot of time, and I'll pay you five dollars for each case." Now that was a horse of a different color. As scarce as money was around that time, if I was going to be paid five dollars for dissecting the brain, I didn't care if he had three or four autopsies each day. From that day on, I looked forward to assisting him.

Just one frightening incident happened during that time. We had just completed autopsies on two infants. The pathologist and secretary had left the room, and Dr. Finch and I were left to sterilize the instruments and leave the place in order. When he left the room to take the instruments to the sterilizer, I told him that I would take the bodies to the morgue. "All right," he said. "If you're going to do that, then I'll just go on up to dinner." He left the room.

I picked up the infants and took them to the morgue. Now the morgue was a large, refrigerated room about twenty by thirty feet in size. The bodies were stacked in tiers, one above the other.

Formaldehyde, a very toxic chemical, was sprayed around the walls, on the trays that held the bodies, and on the floor and ceiling to keep down contamination and counteract the odor emitted by the dead bodies. We also always left the door open when entering the morgue because of the odor. We were in there for only a few minutes, so we took no precautions against strong formaldehyde fumes.

On this particular day, for some reason, the door closed and locked behind me. Try picturing that situation: Here I am, locked inside a vast refrigerated room reeking with formaldehyde fumes, with nobody outside to open the door. To make matters worse, when the door closed, the light automatically went out, and I was in total darkness. I was slightly disoriented, and instead of finding the door that had a safety bar on it, I came in contact with one tier of bodies after another.

I was almost overcome by formaldehyde fumes by the time I finally got myself straightened out and lunged against the door. It flew open, and I staggered out of the room and fell onto the floor.

I lay there for about five minutes trying to catch my breath. I then went straight to the dining room where everyone had assembled.

Dr. Finch looked around and said, "Quig, where in hell have you been?"

"I was locked in the damn morgue," I said. I reported it instantly to the Medical Director, and he issued an order then and there that "whenever any person enters the morgue, a second person must be present in the autopsy room." That was the most terrifying incident during my internship. I was very glad when, after six months, the time came for me to switch over from the medical to the surgical service. After all, I was planning to be a surgeon.

It was my luck to be assigned the easiest services first: urology. We treated gonorrhea and syphilis in all stages and some severe kidney conditions. The next service was eye, ear, nose, and throat. Again, this was very easy for me. At that time, we were doing anywhere from ten to twenty tonsillectomies on children on Tuesdays and Thursdays. The operations were routine, and we rarely had any serious complications. I had some flashbacks to the time my tonsils were removed. Needless to say, a lot of changes and improvements had been made since then.

Following the completion of my tour of duty on eye, ear, nose, and throat, I was transferred to the orthopedic service. Orthopedics was a lively service, especially during the winter months when there were many fractures from people falling on ice and breaking ankles, arms, legs, hips, and even breaking their necks. There were the ever-present automobile accidents and the distasteful mess of treating chronic bone and joint conditions, especially those related to bone and joint tuberculosis.

While I'd been on emergency services, I treated a young man unfortunate enough to be suffering from tuberculosis abscesses along his spine. There was profuse drainage from the abscesses, along with a very offensive odor. This same man turned up in orthopedics with draining abscesses extending all the way from his pelvis to just above his knee. The orthopedic surgeon in charge decided to treat him by exposing the anal fistula, which is a small tunnel that connects the abscesses, and using a type of packing, with the hope that the abscesses would heal completely. We knew that the operation would be long and tedious and, above all, very offensive to the nose. I was not at all interested in the technique involved because making orthopedics my life's work was the farthest thing from my mind. All I wanted was to get out of the operating room that day.

As the operation progressed, Dr. Horowitz, the surgeon, had me holding a retractor so he could get down to the bone and scrape away the infected material. I was looking out the window. All of a sudden, Dr. Horowitz stopped working. Nothing was going on, so I looked around quickly to see him staring intently at me. He said, "Now, doctor, I understand that you are not interested in orthopedics and that this operation is very distasteful to you. However, inasmuch as you are assisting me, I would appreciate it if you'd pay more attention to what you are doing."

I felt like a fool. I realized that my inattentiveness was adding more difficulty to an already complicated operation, so I hastened to apologize. From that moment on, I paid more attention to the surgery at hand.

When we returned to the dressing room following the operation, I spoke to the surgeon again. "Dr. Horowitz, I want to apologize again for my behavior during the operation. Although I am not primarily interested in orthopedic surgery, I realize that you are, and you do the best you can for your patients. I realize also that I should have paid closer attention to what was going on."

Dr. Horowitz said, "Oh, that's all right, doctor. This is not the first time I've had to reprimand an intern assisting me."

I replied, "That very well may be. However, I assure you that your reprimand has indelibly etched a lesson in my mind. From now on I shall give my utmost attention to the job at hand."

Following that incident, I looked upon orthopedic surgery as one of the specialties that I had to undergo in training and did my best to satisfy my superiors and myself that I was doing the best I could for patients under my care.

Male surgery followed orthopedics, and I found myself getting into the part that interested me most of all. We had the usual run of appendectomies, cholecystectomies, intestinal, and colon surgery. We had our share of serious gunshot and knife wounds. Indeed, Friday afternoon through Sunday was designated as the knife and gun period. I remember one case in particular.

A man was struck by an automobile and suffered a ruptured kidney. The accident happened about 2 a.m. Dr. John Thomas, the surgeon on call, was known for his speed and dexterity. We prepared the patient, called in the anesthetist, and Dr. Thomas came in promptly. The patient was anesthetized, and Dr. Thomas said, "Well now, let's get to work." He removed the kidney in about ten minutes. All I could do was stand there and watch.

When he finished, he said, "Now, Quig, this man has lost so much blood we'll have to contact his relatives to see if we can get some blood and transfuse him." At that time, there was no such thing as a blood bank. Following surgery, the relatives in the waiting room were ready for us to answer their questions about the delay involved in the surgery. I tried to explain that the surgery had been carried out as quickly as possible and that the patient was out of danger, except that he was anemic and needed some blood.

One of the brothers said, "Damn it, get him some blood."

I explained to him that we had to find donors and that the blood would have to be typed and matched before it could be given to the patient. The brother insisted that we get the blood right away and give it to him. I said, "Now it's most likely that your blood would be compatible with your brother's, so we could use yours. What about giving about two units of your blood?"

The irate man changed his tune right away. "You see, doctor, I'm very anemic myself. I don't think I could spare the blood, but I'd appreciate your doing the best you could."

I said, "Well, mister, the best thing you could do would be to shut your mouth and get out and help find some donors."

Another night, a patient was brought to the hospital suffering from gunshot wounds to his face. We learned that he had been in a fight. His adversary pulled a .25 caliber pistol and fired several bullets all around the victim's turning head. The last bullet that hit him penetrated the orbit and lodged in his skull. Our x-rays revealed that the bullets were flattened against the skull. In other words, the man's skull was so thick that the only bullet causing damage was one that penetrated his skull through his eye socket. The patient was transferred to another hospital for brain surgery.

X-rays were scary for me. A tragic incident occurred two or three years before my internship in which we were forced to work with deplorable equipment. A violent patient struggled during an x-ray attempt while the current was turned on. His arm came into contact with exposed wiring, causing him to be severely shocked. The intern on duty who attempted to save the man inadvertently came into contact with the victim and was also electrocuted. That same equipment was in use when I went to the hospital as an intern. It goes without saying that I lost no time in the x-ray department.

One Friday night while I was on male surgery service, a man who had been in an altercation with another man was brought to the hospital with several cuts about the upper part of his body, chest, and back. He was bleeding profusely and so his wounds were duly sutured in the receiving room. Because of severe loss of blood, he was persuaded to remain in the hospital. I had to write up his history to present his case to the visiting surgeon the following morning.

After a routine physical exam of his head, neck, chest, abdomen, back, and upper extremities, I wrote my description that all was normal. I then threw the covers back and took one look at his lower extremities and closed my description of his condition by stating that the lower extremities were normal as well. The next morning, I presented the case to the visiting men accompanying Dr. Hampton, who was making rounds and had come to check on the man. I read the patient's history, stating why the man was admitted, and then I described his head, neck, chest, abdomen, upper extremities, and finally, that the lower extremities were normal.

Dr. Hampton said, "Doctor, will you read the latter part of your description again?" I read it to him again, ending with "lower extremities normal." Dr. Hampton pulled the sheets off the bed, exposing the man's lower limbs. One foot was absent. The laugh was on me. I did not know that Dr. Hampton had amputated the man's foot about four years earlier on a previous admission.

During the previous ten months of my internship, I had had occasion to laugh at some of my fellow interns because of mistakes or omissions they had made. The fellows had never had a chance to laugh at my mistakes, and when this incident came up, I could not rest for three or four weeks. Every time I went to bed and tried to sleep, some intern would come in, shake me, and say, "Wake up, Quig, lower extremities are normal." From then on, I took pains to thoroughly examine all of my patients, from head to foot.

It was at about that time that interns were making applications for senior internships and residencies. I had promised the Lord that I would not stay at that hospital more than one year, provided that I was able to finish internship without developing tuberculosis or something worse. So, when I was approached about my application for senior internships and residencies, I turned the idea down emphatically.

Although Dr. Hampton was a graduate of Meharry Medical College, he was reluctant to grant senior internships and residencies to Meharry graduates because he felt their work revealed them to be inferior in training to graduates of other medical schools. Whenever the matter came up, he stated that Dr. So-and-So from Meharry would have been selected if he had only applied for residency. That had gone on for four or five years.

The eight Meharry interns were discussing the matter one day and came up with the idea that all of us would apply for senior internships and residencies. Out of the eight, we thought that at least one would be given the chance at senior internship or residency. I reminded the group that I had promised the Lord that I wouldn't stay there for another year. They immediately jumped on me from all angles. "Now, Quig, you're going to mess up the whole thing. If you fail to apply, it could easily be said that you would have been given either a senior internship or residency if you had applied." I was caught between a rock and a hard place. So, I agreed to apply.

My last tour of duty at the hospital was on female surgery, which was a busy service at that time. There were three to six operations every day. The surgery cases included thyroidectomies, stomach surgery, and intestinal surgery, including surgery of the colon for malignancies and for the care of those unfortunate women who suffered lymphogranuloma inguinale, resulting in complete closure of the rectum and vagina, necessitating colostomies.

One day, a patient was admitted to the hospital because of gallbladder disease, and an operation was indicated. We had several major operations during that day, and I had not performed the pre-operative examination on the patient until after dinner. I took a short nap, returned to the ward about 10 p.m., and did the pre-operative exam. I made notes as I did the examination and returned to the ward station to record my findings. Just then, a patient was rolled in with a tentative diagnosis of appendicitis. So now I had to tend to this new patient.

The intern on duty was required not only to make a pre-operative examination, but to do the laboratory work if the patient was admitted to the hospital after 8 p.m. Whenever the patient was admitted with lower right abdominal pain, especially a female during the childbirth period, the differential diagnosis had to be made between pelvic inflammatory disease, which in most cases was a result of venereal disease, and appendicitis. In order to make a diagnosis, lab work and painstaking exams had to be done.

In this instance, after working up the new appendicitis patient who had interrupted my work on the gallbladder patient, I notified Dr. Bill Sinkler, the surgical resident, the anesthetist, and the surgical team. The appendicitis patient was taken to the operating room and prepared for surgery. Following the operation, the patient was returned to the surgical ward because there were no recovery rooms.

I then went back to the station, intent upon recording my findings on the gallbladder patient.

But at that instant, another patient was rolled into the ward with a tentative diagnosis of acute appendicitis. The same procedure followed that had occurred with the first appendicitis patient. The second operation was done, and the patient was returned to the ward. By that time, it was 2 a.m., and I was very tired. I decided to get forty winks and record my findings on the gallbladder patient before she was taken to the operating room the next morning. I left a request with the switchboard operator to call me at 6 a.m., and guess what—he forgot.

I was rudely awakened about 8 a.m. by one of my roommates who said, "Quig, you'd better get up. I understand that the surgical team is scrubbing for the first operation, which is a cholecystectomy." I ran up to the operating room suite and found everyone scrubbing for surgery. I didn't have time to record my findings then. They went into the operating room, and I felt confident that everything would go along smoothly, and I wouldn't have to worry about not having recorded my findings.

Well, the visiting surgeon from the St. Louis University surgical faculty stated that he was going to perform the operation under spinal anesthesia. It was then the custom for the intern serving on anesthesiology to do the spinal injections. Dr. Gage Moore did the injection, and as anticipated, the spinal anesthesia was effective. The patient stated that she felt numb up to and above her navel. The operation was started by the surgeon, and upon opening the abdomen, extensive gallbladder pathology was observed, and dissection of the gallbladder was done.

About fifteen minutes into the operation, the intern monitoring the vital signs called out that the blood pressure was dropping and the pulse rate increasing. The foot of the operating table was elevated, preventing further ascent of the anesthetic toward the vital centers. The patient's breathing became labored, her blood pressure continued dropping, and her pulse rate accelerated even further. The operating procedure was interrupted when that condition was announced. In three or four minutes, respiratory paralysis ensued, the blood pressure dropped to zero, and her heart went into fibrillation.

At that point, the surgeon asked for the pre-operative blood pressure. As I was the third assistant and positioned next to Dr. Sinkler, I whispered the pressure to Dr. Sinker as I had remembered it—120 over 80—and he informed the surgeon. The surgeon then asked for the pulse rate. I told Dr. Sinkler it was around 86, and he relayed that information as well.

Then, the worst thing in the world happened. The operating surgeon asked one of the observing interns to read the pre-operative findings, none of which were there. At that point, Dr. Sinkler said, "If Quig says the findings are there, you'll find them right where he said you'd find them."

I kicked Dr. Sinkler on the foot and said, "Bill, I examined the patient but didn't get a chance to put down the findings."

He replied, "The hell, you say." Of course, no findings were found in the chart because I hadn't had time to record them. That was all the visiting surgeon wanted to hear.

He said, "Damn it, see what happens if you don't watch everything? We have lost this patient simply because information that should have been recorded on the chart was not there. If I had known this patient was a poor surgical risk before starting surgery, I would have cancelled it."

I knew at that moment that I was in the doghouse. The operating surgeon slammed his instruments down and strode out of the room. I was left there with the second assistant to close the abdomen.

Dr. Sinkler was infuriated. He felt that his staff had let him down, so he scheduled a meeting of the surgical staff for 1 p.m. that day. At the appointed time, all of us were assembled, and everyone looked straight at me. Dr. Sinkler came in cussing, saying that here we were, doing our damnedest to prove ourselves to the visiting staff, and that I was responsible for the death of this patient. Just before the meeting, I had stopped by the switchboard and picked up the record of calls on the night before the incident. There it was—the record of my having asked the switchboard operator to call me at 6 a.m. I freely accepted responsibility for the whole affair and requested that Dr. Sinkler stop upbraiding the entire surgical staff because of my mistake.

The meeting was promptly adjourned, and I was given sympathetic consolation by other members of the surgical staff.

Right then, I knew I would not be selected as a senior intern. The meeting for the selection was slated for two weeks later. After the meeting, I was called to the medical director's office along with a Meharry graduate and a Michigan graduate. I was called in first and informed that I had been selected as the surgical intern. The surgical internship training was the only position carrying a stipend.

I turned to Dr. Sinkler and said, "Just why in the world would you choose me after that terrible mistake I made up in the operating room?"

"Well, after all," he replied, "you admitted the mistake and took blame for the entire thing. That showed guts, and what we need in a surgical trainee is somebody with guts."

I thanked the medical director and his staff but said I was sorry and had to turn the offer down.

"Just why in hell are you turning down this offer, you fool?" he asked. "Fourteen of the sixteen interns applied for this job, and you're turning it down?!"

I informed the gentlemen that when I began my internship and observed three residents on the sixth floor suffering from tuberculosis, I promised the Lord that if he would let me remain at this hospital for one year free of infection, I'd get out of this place. And I was afraid to go back on my promise to God.

Dr. Hampton said, "Well, it's your decision, and if you remained here and anything happened to you in the way of contracting tuberculosis, you'd never forgive yourself. We accept your decision."

I walked out of the room. The other interns were waiting and asked, "What happened?"

I told them, "I was offered the surgical internship with pay and refused it." Every one of them called me a "damn fool." One or two even took a kick at my butt. I told them I would stand by my promise to God. So, the surgical internship there was awarded to a graduate of the University of Michigan Medical School.

About a week after that incident, I received a letter from Dr. Rolf, professor of physiology at Meharry Medical College, offering me a position at Meharry to serve as assistant instructor of physiology. He had not learned that I had already refused the internship in St. Louis, and he did not know that his offer was perfect for my needs. Although I was finishing my internship, I did not feel ready to go into practice yet, as I really did not know quite enough about physiology, the normal mechanisms and functions of the human body. Further training in physiology would better fit me to treat patients once I got into medical practice.

After a week of consideration, I answered Dr. Rolf 's letter, accepting the position. And so, I returned to Meharry Medical

College in Nashville to assist him. I was there with my friend and former classmate, Dr. Ralph Weathers, who assisted Dr. Hernandez in neurology and histology. It was my original intention to teach one year and then find a place to practice medicine. But although teaching was interesting, after being in that position at Meharry for only six months, I began feeling restless. I knew it was time for me to begin planning my venture into the great unknown of practicing medicine. My teaching salary was very meager, so I had to do quite a bit of skimping to amass the money that I would need.

Just about that time, an incident reinforced my desire to get myself prepared to leave Nashville. One of the other teachers at Meharry developed a severe case of gallbladder disease. He knew he had the disease but, as is the case with many, he put off seeking medical attention. This man had a family, and it was hard for him to make ends meet on the sparse teaching salary. He, along with several other teachers, resorted to borrowing money for various reasons at different intervals. Therefore, he had several outstanding loans at banks in and around Nashville, and some of the other teachers had co-signed for him.

When it became generally known that he was in critical condition, his co-signers held a meeting. I happened to be working in the lab during the course of this meeting. All of them were greatly concerned and were trying to figure out just how they would take care of the loans they had co-signed if the doctor died. During all of this, one of the teachers pulled me aside and said, "Quigless, if you have any sense at all, you'd better get out of here before you get embroiled in one of these situations. If that man dies on us, all of us will be in a hell of a fix."

You can believe that everything was done to save the good man's life. Fortunately, the doctor consented to the much-needed surgery, and it was successful. I decided then and there that I had to get out on my own before I became entangled in financial difficulty by attempting to help somebody.

My good friend Weathers and I discussed the situation and decided to leave at the end of the school year, scouting surrounding states for places we thought might offer the best opportunity for initiating practices. It had been my intention to practice in beautiful, green North Carolina from the very first time I visited the state as a trombone player with the minstrel show. So, the first thing I did was pull out a map, locate North Carolina, and begin circling the cities and towns I felt might present an opportunity for me to establish a practice.

CHAPTER 15

PRIVATE PRACTICE

I wrote to the Chambers of Commerce in the cities of Raleigh, Winston-Salem, Charlotte, Elizabeth City, and Fayetteville, requesting information on how many Black doctors and hospitals there were in each city.

I received answers from just about every Chamber. All of them asked me to please come and take a look at their city, and said they hoped I would settle there. Before choosing, however, I wanted a chance to visit these cities. I really wanted to begin a practice in a small town and had decided that if I ran into a smaller town that showed promise, I would settle right there.

About that same time, the president of Meharry started putting pressure on me to remain in the Department of Physiology or any other department they could get me to stay in. He pointed out the fact that the Depression was on, that doctors would probably be starving, and I would be out there among them. One good doctor said, "You'll never find me starving to death, knocking on doors, or ringing doorbells. I'm going to stay here where everything is cozy." But the more I thought about it, the more resolved I became to get out on my own.

I had to take the North Carolina Board to practice in that state, so I decided to kill two birds with one stone—go to Raleigh to take the North Carolina Board and look the state over for a likely place to practice. I talked with Weathers, but he would have nothing to do with North Carolina, because he was from Erie,

Pennsylvania, and could not bring himself to accept Jim Crow with all its ramifications.

Having been born and raised in Mississippi, I knew how painful it was to exist under Jim Crow conditions. And after having lived in Chicago for four or five years, it was hard for me to accept the Jim Crow practices again. I had noted the change as soon as I got off the train along with my friends in Chicago, both of whom had been raised in North Carolina. But when I went to Raleigh to apply for my medical license, I was directed to a hotel and was surprised I did not have to go around to the back door to enter.

At the end of my first school year teaching at Meharry, I had about ninety-five dollars in my pocket to take the train to Raleigh to meet the Board of North Carolina Medical Examiners.

When my name was called to meet the Board, I went in hyped up and ready to answer all sorts of questions. The members, some middle-aged and some elderly, all white, were sitting around a table. They gave me a seat at the end of the table. None of them exhibited any animosity toward me because I was Black. They welcomed me, asked my name, where I was from, and why I wanted to come to North Carolina. I told them, "I have always wanted to come here."

"Where do you think you're going to practice?" they asked.

"I don't know," I said. "I'm looking around now."

"Well, I wish to hell you would come to Charlotte. We need someone there," one said.

"No, come to Raleigh," said another.

"No, come to Greensboro," another said.

Instead of questioning me, everyone put in a bid for my practice in his town. I asked when they were going to question me.

"Question you? No, we just want you to come out here and go to work," one said. "That'll be all. You can go now. We think you're qualified, and we'd like to have you in our state and are glad to give you your license."

I decided to look up some fellows I knew who were practicing in the state. My first stop was in Greensboro to see Dr. George Evans. He had been there for two years and was well established in his practice. There were several doctors there, and they all seemed to be doing very well. However, Greensboro was just a little bit more of a town than what I had in mind. I wanted to be in a small town where a doctor was needed.

Rocky Mount was my next stop. I visited my friend Dr. Frank Avant. He had been in that city a couple of years and seemed to be doing very well. I spent some time getting around with him. I hadn't been out to observe the practice of medicine, so I wanted to see exactly how it was done. After three or four days with Dr. Avant, I was ready to move on to visit Elizabeth City and then Charlotte.

"Where do you think you're going to practice?" Dr. Avant asked.

"Oh, Frank, I'm looking for a place where I think I might be needed."

"Well, I'll show you a place where you'll be needed," he said.

"Where is that?" I asked eagerly.

"I'll take you to Tarboro."

"Tarboro? I don't like the name," I sputtered. "What kind of place is it? I don't want to go to no place with a name like that."

"Wait a minute now," he said calmly. "You said you wanted to find a place where you'd be needed. You'd have a chance to work in Tarboro. Let me take you there so you can take a look around."

Tarboro was only sixteen miles from Rocky Mount. We drove directly to the "colored" drugstore that he had mentioned. Sure enough, it was a well-equipped drugstore with a well-stocked pharmacy, and its fixtures were modern for the time. The owner of the drugstore had his doctorate in pharmacy and was overjoyed to see me, begging me to come to work in that town.

"This is the place for you," he urged, "and you won't have a care in the world. We need you badly here. You'll start making money the very day you open your office."

I met a man who was crippled with arthritis sitting over in the corner at the store. He had severe osteoarthritis—he was unable to move his arms, both of his legs were drawn up, and his spine was so rigid that he had to hold his head in one position at all times. His name was Dr. Jesse Cain.

Dr. Cain had finished pharmacy at Leonard Medical School in Raleigh, gone on to study medicine, and had gotten a degree in medicine as well. He was stricken with arthritis while in medical school. By the time he graduated, he was disabled to such an extent that he could do very little practicing medicine. So, he spent his days at the drugstore where he was able to see a few patients and fill prescriptions.

The owner of the drugstore, Dr. Smith, spent most of his time managing his other drugstore in another city. Since as he happened to be in Tarboro when I was visiting , he used all his persuasive powers to convince me that Tarboro was the place for me to practice. I told Dr. Smith that after paying for my license and buying a roundtrip ticket between Nashville and Raleigh, I only had ten dollars to my name. Dr. Smith reassuringly told me that if I agreed to come to Tarboro right away, he would see to it that I was able to borrow enough money to open an office.

I left Tarboro that afternoon thinking about what I had heard and the men I had met. About two hours later I asked another friend, Dr. Williams, to bring me back to Tarboro. We approached

Dr. Smith again. "Now, Dr. Smith," I questioned, "you said you would be able to help me borrow enough money to begin my practice if I come out here right away?"

"Yes. I am quite sure that I would be able to help you get the money to open your office," he reasserted.

I then told Dr. Smith that my worldly possessions consisted of a wardrobe trunk containing some well-worn clothes, a stethoscope, and a bag full of samples.

"Don't worry about that," he assured me. "Just let me know when you are coming, and I'll be right here to meet you and help you borrow the money."

I made up my mind right then to move to Tarboro.

When I returned to Tennessee and met with Weathers, I told him of my plans. "Do you mean to tell me that you're going to a country town?" he asked, amazed.

"Yes." I was firm. "I feel that Tarboro is the place for me."

"I wouldn't be caught dead in a little old place like that," he shuddered. "Where are you going?"

"I'm going to Portsmouth, Ohio," he said.

"Well, what's so great about Portsmouth, Ohio? What do you have there?" I countered.

"There are two or three factories there, and everyone is employed," he reported. "They are paid by the week or by the month. How do people get paid in North Carolina?"

"Well, most of them are sharecroppers," I said. "The landowners advance them enough money to live on during the year until the crops are harvested in the fall. The landowners then settle up with the sharecroppers, paying them the money they are due for growing the crops."

"What will happen if they don't make any money?"

"Oh well, some of them are going to make some money," I said. "I don't think I'll starve to death with all of the food growing around there."

"If you're going to be a country bumpkin, and there is nothing I can do to persuade you to go elsewhere," he said, "then go ahead, go your way."

"Wait a minute." I couldn't let our talk end like that. "I'm going to a small town, and I may not do too well, but you're going to a small city and may not do too well either. Then again, we both may do all right. Anything can happen. But I want to ask you something. If I get in trouble in North Carolina, will you bail me out?"

"Yes." He did not hesitate.

"If you get in trouble in Portsmouth, Ohio, I'll bail you out. Is that a bargain?" "Yes," he agreed.

"Go your way, brother, and I'll go mine." So, we parted as good friends.

Weathers loaned me money for my train fare back to Tarboro, and I returned one week later. I got off the train at the station in downtown Rocky Mount and decided to stop in to see my good friend Dr. Williams before boarding the bus to Tarboro.

I arrived in Tarboro about 10:30 a.m. on a Sunday and went to Mrs. Jacob's home. She was Dr. Smith's sister and in charge of the drugstore while he was out of town. I rang the doorbell and said, "Good morning, Mrs. Jacobs. I am ready to be introduced to the people of Tarboro." She did not seem overly glad to see me.

She said, "This is not my church Sunday, so I usually take this Sunday to rest. Now you go down to the drugstore, and the clerk will show you around town. I'll see you tomorrow."

To tell you the truth, I felt a little bit rebuffed. I thought that since I was coming to town, the lady would be glad to see me and introduce me to some of the people. However, I went along to the drugstore and found it was just about closing time because most everyone in Tarboro went to church on Sundays.

There was a Mr. Jones at the drugstore who took me to the A.M.E. Church where the service was in progress. We took our places in the rear of the church, and after the sermon, Mr. Jones introduced me to the congregation.

I began the day with seven dollars in my pocket, put one dollar in the collection plate, and wondered how long the remaining six would last. After the service, I strolled around town with Mr. Jones who suggested that we go to the Elks Lodge to meet quite a few people who gathered there after Sunday services. The Elks was a strong organization in Tarboro at that time, and the lodge was situated in a large, well-kept house. We approached the house and saw two men sitting on the porch. I later learned their names were Boisy Porter and Lee Williams. Lee was a loquacious sort of fellow who said whatever came to mind, regardless of how it sounded. As I approached the house, he turned to Boisy and said, "Who is that little skinny nigger coming up here?"

Boisy had been at the church where I had been introduced, so he said, "That's the new doctor coming to town."

"He looks like he's about to fall dead, and you mean to tell me he's a doctor?" Lee said, not caring that I could hear him. "He's so damned skinny, he looks like HE needs a doctor...and soon."

"Don't talk so loud. He can hear you," Boisy said, embarrassed.

"I don't give a damn if he hears me," Lee continued. "He is skinny. He'll probably do just like the last one that came. He'll leave and probably borrow the money to do it with."

I turned to Mr. Jones and said, "You didn't tell me someone had been here and left before me."

Mr. Jones said, "Oh, don't pay that any mind. There was some-one here, but I'm not sure if he was a doctor or not. He was afraid of blood and didn't want anyone disturbing him after five o'clock in the afternoon. Sure, he had to leave town, but it was because he was so irritable that nobody could get along with him."

I said, "If I had known that I probably wouldn't have taken a second look at this town."

"Don't worry. You'll be all right," he assured me.

We chatted awhile, then strolled further on down the street. I saw another house with a well-kept lawn and asked Mr. Jones, "Who lives in that house?"

"That's where Nat Gray lives. He's one of the barbers in town."

As we passed the house, the door was wide open, and I looked back into the dining room where I saw several fellows sitting around the table eating. Nat looked up, saw me, and yelled out, "Hey, Jones, who's that you got with you?"

Mr. Jones said, "This is the new doctor."

"He is? Come on in and have some dinner." I remembered that I only had six dollars in my pocket, so I gladly accepted the dinner invitation. That's when my friendship with Nat began.

I had not arranged for a boarding place and reminded Mr. Jones that I had to find some place to sleep. He immediately thought of a local widow who rented rooms. We went to see her, and she gladly agreed to take me in as a boarder. Two meals a day and a room was thirty-five dollars a month, and I gladly accepted. I asked her if she needed the money in advance, and she said, "Oh, don't worry about that. I know you're going to be all right." That made me feel happy.

Bright and early the next morning, I went to the drugstore, and sure enough, Dr. Smith came in about 10 a.m. So, I started in,

"Now, about borrowing some money to open my office."

"We can attend to that right away," he said, ready to help. "I'll tell you what. I don't have the money myself, but I know a very good man in town who will lend you the money if I recommend you. I'm busy right now, but I'll call him on the phone and tell him you're coming up there."

I asked, "Who is this man?"

"His name is Mr. Clarence Johnson."

I said, "What's his mission on earth?"

"He's a merchant," Dr. Smith replied. "He handles fertilizer for the farmers and loans them money to carry their crops until fall. He's a good man, and if you're trying to help yourself, he'll help you. He came up the hard way. He came to Tarboro as a clerk to work in somebody else's store and advanced to such an extent that he has a business of his own. All you've got to do is talk to him, and I'll call and tell him you're coming. You tell him your mission in town."

Mr. Johnson's office was just off Main Street, across from the Town Hall. When I entered his office, there were several white men and two Black men sitting around. I walked up to his desk.

"What can I do for you?" he asked.

"I came here to borrow two hundred fifty dollars to open my doctor's office," I said.

"Oh, you're a doctor." He was flabbergasted. "Wait a minute, and let's talk this thing over."

I started telling him about myself, starting from when I was a child on up to the present, adding how I happened to come to Tarboro. I told him I had come to the town as a recommendation and saw that the town needed a Black doctor. He agreed. We talked for about an hour, and then I finally said, "I see you've got people waiting for you, so I'll come back tomorrow and talk with you more about this. I don't expect to convince you that I'm worthy of your attention on one visit, so I'll be back tomorrow."

"No, don't stop," he said.

"No, you've got people sitting here," I said again, "and I can wait. I'll come back tomorrow."

"Okay, come back tomorrow, and we'll talk some more about it," he agreed.

I went back the next day and told him more about the story of my life for about another hour. I had been watching the clock, so then I left again when I had taken up his time.

"Okay, come back tomorrow about one o'clock," he said, "and we'll talk some more."

So, I went back to see him on Wednesday. At the end of our talk, he said, "Doc, I believe you are the man all of us needs in this town. Not only your folks, but my folks too, and I'm willing to let you have the money. You tell Smith to come up here and sign the note with you, and you can have the money."

I was so jubilant I ran almost all the way down the street to the drugstore. I found Dr. Smith and said, "Mr. Johnson said if you would sign the note with me that he would let me have the money."

"Okay. Don't worry about it. I'll do it," he said. Just about that time, his sister called him to the back of the store, and I left.

The next morning, I went back to the drugstore, but Dr. Smith was not there. I saw his sister and asked where he was.

She said, "He left town. He's gone to the other store because they needed him there today."

I said, "Gone to his other store? He promised me he would go with me to Mr. Johnson's and sign a note so I could borrow the money to open my office."

She said, "What do you mean? Do you expect him to sign a note for you to get some money? He doesn't know anything about you. He could sign a note for you, and you might leave town the same day."

I said, "But please, Mrs. Jacobs, I'm here to stay."

"Yes, and I've heard that story before and don't believe a word of it. He's not going to sign anything for you. I told him to go back to Durham. He doesn't know anything about you," she repeated.

This was leaving me in quite a mess since I was depending on him. By that time my six dollars had dwindled to three. All my dreams came crashing down around me. Dr. Cain, the Black pharmacist, had been sitting in the corner listening and said, "Wait a minute, Doc. I've got to go home in a few minutes. Will you drive me?"

I said, "Sure, I'll drive you home." He had his own piece of a car. It was about twelve years old, but at least it was still running. We got in and started out.

He said, "Look, Doc, I don't really have to go home for anything. I just wanted to tell you that I knew you were not going to get that money. Dr. Smith's sister has been fussing with him ever since Monday, trying to persuade him not to help you. She went so far as to make him get out of town so he wouldn't be here this morning. What are you going to do now?"

I told Dr. Cain that I would get the money from someone else. I didn't want to be obligated to a lot of different people, and I didn't want to be obligated to Dr. Smith. Here I was—no car, three dollars in my pocket, eating the widow's food and sleeping in her rented bed. She would be looking for her money at the end of the month. What was I going to do?

Dr. Cain said, "I wouldn't want you to be obligated to anyone else either, but I'll tell you what you can do. Come on and drive me down to Mr. Dancy's store. He's a merchant in East Tarboro. That's where all the colored folks live. I know he'll help you. He knows all about Dr. Smith and Mrs. Jacobs, and he knows she wouldn't let him help anybody in this world. That woman is mean as hell."

I told Dr. Cain, "I don't want to be obligated. What is Mr. Dancy going to get out of it? He has a grocery store, but the drugstore people would at least get something out of my presence here because I'd be sending them all the prescriptions."

He said, "Don't worry about that. He'll be glad to help you."

"I can't ask him to help me. I don't know anything about the man, and he surely doesn't know anything about me," I told Dr. Cain.

He kept insisting that I go and see Mr. Dancy, but I had something else on my mind. I decided I'd go back to Rocky Mount and see my former classmate, Dr. Williams, to try to get his help. When I saw him, I explained the situation.

"Well, you know, Bro. Quig," Dr. Williams began, "I realize you're in quite a predicament. However, since you're going to practice medicine in Tarboro, I think you should look there for help. You try in Tarboro again. If it doesn't work out, come back, and I'll recommend somebody who might be able to do something for you. I know you realize that I haven't been here too long myself, and a fellow should have some cash in order to look out for emergencies. If you'd had some cash when you came here, you wouldn't be in this predicament."

"But you know, Dr. Williams, I was promised all kinds of help by someone on whom I thought I could rely, but because of his sister, I'm left swinging out here without any help and no way to get started."

"I repeat, the best thing for you is to go back to Tarboro and find somebody who'll help you," he advised. "You have my sympathy."

I returned to Tarboro and to Dr. Cain's house. He was eager to know what Dr. Williams said.

"He gave me all sorts of excuses and ended up refusing to help me," I concluded.

Dr. Cain said, "I know you hate being obligated to anyone, but suppose we try getting help from Mr. Dancy?"

I was still upset but decided to give it a try.

Mr. Dancy's general store, a two-story cinder block structure, was located in East Tarboro, way down in the colored section of town. I was told that he had made the blocks himself out of cinders and concrete. The store was on the first floor, and he lived on the second. He sold groceries, meats, mops, brooms, galvanized ten-quart buckets, washtubs, rakes, hoes, fans, and just about anything else you could think of.

When we arrived, Dr. Cain had me go in and call him out. Dr. Cain explained the situation to Mr. Dancy, who replied, "I can understand your situation, and I can understand why Dr. Smith didn't help you because I know his sister that well. I'll be glad to sign a note for you so you can get the money. However, I would like for you to get Mr. Pattillo to co-sign your note. He'll be glad to do it."

"Who is Mr. Pattillo?"

"He's the school principal and would do anything to help our town." That didn't set well with me, but Dr. Cain insisted that Mr. Dancy call Mr. Pattillo. In due time, he came to the store where we all discussed the matter again.

"I'll be glad to help you," Mr. Pattillo said. So, Mr. Dancy suggested that we go to Mr. Johnson's office the next morning to finalize it all.

"I think this is a sorry way to get a doctor to this town," I said, letting off some steam. "After being rebuffed as I have by Mrs.

Jacobs, I don't see how in hell they expect me to send them prescriptions."

Mr. Pattillo spoke up. "Well, I'll help you under one condition, and that is that you go ahead and send your prescriptions to Dr. Smith's drugstore." I reluctantly agreed. The next morning, we were at Mr. Johnson's office at 10 a.m.

Mr. Dancy took control. "Mr. Johnson, this man has come to Tarboro to open his office and practice medicine, but he has been fooled. Dr. Smith sent him to you with the understanding that after you talked to Dr. Quigless, he would come up and sign a note for him to borrow the money. Now Dr. Smith has left town, and this man will have to leave if he doesn't get the help he needs. If he leaves Tarboro and spreads the word that the people here cannot be depended on for help, we will never have another chance for getting a doctor here. Mr. Pattillo and I are willing to co-sign a note so he can get two hundred fifty dollars."

Mr. Johnson said, "That's all I wanted to hear. Give me the telephone." He called the Security Bank and asked for someone named Cherry. "Tell Cherry to get on this phone," he said. We waited a moment. "Cherry," he began, "I'm sending a man down there named Dr. Quigless. He wants to borrow two hundred fifty dollars from the bank, and I will sign the note along with C.M. Dancy and Pattillo. Let him have the money and give him a blank note for me to sign."

He turned to me and said, "Doc, you go get the money and take care of what little bills you have. Get the note signed and bring it back to me tomorrow morning."

"Thank you, sir," I said, then tore out of there.

At the bank, Mr. Cherry asked, "How do you want the money? Do you want it in cash, or do you want a check, or what?"

I said, "I want to open an account and deposit the money." He deposited the funds into my new account and gave me the note to have filled out. I went on my merry way.

The next order of business was finding a building suitable enough for me to open an office. That was the first time I went to my new friend Nat Gray for help. "Nat," I confided, "I've been able to borrow enough money to open an office. Now all I have to do is find a suitable place."

He spoke of several locations near the center of town, but most of them were in the portion of town where all of the white businesses were located. He was doubtful as to whether white businesses would allow a colored doctor to locate that close to them. Then he remembered another place, a vacant fish market. We went to look the place over. It was a one-story stucco building located at the foot of Main Street beside the river bridge.

Tarboro is situated on the banks of the Tar River. Main Street begins at the river and extends in a northwesterly direction for roughly one mile. At that time, Main Street was crisscrossed by about twenty streets going east and west. There were about ten streets running parallel to Main Street. There was some paving down Main Street, but if I remember correctly, there was no curbing or guttering. Just about one-third of the other streets were paved the same way, with asphalt in the middle and no curbing or guttering, all in the parts of town occupied by whites.

Panola Street separated the Black and white areas. The Blacks resided east of Panola Street, and the whites were on the west side. The entrance to the fish market building faced Main Street. There had been plate-glass windows on either side of the entrance door and in the front door, but all had been knocked out and the open spaces were boarded up. The front door was nailed shut as well. We pried it open and went inside to find the ceiling sagging, the plaster falling from the walls on all sides, and the entire area a dismal mess. I felt that it possibly could be turned into an office, provided I got some help with cleaning, installing windows, and spreading a little paint.

After a little investigating, we discovered that the building now belonged to the town, so our next stop was Town Hall to see if it was possible to rent the building. The clerk looked up, saw us, and said, "What can I do for you boys?" I told him that I was interested in renting the old fish market building at the end of Main Street to open an office. He said, "Oh, we don't want to bother renting that place. Every time we rent it, somebody stays for three or four months, tears up the building, goes out of business, and leaves, owing us the rent."

"But I'm here to stay," I implored.

"It don't make no difference. We're not going to rent to anybody," he insisted.

Mr. Johnson's office was right across the street from the Town Hall, so we stepped over there. He saw us coming and said, "Doc, what's the trouble?" I told him I wanted to rent the old fish market down by the river, but that the town had refused to rent it to me. He asked, "Who did?"

"The clerk over at the Town Hall," I explained.

He picked up the telephone receiver and turned the crank. Somebody answered, "Number, please?"

"Give me 99." Mr. Johnson then said, "George? Get George Earnhardt on this phone."

It turns out, Mr. Earnhardt was the town clerk. There was a short pause, then Mr. Johnson said, "George, this doctor went over there to rent the building down on the river front. Doggone it, let him have that building, and you're not going to charge him any rent for six months. Have somebody fix it up and let him pay five dollars a week for having it done. Hop to it right away because he needs a place to open his office."

I then went back to the Town Hall, and Mr. Earnhardt was very gracious. I told him there was no lock on the door, and we had to pry it open to get inside. He had somebody hustle around to get me a padlock. The next day Robert Walston, a carpenter, came in and surveyed the wrecked place. He made a list of things he would need, like lumber, glass, cement, and the like, and presented it to Mr. Earnhardt. The building materials arrived that afternoon. I was able to open my office in five days!

Meanwhile, I had not received my license from the examining board in Raleigh. However, on the third day after my arrival, I picked up the *Raleigh News and Observer,* and there on the front page was an account of the procedures of the North Carolina Board of Medical Examiners. All the names of the doctors who had taken the examination and passed were listed in the article. Yes, my name was right there too. I noted with dismay that my address was listed as Port Gibson, Mississippi, so my license had been sent there. I contacted my mother to have her send my license to Tarboro, which she did. It took at least a month from the time I was issued the license before I received it.

While waiting, I met a surgeon, Dr. W. W. Green, and I'd say he was the dean of the physicians in Tarboro. I realized that it could possibly be three or four weeks before I could get my license mailed to me from Mississippi, so I went to Dr. Green, showed him the newspaper, and told him I was ready to practice medicine, even though my license had not yet been delivered. He called the secretary of the Board of Medical Examiners, who verified the fact that my license had been issued.

Dr. Green advised that I could write prescriptions, and in the event I had to write any for narcotics, he would be glad to sign the prescriptions for me until my license arrived. The controlled substances at that time were mostly codeine, morphine, and cocaine. Since Dr. Green was a very busy man, performing all the major operations in addition to seeing patients in his office, I made it a point to write prescriptions for patients that did not include narcotic substances so that I would not have to bother him so often.

The usual fee for doctors' office visits was three dollars at that time. However, many of my patients were so broke they could not afford to pay for their prescriptions, so I found myself treating twenty-five to thirty patients but being paid by only eight to twelve of them. In the beginning, I was only treating Black patients. It would be another ten years before white patients started coming to me as well.

A local insurance agent named Henry Edmonds stopped by my office, inquiring how I was getting along. I said, "I see plenty of patients, but I'm not collecting too much money."

I remembered something Dr. John Hale, professor of surgery at Meharry, said in one of his lectures. Dr. Hale was a master surgeon with an inimitable way of getting across his subject to students. Every now and then, he would stop talking about surgery and get into the subject of practicing medicine. One day he said to us, "Now, fellows, I'm going to tell you something that I want you to remember real well. When you go out and begin practicing medicine, you are going to make some friends. Some friends will be higher-ups, and some will just be ordinary people. I want to tell you about the big shots. They'll come to your parties, invite you to their homes for dinners every now and again and try to get free advice. However, you will not make a living off the big shots. It's going to be the little fellows who'll make or break you. Give that little man due consideration, and he'll take care of you. Go to his church, take time to be friendly to his children, and develop interest in their activities, and in the future, after you've made your way, it will have been with the help of the little man. When you go into a community, go to the church first, make friends with the pastor, and shake hands with all the members of the congregation. The little man will turn up at your office, and the big shot will wait to see how he got along."

I turned to Henry Edmonds. "By the way, Henry, I want to go to some of the country churches and meet the people and the pastors."

He said, "I have a place for you to go this Sunday. We're going to Mount Pilgrim Baptist Church in Hobgood."

Now Hobgood was about eighteen miles from Tarboro. Henry and I got to Mount Pilgrim Church before services started and were greeted by a very intelligent Baptist preacher named Reverend Jeff James. After the sermon, I was introduced to the congregation and allowed to speak a few words. I found that all the members were delighted to have a chance to shake hands with me and talk for a few minutes.

In the succeeding days and weeks, I had several patients come to me from Hobgood. I got the message that Sunday, and from then on, I made it a point to visit all the churches within fifty miles of Tarboro. It is true that I picked up all the old chronic complainers, the neglected leg ulcers, cardiac patients, asthmatics, syphilis in all stages, and cases that puzzled me as well as the rest of the doctors in the community, but I did the best I could with whatever I had to work with. The results must have been pleasing because I immediately found myself with more patients than I could handle.

Finally, I had met all the doctors in the area except for one. I was advised by many who were well-acquainted with this one good doctor that I should write him off and not bother to try and meet him. It so happened, however, that I got a chance. He owned a farm near Tarboro with tenants living on it. One of the tenants came to me one day and said, "Doctor, I got a little boy at home who's been sick about three weeks. My boss has been seeing him and giving him medicine, but he don't seem to get any better. I'd appreciate you going out and taking a look at him."

I went to his house and found a fourteen-year-old boy lying in bed with symptoms of nausea, vomiting, severe weight loss, and high fever. I knew that typhoid fever was endemic in the area, so I drew blood for a Widal test and prescribed some medication. A Widal test is done to test for the presence of the typhoid fever I thought he had. I saw the doctor who owned the farm standing a few feet away when I started to leave. I spoke to him, telling him that his tenant had asked me to see his son, and I thought he had typhoid fever. I further informed him that I had drawn blood for a Widal test.

The good doctor said, "Fine, that's good. I think you have done the right thing."

The next day the tenant came back to my office and seemed upset. I asked, "How is the boy doing?"

"He's doing better already. But, Doctor, you know one thing?"

"What's that?"

"My boss cussed me out. He told me if I ever let a nigger doctor come on his place, he would kick both me and the nigger doctor off his farm."

So, I had no desire to go back on that man's farm. That particular doctor hated my guts, not because I was another doctor, but because I was Black.

I encountered many suffering from syphilis. They went to the county health department for treatment because they didn't have enough money to pay a doctor. I even ran into two or three cases of untreated, tertiary syphilis, which is the final stage of the disease. I asked several why they hadn't gone to the health department for treatment and instead let themselves get into this condition. One or two said they were just too embarrassed. Everyone would know why they were being treated, and they were too ashamed of themselves for having the disease. These people asked about treatment but said they had no money to pay for it. I agreed to treat them for a nominal fee of one dollar per visit. I obtained the medication to treat them from the health department for free.

Among that group of patients was a very nice lady. After opening my office, she came in and did a critical inspection. She said, "Doctor, you sure have got it looking nice around here, but there's one thing that worries me. You don't have any curtains for the windows, and all those folks passing by are peeping in here. I just don't like that. I don't like them looking at me. I'll tell you what I'll do. If you buy the material, I'll make you some curtains and won't charge you a penny."

My office did have several large windows facing the street. When I had opened the office, I was able to paint the interior of the structure. But after going to Simmons Furniture Company and buying some used chairs, lamps, and Congoleum rugs, I didn't have money enough to make a down-payment on draperies. So, when this lady offered to make them, I quickly bought the material for her. Within three days, that nice lady had made curtains and hung them up.

I was living comfortably in the widow Mrs. Deans's home. Her daughter had assured me that I would be satisfied with the food and the room. And she was right. The room was light, airy, and very clean. I could not see how they could afford to give me room and board for just thirty-five dollars a month. I had bacon, eggs, toast, coffee, cornflakes, oatmeal, and anything else I wanted for breakfast. My dinners were excellent—I had appetizers, salads, entrees, and desserts. I wondered how in hell I could get this kind of food at such a price! It was good, and I ate all of it.

Everything was wonderful for about three months. Then Mrs. Deans's daughter took off for New York where she had gotten a job as a live-in maid for a wealthy couple. Shortly after she left, I noticed a change in the meals. The toast was often burned, the grits scorched, the biscuits hard, and the coffee weak as water. The excellent meals usually served at dinner also vanished. I got a routine diet of collard greens, black-eyed peas, pigs' feet, chitterlings, and the like. I made up my mind that it was about time for me to move on.

I had met a young teacher named Miss Prince about two weeks after arriving in Tarboro. I learned that her parents boarded several teachers who were very well satisfied with their accommodations. So, I made it a point to ask Miss Prince, "Do you think your parents would be interested in taking on one more boarder?"

"I don't know," she said. "We have so many in our house now. They're about to run us out. What's the trouble with you at Mrs. Deans's place?" she asked. But then she laughed. "You don't have to answer that question. I know what happened."

She explained that I had been eating out of what was generally known as the "hot pan." That's when the cooks who worked for the white folks were allowed to take their dinners home. They always managed to cook enough so that after the white folks finished their meal, there would be enough left over to take home to their children. The excellent dinners I had been eating had been taken directly from the "hot pan" of the white folks' kitchen where Mrs. Deans's daughter had been cooking. As the saying goes, "It was good while it lasted."

I went around to see Miss Prince's parents. Her father was a retired farmer who had moved to town after managing a farm for a white man. He had saved enough money to build a nice two-story frame home with three or four extra-large bedrooms, so they were able to rent rooms to teachers. Mrs. Prince said, "Doctor, we would be glad to have you around here, but the only place you would be able to sleep would be in my son's room." Their eldest son had sustained a birth injury that had left him partially paralyzed and subject to attacks of epilepsy. I told her that I would be glad to room with him and moved in two days later.

The room was large enough to have two beds, and everything was clean and comfortable. Mrs. Prince was an immaculate housekeeper and an excellent cook, having cooked for a woman for about twenty years before leaving to take care of her own family. Mr. Prince was a very fine man. Although he had stopped farming, he did odd jobs around town. He still had a good relationship with the white family for whom he had worked for many years. I was very comfortable at the Princes' home. Mr. Prince and I became good friends, and he looked upon me as just another member of the family.

CHAPTER 16

OBSTACLES

I was treating several syphilis patients at my office, including one young man about twenty years old suffering from far-advanced syphilis of the central nervous system. In other words, he acted "off " all the time. After treating him for about seven months, he seemed to be doing fairly well. I had noticed, however, that he missed three appointments. I thought nothing of it until one day, Mr. Prince called me aside and asked, "Doctor, what happened to George Martin?"

"I haven't seen him for several weeks. I don't know what happened," I replied.

"I understand that while you were gone to the beach for the weekend, he went crazy and started beating up members of his family," he informed me. "They had to call the police to quiet him down. They took him to another doctor who told them the medicine you had been giving him made him go out of his mind, and that was why he attacked everybody in the house."

I had not heard a word about it. But "Grandpa Prince," as I had begun calling him, said, "Doctor, you're the only one that don't know about it. They're giving you a bad name." That made me feel so bad that I just about went out of business.

"Somebody will find out sooner or later just what's going on with the fellow," I assured him.

About a month later, the young man's mother came to my office and said, "Doctor, I need to see you privately."

"Okay, come on back to the office, and let's see what's the trouble," I said.

"I want to know what you're going to do about my son."

"What do you mean?" I asked.

"That doctor told me the medicine you gave my boy has run him crazy and that you're going to have to do something about it."

I got mad as hell. Trying to control myself, I said, "Listen, dear lady. Let me tell you one thing. I have the laboratory reports on your son, and he is suffering from far-advanced syphilis of the nervous system. That's the reason he acted as he did. As to what I am going to do about it, I'll tell you exactly what I'm going to do. If I ever hear another word about you putting this stuff out about me giving him medicine that ran him crazy, I'm going to take these lab reports to the courthouse and post them on that bulletin board so everybody can see them. That way the whole town will know that he is suffering from far-advanced syphilis. That's the only damn thing I'm going to do about it. I hope you never put your foot in my place again."

She made a hasty retreat, and I made it a point to go all over town talking about it. The people in town were sympathetic toward me and mad as hell with the lady. All in all, I thought I made a good initial impression on the people in the town of Tarboro.

During the middle of the summer of 1937, I had a call to attend to a child about two years old. When I arrived at the house, I found the child suffering from a very high fever, diarrhea, bloody stools, and convulsive seizures. The grandmother stated that the child had eaten a lot of green plums and peaches, the diarrhea had developed about four days before, and the convulsions had started about two days before. My diagnosis was gastroenteritis.

In that day and time, not much specifically could be done for this condition. I advised the grandmother that the child should be hospitalized because he could get dehydrated, and intravenous fluids might get him over the attack. I had learned about intravenous fluids from my internship. She said she couldn't get the child to Raleigh and didn't want him in the hospital here in Tarboro. So, I began treating the child at home.

In spite of everything I did, the child's condition deteriorated. I told the grandmother that I had done everything I could and would appreciate a consultation with another doctor in town.

There was always a group of women in the room whenever I treated the child, and one of them suggested that I call Dr. J. G. Raby. I did, and he came right away, asking what the trouble was and what I'd done for the child so far.

I related everything I had done, and he saw the I.V. fluids running. He turned around and said to the grandmother, "This doctor has done everything that can be done for this child. He has done far more than I could have done because he's just out of medical school and is up on the latest methods and medicines. I don't see any need to interfere. If the condition persists, the child may not survive, but it will not be this doctor's fault. He has done everything I would have done and more." And with that, he put on his hat and left.

The child died. A lot of women from the neighborhood in the room had heard what Dr. Raby had said. So, the word got around that the child had died but that I had done everything I could for him. "Even Dr. Raby said so," they were saying.

I was well aware that just one word of criticism from Dr. Raby would have sealed my fate in Tarboro. I give Dr. Raby credit for my ability to overcome a very difficult period in my relationship with the people there.

There was another important incident that involved a patient I visited in a small town about five miles from Tarboro. When I got to the house, the lady's husband met me at the gate and said, "Doctor, come in and see what's wrong with my wife. She complained of a severe headache before she went to church. After she got to church, she became very excited and started shouting. When we got home, she was still complaining of a severe headache, and all of a sudden, she fell forward. She has not spoken since. We haven't been able to revive her, so I called you."

I went in, checked the lady, and found her comatose. One pupil was widely dilated and the other constricted. Her blood pressure was 280 over 130. Her husband stated that she had been under treatment for hypertension over a period of several years. However, within the last six or eight months she had not taken any medication. After my examination, I concluded that she had suffered a severe cerebral hemorrhage.

About ten minutes later, her blood pressure continued rising. There wasn't any hope of getting her to the hospital. I told her husband what had happened and that his wife would probably die. In retrospect, I should have left the house at that time. However, I sat around talking to the family members. The lady's husband came out of the room and said, "Look here, Doc. Can't you do something for my wife?"

"I will go in and see what I can do," I replied. I checked her blood pressure again and shook my head.

"Now look here, Doctor," he said. "I want you to do something for her and do it right now."

"I'm sorry, sir. I can't do anything more."

He screamed, "Don't let my wife die!!"

The lady died about that time, and the husband and three children all began screaming. I started gathering up my instruments but couldn't get all my junk into my bag fast enough. I was nervous and in a hurry to get away from there, so I opened my shirt, stuck my stethoscope down it, and beat a hasty retreat.

At this time, I had patients coming to my office from all the communities around Tarboro within a radius of twenty-five to fifty miles who were appreciative of my help, and my fame spread.

However, not everyone was satisfied with my progress. In fact, whenever a particular doctor ran into his former patients on the street, he let them know, in no uncertain terms, that he didn't appreciate them coming to me for treatment. These patients came back to my office and told me of the "cussing out" they got from this doctor whenever he saw them. I wondered how the devil that doctor could find out that these people were coming to me.

Mr. Grimes, a teacher in the community, had been taking his wife to this doctor for treatment over two years. However, his wife continued to complain. When Mr. Grimes heard about me, he brought his wife over for treatment. After a while, she began improving. Naturally, he continued bringing her to me. The word spread around the neighborhood, and others asked Mr. Grimes to bring them over to me for treatment, which he was glad to do.

He told me at one point that he had gotten a phone call from the other doctor. "Stop taking my patients," he demanded. "Otherwise, you will have to suffer the consequences." Mr. Grimes disregarded the threat and continued bringing others to me whenever he brought his wife. Later, Mr. Grimes received another call from the doctor advising him, with a good deal of profanity, that if he didn't stop bringing his patients over to me, the doctor would run him out of town. Mr. Grimes passed that incident off as a prank. But about three months later, a group of men in two cars drove up to his house around midnight. They banged on his door and said, "If you don't get the hell out of town by tomorrow morning, we're going to burn you and that damn woman up in this goddam shack."

After they left, Mr. Grimes and his wife dressed and drove to my home. After relating the incident to me, I calmed them and put them to bed in my spare bedroom. The next day they returned to their home, removed their personal belongings, and never returned to that area again.

After that incident, a lady who lived in the same area came to my office. She stated that she was pregnant and didn't want to have the baby. She asked me pointblank if I would give her an abortion. Fortunately for me, one of her friends accompanied her to my office. I flatly refused to give the lady an abortion. She offered me money, but I refused her again. She stated that she had been bothered with indigestion for some time, so I gave her medication to relieve her indigestion, and she left my office. I later learned from her friend that she had thrown the medication away and was going to find a root doctor who would do the abortion.

Three weeks later she developed severe vaginal bleeding and had to call in that other doctor who had threatened Mr. Grimes. When he found her bleeding, he asked which doctor she had seen. She told him that she had been seen by me. That was all the doctor wanted to know. He walked off and left the lady bleeding. Fortunately for her, the bleeding stopped. However, that doctor was not finished with the incident. He reported the lady to law enforcement officers and took out a warrant against her.

She was brought to trial by the local magistrate. When she went to trial, she was accompanied by the same friend who had come with her to my office. The doctor got on the stand and stated that the woman had undergone a criminal abortion and that she had told him that I performed it. He stated further that he wanted me indicted for performing the abortion.

In that instant, the lady's friend spoke up and said, "That woman knows she went to Dr. Quigless, and he refused to do the abortion for her. He gave her medicine for indigestion. She knows she threw the medicine in the river after leaving his office and asked me where she could find a root doctor. I don't know who did the abortion, but I do know that Dr. Quigless didn't do it." That ended the trial right there. The entire case was dismissed. I realized then that the other doctor was after my scalp.

There was a service station right across the street from my office where I usually bought gas and had my car serviced. One day when I went to the station, the owner began talking with me while he filled up my gas tank. "Doc, do you know Dr. _____?" he asked, naming the doctor who was after me, and whom I do not wish to identify by name.

"Yes," I answered.

"He comes to my place," he said, "and we sit and talk for hours at a time. He really is a fine man."

"When was the last time he came to your station?" I asked.

"He was here about two weeks ago."

"What time was he here?" I asked further.

"Oh, he comes in around one o'clock in the afternoon and stays for two or three hours," he said. "I don't know when he does his practice because he's always over here."

I knew right away what was happening. This doctor was sitting at the service station watching patients come into my office.

Despite his threats, the people of that community did not stop coming to me. I advised them to stay clear of that doctor, and whenever he approached them concerning their present-day treatment and who they were seeing, I told them that all they had to say was, "Where I go is my business. It is my money I'm spending, and if I ever need you, I'll call. Thank you." That doctor continued harassing my patients for at least another year.

A satellite clinic bearing his name was established in that area after he passed away. The Grimes couple moved to another area and resumed their teaching careers. I continued treating Mrs. Grimes, and their union was blessed by the birth of two girls. They retired and lived happily ever after.

***

I had been in Tarboro about a year and a half when I was called to the farmhouse of Mr. Walter Plemmer, which was located about a mile out of town. When I got to the house, I found Walter, Jr., who was about eight years old, complaining of severe pain in both ankles. I examined the boy, and indeed, his joints were greatly swollen. He was in such severe pain that he was unable to move without screaming. Young Walter loved music. However, when he attempted to practice on the piano, the joints on his fingers became swollen, and he had to stop. His father stated he had been seen by several doctors who diagnosed hemophilia, and he had been treated at the children's hospital in Gastonia, North Carolina, on several occasions. He further stated that the Edgecombe County Welfare Superintendent, Mrs. Mary Ellen Forbes, had become very interested in young Walter's predicament.

From his case history I concluded that he was indeed suffering from hemophilia. At that time, very little could be done in a definitive way for people suffering that severe malady. On several occasions, Mrs. Forbes volunteered to take Walter to the children's hospital in Gastonia on her own time. Gastonia was about ninety-five miles from Tarboro, and, as far as I knew, that was the only hospital for treating children in the state. They didn't really have an effective treatment for hemophilia at that hospital, and though I had studied hemophilia in medical school, I knew there was nothing in the way of treatment that would help.

At that time, I subscribed to the Pryor Publication. This organization furnished any subscribing physician with requested abstracts of recent advances in diagnosis and treatment of diseases. The cost was twenty-five to thirty dollars per year, which was costly but well worth the price. So, I had the service abstract all the articles they could find on the treatment of hemophilia and forward them to me. When reading the abstracts, I found nothing applicable to Walter's condition. However, one of the investigators did advance that hemophilia, in most instances, was observed in males. The investigator's opinion was that there was probably some factor in the blood of females that prevented the disease from developing in them.

A few years prior, female sex hormones had been identified and isolated so that they could be used in treating conditions associated with low estrogen levels in women, common during menopause. Inasmuch as enterogenic substances were available, I conceived the idea of treating young Walter with female sex hormones in the form of theelin. I talked to Walter's father, explaining that there might be some untoward effects in the treatment before puberty, and there was danger of feminine characteristics developing. But he signed a statement to the effect that I would not be held responsible if those effects developed as a result of the treatment.

I began injecting Walter, Jr., with theelin at the rate of .4 cc every three days. I used a 25-gauge hypodermic needle and made injections into his deltoid muscle. Luckily for me and Walter, there was no bleeding. After three weeks, the joint swelling failed to develop further, and blood was absorbed from the affected joints. Walter was able to practice the piano without developing any swelling in his fingers. I continued these injections for two months. Although the results were gratifying, Walter complained of pain incidental to the injections and begged me to give him the medication by mouth. So, I tried treatments by mouth for a period of two months. However, his joints began swelling and bleeding again.

I sat down and talked to him. "Which would you rather have," I asked, "a slight pain in your shoulder or your joints swelling so badly you can't play the piano?" He agreed to continue with the injections. Subsequently, I reduced the injections to .5 cc of theelin every week—still no bleeding! Then I reduced to .5 cc every other week with no bleeding! I reduced the injections to once a month for several years, and all during that time, there was no intra-articular bleeding—no bleeding into his joints.

In the meantime, Walter continued his piano studies. By this time, he was about sixteen years old and was featured on the local radio station. But he started missing his injections; for a period of three or four months, he failed to come in for a single one. Then one night about 11:30 p.m., as he was leaving the radio station, three or four boys jumped him and beat him up. He sustained a cut above his eye and began bleeding profusely. I sutured the wound and applied a pressure bandage, but it did not stop the bleeding. I realized then that we were in for some trouble. I took him into the hospital and started blood transfusions with an injection of theelin every other day. It must be remembered that at that time there were no blood banks, so it was necessary for me to crossmatch the blood before administering it. I used eighteen donors before the bleeding subsided. After that, Walter did not require a single blood transfusion.

After that bleeding episode, I decided to publish my findings and results. But first of all, I needed his early history, so I contacted the hospital where he was treated. I received no cooperation. I talked to Mrs. Forbes, and she made a trip to Gastonia in an effort to secure copies of his early history. And she received no cooperation. In fact, I understand that the physician in charge told her that if Walter Plemmer, Jr., was still alive, he did not have hemophilia, and he had made a card to that effect.

Since I had started treating Walter during his childhood, I wondered what effect the female sex hormones would have on the development of his secondary sexual characteristics which identify him as male. No hematologist agreed to do further work on the problem. I wish that someone would investigate the phenomenon. Walter went to college, majored in music, and returned to Edgecombe County to teach in one of the county schools. All the while he continued to take intramuscular injections at intervals of two to three weeks.

My practice continued thriving, and I saw many patients who required hospitalization. I felt the time was right for me, so I applied for staff privileges at Edgecombe General Hospital. My application was refused. I was called to the Medical Director's office, and he explained the reason for my denial. It seems it was not an issue of my competence but rather because the white patients in the hospital would object to the presence of a Black doctor. Because there were only a few beds allocated for Black patients, I found it necessary to refer many of my patients to hospitals in Rocky Mount or to send them to Raleigh where they could be treated at the all-Black St. Agnes Hospital.

At Old North State Medical Society meetings, usually held in June of each year, I was able to meet Black doctors from all over the state. About 95 percent of the Black practicing physicians in North Carolina at that time were graduates of Meharry Medical College or Howard University Medical School. One notable exception was Dr. Clyde Donell, who was a graduate of Harvard Medical School. He was the Medical Director of the NC Mutual Insurance Company, a Black insurance company headquartered in Durham. Other exceptions were a few elderly physicians who had trained at Leonard Medical School, a department of Shaw University in Raleigh. In those days, the Old North State Medical Society and all local Black societies had to hold their meetings in different cities throughout the state.

We were not allowed to meet in hotels, so our first meetings were held in churches in the larger cities. Our lodgings were found in the homes of Black townspeople, who were gracious enough to let us stay with them. After a while, we were not satisfied with these arrangements and began talking with principals of Black schools in areas such as Elizabeth City, Fayetteville, and Greensboro about using their school auditoriums, to which they agreed. In most instances, the school cafeterias opened so we could eat our meals there as well. This arrangement continued until after desegregation came into being.

There were three Black doctors in Wilson. One of them attended meetings of the white medical society in Wilson where he listened in on discussions and gained valuable information. He asked me, along with some of the other Black doctors in the area, to attend the meetings with him. We all agreed to go as guests of our host doctor. The meetings were held at the Cherry Hotel, and when we arrived, the men were having a dinner meeting.

They had not yet finished eating, so we were advised that to wait outside until dinner was finished. I did not like that at all. When we were finally admitted to the meeting, our host doctor went around introducing us to the white doctors present.

"Quig, I want you to meet our chief surgeon," he said. I extended my hand for a handshake, and the doctor put his hand in his pocket.

I started to leave, but one of the Black doctors asked me to stay, saying, "Oh, Quig, don't go. The information we'll gain is more important than any handshake." I felt very uncomfortable throughout the entire meeting. I vowed that I'd never leave myself open to another embarrassing snub like that. I was so steamed that I never heard a word any of the speakers said that night.

***

When I was studying to be a doctor, during Dr. Hale's lectures he sometimes digressed from his main subject to talk to students about the pitfalls and disappointing situations we would no doubt encounter, especially at the beginning of our practices. He reminded us that whenever we started practicing in a neighborhood, we would be confronted by all the chronic cases that had failed to improve under the treatment they had been exposed to prior to our arrival. He was so right.

I saw several patients who suffered from chronic rheumatoid arthritis. They came in on crutches, in wheelchairs, and in one or two instances, on stretchers. In medical school, I had been taught that aspirin and sodium salicylate were drugs affording more relief to arthritic patients than anything else in use at that time.

However, by the time I began practicing, an intravenous injection composed of sodium salicylate, sodium iodide, and colchicine was in use. Upon giving the intravenous injections of that substance, I found that most patients were relieved of their arthritic pain in one to six days. Patients suffering from gout also received much welcomed relief from these injections.

But the medication had one particular drawback—many patients were allergic to iodides. The symptoms of iodism were nausea, sometimes vomiting, redness of the eyes, and congestion of the nose. On one or two occasions, patients developed respiratory difficulties because of severe swelling of the throat due to the iodide in the injected medication. Whenever I treated an arthritic patient, I would normally give him one-fourth of the recommended dosage intravenously and watch for reactions to the iodide. If any reactions developed, I found that sodium chloride tablets (plain salt) given by mouth would tend to correct the allergic symptoms. I would know then that I could not treat that patient with the salicylate, colchicine, and sodium iodide. I then resorted to heavy doses of aspirin and at the same time allowed the patient to use time-honored remedies such as liniments, plasters, and poultices.

A local minister, Reverend Riddick, who suffered from arthritis needed my help. I was persuaded to visit the gentleman and was shown the way to his house, a simple four-room tenant house. When I got there, I found his four children running and playing in the yard. One of them took me to a room where I found the man lying in bed, apparently in a great deal of pain. I introduced myself, and he began telling me about himself. I had already heard about his activities in the educational field from others. However, I was deeply touched when he told me of the incidents that led to his present condition.

Four years after he had been stricken with arthritis, he married and proceeded to raise a family—three daughters and one son. His first wife had died some years before, after the birth of their fourth child. Here was this elderly man left with his four children and no one to look after them! Kindly neighbors brought him food and gave whatever medical attention they could. As long as he was able to travel, they also took him to physicians in the surrounding area and paid for his treatments.

Within the last eight to ten months, he told me he had become completely bedridden and was entirely dependent upon his neighbors to care for, clothe, and feed him and his family. "Doctor," he concluded, "I have no money to offer you, but if you can do something to get me out of this bed, you nor anyone else will ever hear the last of it."

I examined him. He was very weak. He had lost weight, and his muscles had just about completely disappeared. His knees were drawn up; he couldn't straighten his legs and was unable to move his head from side to side. He depended on his neighbors to come in two or three times a day to change his position and keep him as clean as possible. I decided to start treating him, even furnishing his medication.

I went out to see him as often as I could. After about three or four weeks of treatment, his pain subsided to a certain extent. I instructed his neighbors in the fundamentals of passive exercises. After about six weeks of this, he was able to sit up without severe pain. After two months, his neighbors were able to bring him to my office for treatment. Reverend Riddick continued improving to the extent that he was able to walk with assistance.

Later, he was able to walk with crutches. It was then that he begged his neighbors to take him to church. And they took him. He sat in the pulpit and started preaching again. He always ended his sermon by saying, "Now if you are sick, you go and see that Dr. Quigless in Tarboro, and he'll get you going again, just as he got me going."

One day, Reverend Riddick came to my office and picked up a handful of my business cards. One of his church members came in the following week and said, "You know something? Reverend Riddick started passing out your cards, just like somebody dealing out cards in a poker game." The publicity did me no harm whatsoever. In fact, it increased my practice by about 20 percent. To tell you the truth, I think my treatment of Reverend Riddick was the best business investment I ever made.

***

My phone rang about two o'clock one morning. When I answered it, the man on the other end was just about incoherent. He told me, "Doctor, please come and see about my wife. She is having a baby and is about to bleed to death. The baby is here, but she is bleeding something terrible. Please try to do something for her."

I dressed hastily and drove about six miles to the man's house. I found the room full of neighboring women and a woman lying in bed gasping. Blood was everywhere. This was her first pregnancy. She had had very strong pains, and when the baby was finally born, she had a severe pain that ruptured everything. She had what doctors call a third-degree laceration extending deep into her pelvis.

The first thing I had to do was stop the bleeding, which was simple—I inserted a packing of towels. I then called the hospital, but there was no room for her. Next, I called my receptionist and had her come out and bring two cans of ether. This was an emergency situation, and I had no time for sterility or anything else.

Because I was using ether, it was necessary to have the people in the house go around and put out all the fires to prevent an explosion. I repaired the lacerations as well as I could. There was no thought of a blood transfusion. We just had to depend on nature to keep the lady alive. Luckily, the patient survived, but one area of her wound did not heal completely.

I wrote to Dr. F. Bayard Carter, Professor of Gynecology at Duke University, explaining the woman's situation. He gave me an appointment, and I sent her to Duke. He examined her and immediately called me on the phone. "Doctor," he said, "how in the world did you ever repair that laceration in the country in an unsterile environment and get the type of results you did? How in the world did it happen? I have never heard of anything like this before. I'm going to keep this nice lady here and finish the job for you, but I want to tell you right now, if you ever run into anything like this again, and you can't get any help locally, just load up the patient and send her over to me, and, by golly, I'll attend to her." That incident was the beginning of a long friendship between Dr. Carter and me that lasted until his death. As for the patient, I was able to deliver three more babies for her before I insisted on a tubal ligation, to close her fallopian tubes and prevent another pregnancy.

***

Right after arriving in the Tarboro area, I also started running into cases of skin diseases, which were very puzzling. I treated them as well as I could with what I knew, but when I found that I was not making any headway, I sent the patients to Dr. J. Lamar Callaway, chief of Duke's dermatology service. Whenever I sent him a patient, I would write a note explaining the patient's condition and that I didn't know what else to do for them. When he received one of my patients and my note, he called me on the phone and gave me a lecture on dermatology. I took notes while he talked. We did that for many years.

Much later when I was getting older, he decided to give a post-graduate course to general practitioners interested in skin diseases, and I signed up for the course, traveling to Charleston, South Carolina, to hear him. When I showed up, Dr. Callaway looked around, saw me, and said, "What in the hell are you doing here? You already know everything I'm going to teach these guys. Hell, you could teach the course yourself." I told him that I wanted to learn all I could about dermatology because my eyes were getting bad, and I would soon have to get out of surgery. After the first lecture, he pointed me out to those present and told them, "Now here is a doctor who should not be here because he already knows everything I'm going to teach."

I had never been to Charleston, so while I was there, I signed up for a tour of the city, planned for the third day of the course. During the last lecture, Dr. Callaway said he had about two thousand slides he wanted to show if any of us wanted to stay and see them. I had paid forty-five dollars for the tour, but I was glad to lose that money so I could stay and see those slides. After he retired, he was always available for advice, just a phone call away at his home. I am forever grateful to him for his assistance.

***

In the early years of my practice, eastern North Carolina was primarily an agricultural area. We had county fairs for farmers to exhibit their livestock and women to exhibit needlecrafts, canning products and the like. White farmers exhibited their wares in big pavilions, and there was space set aside in smaller buildings for Black farmers to exhibit theirs.

Mr. Neil McLean, from the Bricks Normal Institute, came to Tarboro to help Black teachers and farmers arrange their exhibits in the fair. The American Missionary Association had established this institute about fifteen miles from Tarboro, in a Halifax County community called Bricks. There were few, if any, high schools for Black students, and in order for them to get a high school education, they had to go to normal institutes situated throughout the area.

The Association had gone to great expense to establish the school in Bricks. They constructed several large buildings, including an administrative building, a classroom building, a dormitory for men and one for women, along with teachers' cottages. They also bought a large farm connected with the school. Mr. McLean was the resident manager of their school's farm in Bricks.

He became ill while helping the farmers at the fair one year and was rushed to my office. He complained of nausea, vomiting, and severe abdominal pain. When I questioned him, I found that he had left home early in the morning and didn't get a chance to eat breakfast. He came to Tarboro and worked until 2 p.m. before eating any food. He had been so hungry that he overate on hot dogs and hamburgers. He then developed a full-fledged case of indigestion and was, of course, very much frightened. I gave him medication to relieve his indigestion and had him lie down in my office and rest. Later, he felt much better, and I let him go back to work. It was simple, really, but he never forgot that incident.

***

By 1936, the NC Department of Education had gotten busy establishing Black high schools, with at least two or three in each county. Students could then get a high school education near home, so there was no further need for a boarding school in the Bricks community. But the Halifax County Board of Education saw fit to continue using the school facilities at Bricks as a community high school for the neighboring town of Enfield. Mr. McLean looked after the unoccupied buildings on the grounds.

The federal government initiated a program of summer camps for Black children aged ten to sixteen. Luckily for our area, one of the camps was located at the Bricks complex, which was well suited for that type of program. A Black supervisor, Mrs. Yancey, headed the project and selected several teachers to work there. The summer camps plan also called for a full-time registered nurse and a physician to be on call. When Mr. McLean heard of this and was asked to recommend a local registered nurse and physician, he recommended me, much to the chagrin of other Black physicians in the area.

We set to work. The children came to me for their physical examinations, and I took care of their serious complaints whenever they had them. I also administered typhoid and tetanus vaccines. These responsibilities were very easy. I was seldom called to make emergency trips to Bricks. I started thinking: Here were all these substantial brick buildings with their facilities in place, operational, not too far removed from a small town on a paved highway, and in an area where we needed a hospital.

At that time, I belonged to a regional medical association for Black doctors, which met monthly to discuss problems and host lectures by authorities in different fields. At one such meeting, I proposed that we, as a group, undertake to establish a hospital in Bricks. I was questioned at length by some of the members who wanted to know how the hospital would be financed. I answered that perhaps we could receive help from the American Missionary Association. I further challenged them, saying we could get off our butts and go to work in the community to try to raise enough money to open the hospital.

One of the doctors said, "It is quite evident that if we build a hospital, you're the one that will make all the money out of it."

"No," I said, "it would be for all of us. We all could practice there. We can't get privileges in the hospitals around here, so it's time we did something for ourselves."

"No, you're the one that's going to make the money out of it," one good brother insisted, "so you build the hospital." The other doctors agreed with him.

That made me mad, so I said, "Okay, if you say I'm the one that's going to make all the money, then I'll build the damn hospital. Just give me time."

I hadn't known it before, but I found that there was quite a lot of jealousy among these good brothers—jealousy toward me and all I was trying to do for the good of the community. I passed it off, but in the back of my mind I knew that one day, I would build that damn hospital.

***

After rooming with the Prince family for almost a year, I was approached by a real estate man who said, "Doctor, I have a good house for you to buy. You need a place, don't you?"

"Yes," I quickly agreed.

"I have a nice two-story house I think you would like." And he took me around to see the house.

It was in a good neighborhood; that is, Blacks and whites had been living there for many years. The asking price was just two thousand dollars, which sounded pretty good to me! However, I was interested in knowing how and why the house was up for sale and who the previous owners had been. I turned to my friend Nat Gray to find out the story of this house, and it turned out to be a very interesting one.

The house was built by Mr. Williams, a barber, who had a very good business in town and was also a very devout churchman. He was so proud of his church that he built his house right across the street from it. In the early 1920s, the church members decided to buy a pipe organ. In order to get it, they needed to borrow the money from the bank, so the trustees had to sign a note guaranteeing payment. They received credit, made a down payment, and had to make monthly payments. Along about 1931, the trustees found themselves in the red on the note every month, and the organ company came back to them. They later found that among the trustees, only Mr. Williams had money in the bank. The trustees appealed to him to help them out of this difficulty. To do that, he had to mortgage his home for nine hundred dollars. Things got so tough that the trustees couldn't keep up the payments to the bank.

The bank advised Mr. Williams that they were going to have to take foreclosure action. He didn't have the money, but he had some friends who he was sure could help him out of this difficulty. The mortgage was advertised, and the house was to be sold at the courthouse door at noon on a certain day. Mr. Williams's friends were there, ready to bid on the house for him. However, they stood around the courthouse door until 2 p.m. that afternoon, and nobody came to auction off the house.

Finally, the real estate agent came out and saw the man's son-in-law and said, "Jim, are you here to bid on Mr. Williams's house?"

"Yes, sir. That's what we're here for," he said.

The agent said, "I'll tell you what. I have already bid the house in, and you can buy it for two thousand dollars."

"What in hell is going on here?" Jim asked. "It was supposed to have been sold at the courthouse door."

"No, it was sold at the court*room* door," the agent explained, "and that is upstairs. I bought it, and you can get it for two thousand dollars."

Jim got mad, turned around, and said, "You can keep the damn house as far as I'm concerned. I wasn't buying it for myself anyway. I just wanted to help Mr. Williams, but if you are going to do like that, to hell with the damn house."

That just shows you the way things were done in this area. Instead of selling at the courthouse door, it was sold at the courtroom door upstairs where nobody would be able to bid on it except the real estate agent. So, the agent was stuck with a house in the "fringe" neighborhood. No Black man would buy it, and since it was built and occupied by a Black family, no white man would buy it.

The agent had it for three or four years before I came to town, and he finally found somebody who may be willing to pay for it. It was a bargain at two thousand dollars, so I bought the house and moved in. My sister, Ruth, then came out to keep house for me temporarily.

CHAPTER 17

RACIAL SHENANIGANS

By 1938, I had been in Tarboro about two and a half years, and that winter, we had very severe weather. There were record snows in the Midwest and east, and naturally, when the spring came along and the snow began melting, the papers and airways were filled with details of severe flooding, with emphasis on the Ohio and Mississippi rivers. I became particularly interested in the accounts of floods in the Ohio area since my friend, Weathers, had gone to Portsmouth.

I followed the reports from day to day, noting that the flooding was severe in and around Portsmouth. The media reported that the city was inundated completely, and people were advised to leave their homes for higher ground. I immediately began worrying about Weathers and tried contacting him. All the phone services were out, but I finally was able to contact him through the Red Cross. He told me that he had had to abandon the first floor of his home and take his wife and baby up to the second. That was how they were living, just trying to wait out the flood.

I wanted to help Weathers because I owed him much gratitude for helping me out a few years earlier. I had been assisting Dr. Rolf at Meharry when my sister, Virgie, died of thyrotoxicosis, a disease of the thyroid gland, which is treatable if caught in time. She had become ill while in Mississippi, and the doctors there had misdiagnosed her case, saying that she had "bad kidneys, a bad heart, and a swollen liver." I was able to get her to Chicago where she received proper care. However, the toxic goiter had done its dirty work, and in 1935, she died. At the time of her death, I did not have enough money to go to Mississippi for her funeral, so Weathers loaned me forty dollars to make the trip. That was one of the reasons I owed him.

Another reason was because of his support during a time when I desperately needed help and had a hard time finding any. I remembered well how let down I was upon arriving in Tarboro, expecting help, and being refused by the drugstore owner. When I had appealed my friend Dr. Williams in Rocky Mount, he sidestepped me too.

So, I invited Weathers and his wife to come to Tarboro. The day before he arrived, I made it a point to see Dr. Williams and inform him that Weathers was coming the next day.

He asked, "What's happening?"

"You know the flood wiped out everything he had," I explained, "and I told him to come down here, and I'd see to it that he had a place to practice."

"Well, where in hell is he going to get the money?" Dr. Williams asked me. "I know he doesn't have a change of clothing because the flood destroyed everything he owned."

"You know," I began, "I had it pretty tough when I got here. Nobody helped me, but I'll be damned if Weathers is going to have to go through all the hell I did to get started. Don't worry about who is going to help him. I'm going to help him!"

The next day, Weathers arrived with his wife, Jewel, their one-year-old son, and all their earthly belongings packed in a Chevrolet coupe. I was glad to see them. My sister Ruth had gone out of town, and I had been eating in a restaurant. "Come on in," I welcomed them, "and we'll go to the restaurant and get some dinner."

"No," Jewel said, "I'm going to fix dinner." And she proceeded into the kitchen and began cooking steaks in the inimitable manner which Texas gals can cook.

After riding around with them for a few days, I encouraged Weathers to look at some of the other towns in the vicinity for a place to begin a practice. He looked at Enfield but thought that town was too small. He said he would rather be in a larger place, and after looking at several towns, he settled on Goldsboro. I saw to it that he had enough capital to set up an office and paid his expenses until his practice picked up and he could look out for himself. His practice grew by leaps and bounds. There was another Black physician in Goldsboro who said he was satisfied with his practice and felt that there was plenty for Weathers to do as well. Within six months Weathers had paid me back every penny I had loaned him.

***

When I arrived in Tarboro, the health department was conducting maternity and infant welfare clinics. The main clinic was held in the courthouse with the county health officer, Dr. Parks, in charge. In addition, there were four other clinics held in different parts of the county. I was introduced to a lot of folk medicine at those clinics.

One lady came in with a string of needles around her neck. There were about seven needles with the points encased in a cork stopper. I said, "Mrs. Jones, what in the devil are you doing with those needles around your neck?"

A woman named Mrs. Sue Pender spoke up right away and said, "You don't know, Doctor? Those needles help cut the pain.

That's why she put them around her neck, so they can cut the pain when she goes into labor."

That's the first time I had heard that. Another neighboring lady came along with her child and said, "Doctor, this child doesn't seem to be able to talk. I don't know what's the matter with him." I checked him and discovered that he was tongue-tied. This happens when a fold of tissue on the underside of the tongue is very tight and prevents the person from protruding his tongue, thereby making it difficult to enunciate words correctly.

Mrs. Pender spoke up with a remedy for that as well. "All you have to do is put a peanut under the tongue, stretch that thing, and he will be able to talk next week."

"Now, how in hell are you going to put a peanut under a baby's tongue?" I asked.

"That's all you need to do," she asserted. "It'll take care of itself."

Another lady came in and asked what we could do for her child, who was slow to speak. I told her that it just took time, that the child would straighten out after a while.

But Mrs. Pender said, "You don't know what to do for that? Now, if the child comes in and is slow in speaking, all you have to do is write the child's name on an egg, put the egg up over the door, and carry that child in and out of that door about ten times every day for about two weeks. That child will start talking just like a lawyer."

I had to put up with all sorts of stuff like that. You couldn't just laugh and go on because they'd get angry. Those were all time-honored remedies, so you had to put up with them.

One of the clinics was held in the school near a little town called Old Sparta. To get to this clinic, patients had to cross a bridge spanning the river. There were about fifty women at the clinic on one particular day. I finished my work and helped the nurse pack up our equipment. I started back about half an hour after the last women in the clinic had left in a wagon. When I got to the bridge, I saw that the wagon was stopped midway over the bridge, and the driver seemed to be having trouble controlling his pair of mules. There were six pregnant, frightened women in the wagon.

I drove up and said, "Just what's the trouble here?"

The driver said, "Doctor, that white man over there in the car said he ain't going to get off the bridge, and my mules is scared, and I'm scared for these here women folks."

I went around the wagon to talk to the man in the car. The white driver was drunk. I said, "Mister, what's the trouble? Can't you back off, and let these people over this bridge? The mules are afraid and may panic, and these women could get hurt."

"I don't give a damn what goes on," he argued like a child. "I ain't backing off. I was on this bridge first."

"But, sir," I pressed, "these women are with babies, and somebody may get hurt if this goes on like this."

"Let him back the damn mules off," he continued. "I ain't going to back off nothing."

"I'm sorry, sir. If you don't back this car off, I will have to report you to the sheriff when I get back to Tarboro," I said.

"Who in the hell are you?" he countered.

"I'm Dr. Quigless," I informed him.

"You're a what? You're a doctor?" he said incredulously.

"Yes, I'm Dr. Quigless," I repeated.

"I'll do it this time," he decided reluctantly, "but, damn it, I don't want to."

He then backed his car off, and the wagon proceeded without any more trouble. That was the attitude that so many white people in and around Tarboro assumed when it came to Black people in general.

We continued holding maternity and infant welfare clinics in different areas of the county for many years. That is, until a new public health building was erected. When that building was completed, a plaque was attached to it with the inscription stating the year and the doctor's name who was health officer at that time. The white nursing staff was listed as: Mrs. Julia Jones, RN; Mrs. Mary Smith, RN; Mrs. Sallie Williams, RN; and beneath that the Black nurses were listed, not as Mrs. Carter, RN, but as Nurse Carter and Nurse Mebane, with no mention of RN behind their names, although both whites and Blacks listed were all registered nurses. They were listed in that manner so as not to have a prefix, such as "Mrs." or "Miss," with their names. Much later when many additions were made to the structure, I don't know where that ridiculous plaque went.

***

I was called one early morning, about 2 a.m., by the overseer of Mr. Owens's farm. "Dr. Quigless," he said, "one of the tenants out at the farm is having some trouble. She's in labor and the midwife asked me to call you. Please go out and see what's wrong with her and what you can do for her."

I dressed, drove out to the farm, and found the woman in labor with very intense pain. Upon examination, I found the infant in the wrong position with one hand protruding from the mouth of the womb. I realized immediately that the baby could not be delivered in that condition. I called the hospital, but no beds were available. I rushed back to town and got my receptionist, whom I had taught how to administer ether. We returned and extinguished all the fires in the house for safety.

Fortunately, there was electricity in the house that gave us light. My receptionist proceeded giving ether to the patient. While she was anesthetized, I was able to manipulate the baby into another position so it could be delivered without damage to it. About one week later, after I was sure that the infant and the mother were doing well, I took the bill for twenty-five dollars to the landowner, Mr. Owens. In addition to his farming interests, he conducted a stable business in Tarboro where he sold and bought horses, mules, and cattle. I found him standing at the door of the stable where he was usually found during business hours. I approached him, saying, "Mr. Owens, I'm Dr. Quigless. I was called to your farm a few nights ago to deliver a baby, and I have a bill here for my services."

"You are Dr. Who?"

"Quigless, Dr. Quigless." I repeated.

"You look like a yellow bastard to me," he said. "How in the hell did you get to be a damn doctor?"

I didn't know what to say, so I stood there with my mouth agape in amazement.

The fellow continued! "You ain't no goddam doctor. You're just a yellow bastard. You get the hell away from here and out of my sight. I ain't going to give you a damn thing."

He had a walking stick in his hand that he used to poke livestock while showing them off to customers. "If you don't get the hell out of my sight," he said, "I'm going to take this stick and knock your damn brains out. What in the hell you mean coming here and talking about being a goddam doctor?"

I didn't know what to say and wondered why he was so angry with me. I stood there looking at him with my mouth still wide open.

He spoke again. "I said get the hell out of here before I take this stick and knock your damn brains out."

I wasn't standing too far from him, but he wasn't making a move toward me. We just stood there looking at each other. I had my little pistol in my pocket, which I had been carrying around as protection for several years. I did not intend to let him hit me in the head with his stick. I guess I stood there for a full minute before I decided that I didn't want any trouble, so I turned around to leave. When I had walked two or three steps, he repeated his same threat.

I stopped, turned around, looked at him, and he stopped talking. I started walking away again when he continued. "I said get the hell out of here, you goddam yellow bastard."

Again, I turned around, faced him, and he said nothing. Finally, I decided the man didn't mean anything. I thought, He's just crazy as hell or drunk. There was no need for me to get into trouble, so I just turned around and walked off.

Just as I turned the corner, I heard him say, "I said, nigger, get the hell out of here, and don't you ever come back anymore."

I didn't know what to say, but I was determined that I would get my money. I went to the sheriff's office and told him what had transpired. He said, "What time was it, Doctor?"

"About two in the afternoon," I said.

"Two o'clock in the afternoon? Oh hell, everybody around here knows better than to go there at that time of day," he said.

"Why?" I asked.

"That man gets drunk every day about noon," he explained, "and when he's drunk, he doesn't give a damn about what he says or does. I've seen him pick up a friend and throw him halfway across the street. He's basically a good fellow though when he's sober."

That did not make me feel any better, so I said, "I've done the work, and I need my money."

"I'll tell you what to do," the sheriff advised. "Rather than have any trouble, you just give me the bill, and I'll collect it for you. But I'm going to give you some advice. Stay away from that man because he's bad when he gets drunk."

All of this reminds me of another incident. I had been in Tarboro for about eight months when a landowner, who owned several farms in the county, called me. He said, "Doctor, I'm glad that you are in Tarboro. I heard about your good work and want to get acquainted with you. Sometime when you get a chance, you come around to my office, and we'll have a talk."

When I went to his office, he started out by saying, "You know, I have some farms around here, and I have a lot of tenants. Of course, I don't have time to look after the farms myself, so I've got overseers to run the farms for me. If any of them call you to come and look after any of my tenants, you go ahead and just keep a record of the charges. In the fall, you bring them in, and when we are settling up our accounts, I will be able to pay you anything that I owe you."

I thanked the man and left. Shortly thereafter, I began getting calls from his overseers, asking if I would come out to such-and-such farm and see such-and-such tenant. I made the house calls, and some of the tenants came to my office for treatment. I kept a record of the patients' names, diagnoses, and types of treatment, along with the charges.

About three weeks later, a white man came to my office. At that time, white patients would never come in the front. They would come in through the back door so as not to be seen coming to me.

But this man came in through the front door and stated that he was suffering from severe arthritis and had been under treatment for several years, but his condition was getting worse. He asked me if I would treat him, and I said yes, I would be glad to.

About three weeks after I started treatments, he became much improved and was able to go back to work. One day he said, "Doctor, I see you're doing treatment for different tenants around the county. I just want to tell you one thing. What you are doing is all right, but when the time comes for them to pay off, I want to give you a little warning. There are some of these folks that will try to intimidate you. When it comes time to collect your money, they'll try and get you to come down on what they owe you. I hope you won't let them intimidate you to the extent you won't be getting half-way paid for the treatment you are giving their tenants."

"Just who are you referring to?" I queried.

"Now listen, I'm not going to tell you any more than I've already told you," he said. "If you don't know what to tell these folks when you come in contact with them, then shame on you. That is all I've got to say."

I thanked him, and he left.

About the latter part of November, I made up an itemized statement for this particular landowner, showing the name of his tenants, the diagnoses, treatments, and charges. When I added up the charges, the bill came to $960. I took the statement, as he had requested earlier that year, and went to see him. When I got there, he said, "Come in, Doctor. What can we do for you?"

"I have an itemized statement of the services I rendered to your tenants during the year," I said.

"Well, let's see what we've got here," he said, looking at my bill.

"Oh yes, it comes to nine hundred sixty dollars. That's a lot of money, isn't it?"

"I don't think it's too much for the services I've rendered."

"I don't take care of these things myself since I turned all that over to my son," he said. "You take this bill to him, and he'll pay you."

I then took the bill to the landowner's son, and he said, "What have you got here, Doctor?"

"This is my bill."

"Gee whiz. That's over nine hundred dollars," he said.

"I've worked day and night in the office and in their homes," I explained. "It all adds up, and I don't think I've overcharged you at all."

"Well, that's a lot of money, you know," he continued. "I'm going to give it to you in cash. You do know that we require ten percent of the bill for paying you in cash?"

I had heard this before and told him I understood.

"Now this bill is big and is a whole lot of cash," he said. "Can't we do a little better on it?"

"What do you mean?"

"Since you're getting paid cash..." He kept repeating about getting paid cash, but I held my ground and kept interrupting him, "Mister, I have been carrying these accounts for over ten or twelve months in some instances, and I don't consider it cash."

"Well, I do," he argued. "It's over nine hundred dollars. I'll tell you what we'll do. Since you are getting paid in cash, why don't we cut it about thirty percent, and I'll pay you on that basis. We'll call it a deal and go for another year."

It then came to me just what I had been told about a particular landowner who would try to cut my bill. I slapped the bill down on his desk and said, "I'll tell you what. You just give me any damn thing you want, and we'll call it quits. You're asking for ten percent for collecting, and now you're asking me to cut my charges thirty percent. I can't accept that. If you want to terminate this deal right here and now, just give me what you want, and you won't have to worry about me bothering you anymore. And don't have your overseers call me anymore."

"Oh, I don't mean to have any trouble here," he said. "I just thought that since this is cash, you would be glad to get what you could."

I repeated, "It is not cash, and I'm not glad to get what I can get. If you don't feel you are supposed to pay me what I'm owed, I'll understand and won't look forward to treating any more of your tenants."

"Doc, I'll pay whatever you say," he backed off.

He paid me, deducting his 10 percent.

I had no further trouble with that landowner. I continued treating his tenants for many years, and we never had another run-in about my bill.

***

There were difficult landowners, but I want to set the record straight by relating some stories relative to some of the area's good landowners.

Robert Shaw, Jr., was born and raised on the Mayo Farm, owned and managed by Columbus Mayo. Mr. Mayo saw to it that his tenants had cows so the children could always have plenty of milk. He also encouraged them to have large gardens and saw to it that they always had medical attention. Mr. Shaw informed me that when Mr. Mayo's two boys were old enough and large enough to work, he put them doing farm work right along with the tenants' children. They worked and played together. He said it wasn't unusual for either boy to spend the night with him at his mother's house.

When Mr. Mayo married a lady from Georgia, they all trembled in their boots, fearing she would change their ideal conditions on the farm. Their fear was soon dispelled—Mrs. Mayo was the same type of person as Mr. Mayo.

In addition to the farming project, Mr. Mayo and his brother operated a hosiery mill in Tarboro. Mr. Mayo's boys finished high school, went to college, and returned to the area. By that time, the farming operation was not profitable. But Mr. Mayo kept his tenants if they wanted to stay. Because that was the only home they knew, they felt lucky not to have to leave. When the boys returned from college, they took over management of the hosiery mill and continued the same relationship with the Black employees they had learned and practiced on their father's farm. I was fortunate to have met the boys when they were ten or eleven years old. They showed me the same respect as they grew into manhood. I consider Columbus "Lum," Jr., and Ben Mayo to be among my best friends.

Mr. Shaw told me that not only did Mr. and Mrs. Mayo look after their comfort, but it was also customary for them to advance them money to buy cars. They allowed them to have car titles in their names and didn't charge interest on the money they loaned. Many other landowners also lent their tenants money to buy cars, but they retained the titles until the tenants had paid back the loans with interest.

Mr. Shaw was a big churchman, devoted to his country church. Once a year he invited the Mayo brothers to his church to take part in the services. He said they always came and waited around with the congregation until dinner was served and would then sit and have dinner with the members.

Some members of Mr. Shaw's family lived on the Mayo Farm for years and years even after they began working at different places in town. Lum and Ben both continued good relationships with the Black people just as their father had and as they had growing up. I feel it necessary to let the world know that such a family in Tarboro existed during those times.

Another man who exemplified the ideal farm manager was Mr. Thomas Pearsall, who managed an extensive farming operation for the Braswell family. He got along very well with tenants and encouraged them in every way to make life better for themselves and their families. During the latter part of August when all the tobacco had been harvested, it was customary for Mr. Pearsall to organize a field day on which all the tenants gathered at the farm clubhouse for fun and education, which included the County Extension Agent.

For many years, it was the custom of the County Commissioners to have women trained in home economics as County Extension Agents. There was one white agent and one Black agent. Agents taught women the proper selection of food materials, food preparation, sewing, proper hygiene, gardening, landscaping, and many other basic principles that made for better living for their families.

Mrs. Hazel Parker, the Black agent, went into the tenant homes and taught housewives the fundamentals of good housekeeping. Mrs. Parker always encouraged them to do their best at providing for their families and to prepare exhibits for the county fair.

One year, Mrs. Parker invited me to the Pearsall field day exercises. I made a short talk emphasizing health and the practice of medicine. In the afternoon, there was a picnic, boat rides on the lakes, games, and baseball. Following those events, a huge barbecue dinner was laid out for everyone. All the tenants, white and Black, adults and children, formed one single line. Everyone was served as much barbecue as they could possibly consume. No segregation was practiced that day! I was glad to witness such camaraderie and be a part of this annual celebration.

Mr. Pearsall's outstanding treatment of tenants was not limited to the annual field day. He also employed a registered nurse to look after the tenants. She visited them, gave instruction for maintaining proper hygiene, and saw to it that every family received necessary medical care. She also made sure they all had refrigerators that were in working order at all times. Mr. Pearsall also saw to it that their houses were kept painted and well-secured from the cold of the winter and the heat of the summer.

Mr. Pearsall's reputation for fairness was known throughout the community. In fact, in later years, Mr. Pearsall was named chairman of the committee established to implement desegregation of the Edgecombe County Schools. He received flack from many angles but stood fast in his determination to have the desegregation of the schools handled with as much fairness and as little friction as possible.

It goes without saying that good landlords were rewarded in the form of lasting gratitude and had no trouble with tenants leaving their farms. In fact, the tenants could not be persuaded to leave.

***

Until mandated otherwise, segregation was adhered to in Tarboro. The white physicians, with two exceptions, organized the Tarboro Clinic located on St. James Street. When I went to meet the white doctors, I found two entrances—one marked "White," and the other, "Colored." The day I came to the clinic, I entered the building through the "Colored" entrance and was met by the manager who said, "What can I do for you?"

"I'm Dr. Quigless," I answered. "I've come to meet the other doctors."

"Oh, you're a doctor," he said. "Are you coming to Tarboro to practice?"

"Yes sir, I am."

"Well, let me see who is here," he checked. "Oh yes, Dr. Roberson is here, and I'm quite sure he'll be glad to meet you."

"Dr. Roberson," he called. "Come on out here. I want you to meet a colored doctor who is coming to town."

That was my first meeting with Dr. Roberson. We became good friends from that very first meeting. I began practicing in Tarboro in July 1936, and Dr. Roberson started practicing here the same month. We talked for a while about some problems we had encountered when we first started our practices.

About two weeks later, I went back to the Tarboro Clinic, and again used the "Colored" entrance. When the manager saw me come in this time, he said, "You don't have to come in through that entrance. You can use the other door."

"As long as you have it, and it's the custom to have this entrance," I said, "I'll use this door along with your colored patients."

"You can if you want to but understand that you don't have to go through that door unless you want to," he said.

"Thank you very much," I told him.

It was the custom, and the physicians had to follow it or else be chased out of town by people, as they did not feel as kindly toward Blacks as the physicians did.

On one occasion, I met a white dentist. I went to his office and saw that he had one waiting room for whites and a different one for Blacks. He had an operating room for whites with up-to-date equipment. He also had an operating room for Blacks, the same room in which the brooms and mops were kept along with equipment that wasn't in such good condition. Lucky for me, I didn't need the services of a dentist at that time.

But I was having trouble with my eyes. I inquired as to where I might find a good ophthalmologist and was directed to the town of Wilson. I made an appointment, only to find the same conditions existing there that I found in Tarboro.

I gave the receptionist my name, and she wrote it down on a card and directed me toward the "colored" waiting room. When it was my turn to see the doctor, he said, "I will see you in here." He checked my eyesight in the "white" treatment room. I looked across the hall, and there was a "colored" treatment room with a chair, some charts on the wall, and instruments. I could easily see that the instruments in that room had been in use for a long time, and the patient's treatment chair was frayed.

I made up my mind then and there that I would go as far as I could to see a Black ophthalmologist, so I would not have to be confronted with the embarrassing situation of being directed into a "colored" treatment room.

CHAPTER 18

SETTLING DOWN & MY FAMILY

When I had been in Tarboro at least four and a half years, I was so busy developing a practice and treating patients that I had little time for a social life. Tarboro had many congenial people, and everyone tried to make it pleasant for me. At that time, I socialized with the teachers. However, I didn't become romantically involved with any of them. In my practice I met Mrs. James, a teacher in the Tarboro schools, with several relatives in Washington, D.C. One day, I saw her at a reception, and she said, "Doctor, isn't it about time that you were thinking of getting married?"

"Mrs. James," I smiled, "I haven't thought much about it up to now, but I think I had better start looking around and see who's available in the community."

"I have a sister in Washington, D.C., and I go there frequently. I know a nice young lady there that I would love for you to meet. I think you would like her."

"Washington, D.C.? I think that a D.C. girl would be a little bit too fast for me," I said.

"Oh, I don't know. This is a nice young lady who is very shy. Anyway, I would like for you to meet her."

About two weeks later, I happened to be in Washington, D.C., and Mrs. James's sister, Mrs. Cooper, saw to it that I met this "nice young lady" in person. Her name was Miss Helen Gordon, a teacher in the public school system in Washington, D.C. She had a younger brother and sister, all of whom lived with their father and stepmother. Her father was in government service.

Her mother had died several years prior, and her father had remarried. Her stepmother was a professional seamstress, sewing clothes for many influential families in Washington, D.C. All in all, they were a very happy, congenial family.

I was greatly impressed at our first meeting. In fact, I was so impressed that I went back to Washington, D.C., two weeks later for further contact with Miss Gordon. I found that we had many things in common, and our relationship progressed rather quickly. In a short while, I found myself returning to Washington, D.C., more often.

Our courtship lasted but about six months. We went to shows, museums, and other points of interest in the capitol city. When she came to Tarboro, we visited friends, I'd show her the countryside, introduce her around town, and get her better acquainted with some of the townspeople. She was enthusiastic about Tarboro and its people, so it wasn't hard for me to pop the question. We made a pretty good team.

To make our romance story short, by midsummer we were engaged, with the wedding planned for September 1. The wedding was really something. It was held at Helen's home, and everything about the wedding was very formal. There was a harpist who played music before, during, and after the wedding. William "Sky" Parker was my best man. Sky was the leading mortician in Tarboro, and we had become fast friends. I wouldn't think of having anyone else as my best man.

So, there we were in Washington, me in my full-dress outfit, waiting around for the ceremony to begin with Sky. I didn't feel ill-at-ease in the least. Sky was sort of nervous, and I looked at him and said, "Sky, what the hell? I'm the one getting married."

"Well, Quig, these things make me sort of nervous anyway," he said.

"Look at me," I said again. "I'm not nervous. What is all the shaking about?"

The wedding started. The bridesmaids came out. We were standing, waiting for Mr. Gordon to escort Helen down the aisle. I looked around and only saw a few familiar faces. The stony-faced Washingtonians were giving me the once-over. Then I began to shake. My knees wobbled. I thought, "This is very foolish. I can stop my knees from shaking." So, I braced them to make them stop. Then my head started shaking. I agonized through the wedding and was very glad when it was over.

We had our honeymoon in Niagara Falls, which was my first trip there. I had heard about the resort and wanted to go there very much with my new bride. Helen and I took a train from Washington, D.C., to New York City and changed trains there. We had reservations on a parlor car, the type with reserved seats that most people used if they did not want to be crowded in a day coach. It turned out that we were the only Blacks in the parlor car. These seats were not assigned to the passengers—they were first come, first served. As the other parlor car passengers filed in, they took their seats all around—anywhere except on either side of us.

The train left the station, and as we proceeded toward Niagara Falls, more passengers boarded the train. It was Monday morning, and several of the passengers were teachers heading for Buffalo, New York. They appeared to be surprised and curious as to who we were and where we were going. The last man to board the car looked around in desperation and took the seat next to me. Nobody said anything to us. It was quite evident that they were not accustomed to seeing Black passengers in a parlor car. Both

Helen and I were amazed, just watching the reactions of our fellow passengers.

On arriving in Niagara Falls, we went immediately to the Fox Head Hotel where we claimed our reservations without incident. We spent a very pleasant one-week honeymoon at the hotel, receiving first-class treatment. We survived the inspection of the hotel guests, which varied all the way from overt glances to downright staring inspections. The hotel employees were very courteous and made an extra effort to see that we were comfortable and carefree. We took a sightseeing trip to the base of the Falls on the "Maid of the Mist," where we passed so close to the falls that we were wet from the spray. When we returned to our room, we found three maids busily inspecting our wardrobes.

At that time, meat was being rationed on the American side of the Falls. Beginning at 4:30 p.m. in the afternoon, couples from the American side lined up at the dining room for dinner. At one time, we counted sixty couples waiting to be admitted. When we approached the line, the waiters, who recognized us as guests, beckoned us to proceed to the head of the line. One impatient, and probably hungry, couple called out to the waiter, "Why is it that you let that couple come ahead of us? They should be at the end of the line." The waiter smiled and reminded the inquiring couple that we were guests of the hotel, and it was their job to see to it that we were served before the other dinner patrons.

At the end of the week, we were both reluctant to leave the idealistic surroundings of Niagara Falls. Because the return trip to Washington, D.C., was not long enough to require Pullman accommodations, we used the parlor car again. Not much attention was paid to us from Niagara Falls to New York City, and there were not many people on the car going to Baltimore. However, as soon as the train stopped in Baltimore, there was a great rush of passengers to obtain good seats to get to D.C. The car filled quickly, all except for the chair nearest me. Two men rushed into the car and took one look at the situation. The man who was ahead stepped back and told his companion, "That's all right. You take the seat. I'll go back to the day coach." He talked with a very loud voice, obviously so everyone else could hear him. However, no one seemed to have paid him any mind.

Helen and I went to her home upon arriving back in Washington, D.C., and found a room full of wedding presents. I was wondering how we would get all of those presents back to Tarboro.

Then I remembered that before leaving Tarboro to be married and go on our honeymoon, I had made arrangements for a patient to go to Freedman's Hospital for a gallbladder operation in Washington, D.C. In those days there were few, if any, ambulances in small towns in North Carolina. Severely ill patients were transported from their homes to the hospital in funeral cars. This patient, however, was to make the trip from Tarboro in an ambulance, so I called the hospital and had the driver contact me before leaving. He came by, picked up our wedding presents, and transported them to Tarboro in the empty ambulance. When he arrived in Tarboro and pulled up in front of my house, my good friends there thought the wedding had been a little too much for me, and they were bringing me back home on a stretcher!

Prior to my marriage, my sister Ruth had been taking care of me. She agreed to stay on awhile until we got settled in our home and organized so Helen could take over. A few days after we arrived in Tarboro, we had a reception and invited the people of Tarboro to meet my new bride. Helen was welcomed by most, however, not all were satisfied with my selection of the Washington, D.C., schoolteacher. Helen got some dirty looks and quite a few snide remarks from some of the guests at the reception.

But for the most part, everything was going along smoothly for us. Then Helen missed her first period in January. Both of us were elated when it became evident that there was going to be an addition to our family. Along about the fourth month of her pregnancy, we took a trip to Chicago. We were looking forward to the birth of the child, so we went to one of the big stores there that specialized in maternity and infant clothing. We bought a bunch of infant wear. As we started out of the store, I realized that we had bought all blue, so I said, "Wait a minute. We don't have anything pink." So, we went back to the saleslady and bought a cotton blanket, blue on one side and pink on the other.

When Helen was eight-and-a-half months pregnant, I took her to Washington, D.C., so she would have the care of a gynecologist. Finally, the long-awaited day arrived. Our baby girl, Helen Gordon Quigless, Jr., was born. She was a pretty little thing, and I didn't mind that she was a girl. The birth had some complications, but everything turned out beautifully.

I was now a bona fide family man, which made me begin seeing life in a different light.

I realized that I was in Tarboro for life and that my family would have to be faced with the frustrations and inconveniences usually found in a segregated community. We were so happy to have Helen, Jr., and to be married that I didn't give too much thought to my misgivings at that time.

When Helen was about nine months old, it became apparent that my dear wife was pregnant a second time. I remembered the complications with the first delivery and called my good friend, Dr. Bayard Carter, who advised that I bring her to see him at

Duke University Hospital right away. After examining her, he said, "Well, Dr. Quigless, I don't think you need to worry about any complications with this pregnancy."

I asked, "Do you think she could be safely delivered in Tarboro?"

He turned around, looked me straight in the eye, and said, "Just what do you mean by that? You bring me a patient and then ask me to let you take her away from me? I consider Mrs. Quigless my patient from this moment until this child is delivered. Now I want to see her monthly, but when the time comes for delivery, I want her in this hospital."

Dr. Carter watched her closely throughout the rest of her pregnancy. When time for delivery drew near, I took her to Durham to await labor pains. She hadn't been in Durham for more than twelve hours before the onset of labor began. The next morning, Dr. Carter called me and said, "Doctor, congratulations! You have a fine son, and I hope he becomes as good a doctor as you are."

I lost no time getting back to Durham and found my wife in good spirits. I zoomed around to the nursery, and the nurse held up this long, red, seven-pound boy. His eyes were wide open and looked straight at me. He didn't cry. He just looked in the other direction. I said to him, "That's all right, young fellow. I think we will mix together pretty well."

Three days later I returned to Duke University Hospital with all those blue clothes. When we got back home with Milton, Jr., his little sister Helen said, "What is that?"

"That's your little brother!" I said.

"Oh, brother. Huh!" she said. She looked downcast and a little disappointed. She had been queen of the realm until his arrival. Maybe she thought she would automatically be relegated to second place.

"Hi, Bro," she said. And after that, everyone in the household called him "Bro."

Helen's stepmother came to visit after baby Milton was born and remained with us about six weeks. By that time, Helen had learned to cope with two babies. Everything was going along fine with the help of Rose Bottoms, who came in to help look after the babies.

With two children, I became even more interested in the quality of life our family would have in Tarboro. I had heard a lot about "separate but equal" school systems, and as far as I could learn, the Black school system was separate and very much unequal. The elementary school had some very good teachers. However, everything at the high school was substandard. Some of the teachers were inefficient, and students were passed from one grade to the next without regard to their ability to grasp the subjects. The school administration also turned a deaf ear to any suggestions for upgrading high school facilities.

From talking with students at different grade levels, I could see that their training was substandard, and in my own several trips to the high school, I noted some deficiencies. For instance, there was very little attention paid to the sciences. One year they were taught elementary chemistry and the next year elementary physics. There was one science teacher for these subjects. Students studying two subjects were never taught in the same year and they were not required to do laboratory work. The teacher performed the experiments—students would watch and then write them up. As far as biology was concerned, the students would go out and collect leaves and write the descriptions in their notebooks. No attention was given to the zoological aspects of biology.

These deficiencies were brought to the attention of the principal. He assured the parents that the students were getting just what they needed. "After all," he was noted for saying, "they don't need all that fancy stuff."

The PTA was organized, but the school administration did whatever it could to discourage parents' participation. In a couple of instances, the meeting was scheduled at the school, but the janitor could not be found to open the doors. As a matter of fact, I ran into the janitor one day and asked, "Just why is it that the parents were locked out of school on the night they were supposed to be having a PTA meeting?"

"Look, Doc," he said pulling me aside. "I don't want you to say anything about it, but the principal told me to lock up the school and get lost."

It was about that time that we started attending PTA meetings. I brought discrepancies to the attention of the school administration and was advised, "Here you are, a newcomer to town, trying to change everything overnight. If I were you, I'd just attend to my business. All these matters will be cleared up in due time."

I was further advised that the administration had been in place for years, had fought hard to get a high school established and to get things going as well as they currently were. If I came in there running my big mouth, they would not be able to get anything else done. The fact of the matter was that the school administration had come up through hard times because the Board of Education was racist, and whenever the PTA took proposals to them, they were tabled and nothing else was heard of them.

Well, parents got fed up and gave up on their ideas of trying to get conditions improved in the schools. But when I came along, I just couldn't stand for that. I remembered down in Mississippi, where I went to school, that two years of Latin, at least one year of chemistry or physics, and a second foreign language was required before you could expect to graduate from high school. But in Tarboro, if you went down to the colored high school for four years, you would graduate whether you could read, or not. I ran into several of these illiterate graduates of the colored school in Tarboro. I began questioning teaching methods and was reminded that several students had gone to college and had made really high marks. In fact, some of them were honor students. I said "several"—that is, three or four—but I reminded the school administration that students who left the colored high school in Tarboro and went to college made good not because of the school, but in spite of it.

I became more and more interested in the school situation. We organized a civic league. Parents of the school children were very glad to participate, and we started making demands on the school board. We presented proposals and propositions at every meeting, only to be discouraged. At that time, the board was self-perpetuating and was strictly anti-Negro. The chairman of the board got in touch with two or three of the old "Uncle Toms" in Tarboro and told them to advise me to stop, and they obliged. They would not allow me to do anything to start trouble.

Among other things, we asked that a library be established for our children. The school board appointed the governing body for the East Tarboro Library. I was not put on the board, but Helen, my wife, was. Most of the members of the governing board for the East Tarboro Library were influenced and in accord with the thinking of the administration of the colored high school. That was the best that we could do at that time.

The East Tarboro branch of the library, consisting of two rooms heated by a potbelly stove, was situated above a beauty shop. The books consisted mostly of encyclopedias, a few books on Negro history, and some worn school textbooks. Whenever a

Black person went to the library and requested a book that was not on the shelves, the request had to be made in writing to the white library, and two or three days later, he would be able to pick up the requested book—that is, if the white library thought it proper to let him use the book. As to the high school textbooks, most of the time the students were issued books that had been used in the white high schools. Some were in bad shape with pages missing or the backs falling off.

While visiting the colored high school one day, I noted that the students were writing on blackboards with short pieces of chalk. The longest pieces were not more than one and a half inches long. I asked the teacher why.

She said, "We sent in requisitions for chalk. However, the chalk that was delivered was brought from the white school. Those white students got new chalk and sent used pieces down to our colored school."

One day, I passed by the colored school during the summer and noticed one of the teachers replacing some windowpanes. I stopped to talk and asked him, "Is the school board paying you to replace those windowpanes?"

"No," he said, "they're not paying me. I'm just doing this to save the town some money."

"You're not getting paid for it?" I asked. "Then why the devil are you doing it?"

"You know, you have to keep in good with those white folks. I do these little things in the summertime, so I won't have to worry about losing my job," he explained.

I became indignant. "What in hell are you trying to do? You're saving the white folks money, and they're not giving you a damn thing. You're just cutting someone else out of a job," I said. "You get paid for teaching school, but you don't get paid for putting in windows."

"Doc, you don't understand things around here," he said. "You have to do things to please the white folks. If you don't, the school administration will have your job taken away, and I need my job. But you are right. I'm knocking somebody else out of a job by putting in these windowpanes or by painting ceilings and walls during the summer. But I just have to do it. I have to try and safeguard my job."

"You are just another Uncle Tom," I said insultingly, "but you're too old for me to try and change your ways."

We continued to have trouble with the school administration. Finally, it was rumored that the principal, Mr. Pattillo, would retire. The school board had decided to appoint his son as principal of the school. Now that really upset me. Since the son had been the principal at another school for about twenty years, I knew he would be carrying on the same old "Uncle Tom" tactics whenever he got to Tarboro. I talked with some of the other parents about this.

"We need to find out if this rumor is true, and if it is, what do we want to do about it?" I asked.

The chairman of the school board was a physician—the same one who had given his tenant a hard time when he found out that I had gone to his farm to treat the tenant's son. He was the same one who had harassed his former patients who came to me for treatment. After about a week of thinking and discussing, we decided that the only thing to do was go to the chairman of the school board and ask whether the rumor was true. I made an appointment to see the gentleman. When I saw him, I said, "Sir, I understand that the principal, Mr. Pattillo, is retiring and that the board has decided to appoint his son as the new principal."

He looked at me and turned a little red in the face. I had forgotten that he resented prefixing a Black man's name with "Mister." He looked at me and said, "MISTER Pattillo is retiring, and we have decided to have his son as his replacement. What are you going to say about it?"

"Mr. Pattillo's son has been principal for twenty years at another school," I said. "His ideas are the same as his father's. Now here is a good chance to improve the colored high school. I am quite sure that if you advertised that the position was open, you would have applicants from all over with PhDs and master's degrees who might apply. But if you just turn around and appoint someone without giving anyone else a chance, I don't think our interest would best be served."

"Well, DOCTOR," he said, irritated, "we HAVE let it be known, and we HAVE received applications, which were considered before appointing Mr. Pattillo's son. We found him to be fitted for the job."

"Now sir," I continued, "how could you have applications from others when it isn't generally known that Mr. Pattillo is retiring?"

"Well, we have had them anyway," he said, dismissing my question, "and further, we decided to appoint Mr. Pattillo's son as our new principal. The school board has done that, and that is our job. If you think you could do the job better than we have, then you can have the job. We are not getting paid for it."

"Sir, I don't mind taking the job if it would improve the conditions under which colored children go to school in Tarboro," I answered.

"Well, that's the way it is, and the way it's going to have to be," he said. "Good day." He then pushed me out of his office.

And so it was. We had to go along with their decision. When Mr. Pattillo retired, his son was installed as principal. Things rocked along at the same speed. Nothing changed at the school. No improvements were made. Then something happened that turned me around a little bit.

In that day and time, children could not be enrolled in public school if their sixth birthday occurred after October 1 of that year. That was the rule. However, it was not adhered to very strictly. There were ways of getting around it. It just so happened that one of Carey Bullock's daughters was born on October 15, and she was a very bright child for her age.

Carey came to me one day and said, "Doc, you know that because this child was born after October 1, she can't go to school this year. You have to be born before October first, according to the rules. I know a lot of other folks who have gotten their children in anyway. All they have to do is get a certificate from a doctor stating that they were born before October first. Can't you do that for me?"

"Carey," I replied, "I don't think it would be a good idea for me to try anything like that because I'm not on good terms with the school board as it is. They could give me some trouble if they found out that I was doing something like that."

"Well, Doc, everyone else is doing it," he insisted. He then recited two or three cases, so I went along and gave him a certificate stating that his child had been born on September 20.

Things went along fine until it was time for children to be enrolled in school. Carey's wife took her daughter to the school, and she was enrolled. There was a long line of mothers and children waiting to be registered. Then there came another lady who had moved into Tarboro from out of town. She had a photocopy of her child's birth certificate on which she had scratched out the date of birth and inserted a date prior to the October 1 deadline.

She presented the certificate to the teacher assigned the responsibility of registering the children. The teacher was new to the area and didn't really know the procedures and customs around here. When she spotted the altered birth certificate, she called it to the mother's attention. The mother told the teacher that they had made a mistake about when the child was born, and she had corrected it herself. The teacher advised the mother that she could not accept that certificate.

The mother became angry and started talking very loudly. The teacher then called the principal to help with the situation. A big argument ensued, and the principal told the mother that he was very sorry, but they would not be able to enroll the child. The mother retorted that if her child couldn't be admitted to the school, then she knew a lot more children who had been born after October 1 who had been admitted. She then began naming about ten children who had been born after October 1 who had already been enrolled.

The principal took their names and called those mothers in, telling them that they could not enroll their children at this time. He gave each of the mothers back the certificates they had brought in—that is, all except the one I had given to Carey Bullock. The principal kept that one. When Carey told me about it, I thought to myself, "Uh-oh, I am in trouble now." I hoped nothing would come of it. However, that hope was soon crushed.

About two weeks later I received a letter from the NC Board of Medical Examiners advising me that I had to meet with them the following Tuesday at 9 a.m. I called Carey Bullock and said, "Look here, fellow. I am getting into trouble over this thing. The Board of Medical Examiners has called me in for a meeting, and they may take away my license."

I called the Secretary of the Board of Medical Examiners and asked what I was being charged with. He said that it wasn't anything bad or much of anything at all. He said he felt we could get it all straightened out at the meeting; it was just something they needed to call to my attention. I knew then that something was up. I wanted to have something in my favor when I went to Raleigh, so I asked Carey to have his wife get me a list of children's names, their parents, and the doctors who signed the certificates for those who were enrolling at the same time she had been. Mrs. Bullock did what I asked. I had the list in my pocket when I went for my meeting.

Evidently, the Board of Medical Examiners knew something about me. The first Board member said, "Doctor, you have been accused of giving false certificates allowing children born after October first to be admitted into the Tarboro colored schools. Every time you do that you are defrauding the State of North Carolina. That is against the law and is not going to be tolerated."

"Doctors," I answered, "I don't see any other doctors here today."

"What do you mean by that?" he asked.

"I am not the only doctor in Tarboro who has been issuing those certificates," I said. I then reached into my pocket and pulled out the list I had gotten from Mrs. Bullock. "I've got a list here with names of children, their parents, and the doctors who issued the certificates. There are nine doctors' names on this list besides mine. It looks to me like you should have some others in here with me if you are going to give punishment for falsifying certificates."

"Wait a minute. We are investigating you, not them," he said.

"Why don't you investigate them along with me?" I asked.

"That's not the question," he said.

Another doctor spoke up. "Wait a minute. Tell us just what is going on in Tarboro."

I told them about the run-in I had had with the Chairman of the Tarboro School Board. I told them about the retiring principal and the appointment of his son and my objection to how the matter was handled.

When I finished, the Chairman of the Board of Medical Examiners spoke up and said, "This is your hearing. You knew you were breaking the law when you signed the certificate. If you didn't know it then, you know it now. You go on back to Tarboro and do whatever you have to do to improve the conditions of your schools, but don't ever sign your name on anything that can be used against you. Good day." That ended my hearing before the Board of Medical Examiners.

***

When World War II ended, a great wave of patriotism swept the country, and everyone was grateful to the soldiers who had gone to Europe to help defeat Hitler and his army. Following the end of the war, a white American Legion Post, the Eason-Tiney Post, was organized in this area. The Post was named for the first white soldier from Edgecombe County who had died during the war. Shortly thereafter a colored American Legion Post was organized and named for Exum Lewis, the first Black soldier from Edgecombe County to be killed during the war, a young man whom I knew very well.

Everyone was glad when the war ended. A big celebration was held on the Town Common. There were speeches and bands.

About two years later, a proposal was made to build a library as a memorial to the white soldiers who fought in that war. The proposed building would be large enough to serve the needs of all the citizens of Tarboro and Edgecombe County. However, it was to be a memorial to the white soldiers, and there we were with the little East Tarboro Library—two small rooms above a beauty shop.

I did not see any way to change that set-up, so I proposed that, since they wanted to build a library as a memorial to the white soldiers, which would be financed by a bond issue paid for by taxpayers, we felt the commissioners should build something as a memorial to the Black soldiers as well. We had the beginnings of a playground in East Tarboro, and we petitioned the Town Council to build a field-house for the East Tarboro playground. We set about trying to think of how this field-house should be constructed. Someone came up with the idea that the brick building should be large enough to contain a basketball court with space around the court to be used as meeting rooms, conference rooms, and classrooms; it would have a snack bar and even a banquet room with kitchen facilities. For four hundred dollars, we had an architect from NC Central University draw up plans incorporating our suggestions. The citizens league had no money, except for little contributions made at each meeting, so I advanced the money. He took our suggestions and came back with a satisfactory floor plan.

When I took our plan to the Town Council, I was in for a great surprise. The Council listened, and after finishing my presentation, the Chairman turned and said, "Doctor, there is something about this I don't understand. You brought the plans and petition to us, and another group has brought these same plans and petition, saying they're representing the colored people."

I responded by saying I was chairman of the civic league, and no one else had the authority to bring the petition in the league's name. The Chairman showed me the other group's plan. In fact, some of the same men who were on my petition were listed as supporting their petition. This group, which I called "Uncle Tom's Cabinet," who had fought me all along, had developed plans so they could create confusion in the minds of the Council and give them a basis for denying our request.

The Chairman added, "We do not know who to believe, so with both of you having the same proposal, you need to get together and settle the matter before bringing anything else to us."

Well, that took care of the field-house idea for us. Those "Uncle Toms" used the same maneuver when it came to proposals being presented to the Board of Education. It was quite evident that I failed to remedy the situation. "Separate but equal" was apparently going to be in Tarboro for a long time to come.

The Board of the East Tarboro branch of the public library held a meeting in which one of the members objected to my efforts to build a field-house and suggested that a permanent branch of the library be built in East Tarboro instead. The person's father had done work in education in the area some years prior, and she offered to donate land for the branch with the stipulation that the new building be dedicated to the memory of her father. My wife Helen, a member of this board, reminded the group that building a branch library tended to perpetuate the segregated system of that service to the community. She suggested that the offer of the land be refused. Her suggestion was opposed by every other member of the board. She insisted that the proposal be tabled, and she argued so vehemently that it was. She was labeled as one of the newcomers to the community who was dead set on disturbing the good relationship between the white and colored citizens.

This turn of events was very depressing to me. In fact, one of my friends asked, "Doctor, what are you going to do now?"

"I'm going to stop trying to do anything for these people. Maybe someone else will come along, and these damn fools will be willing to listen to what they have to say."

I decided to discontinue efforts toward problem-solving in Tarboro and just stick to practicing medicine and raising my family. I had enough work in my medical practice to keep me busy, including getting my own hospital underway.

CHAPTER 19

QUIGLESS CLINIC-HOSPITAL

I was still delivering babies all over the county and even in some surrounding towns. One night, I got a call from a family living about eight miles from Tarboro. I went out to find that the lady had been in labor for three days. It was quite evident that the baby was dead and must have weighed about seven to eight pounds. The mother's pains had ceased completely, and she was developing symptoms of infection.

The family had no money, and even if they had, I doubt that I could have gotten her into a hospital anywhere in the vicinity. So, it was up to me to do whatever I could to save her life. I went back to Tarboro, picked up my receptionist and a couple of cans of ether, and drove back out to the country. It was mid-July and hot. There were no screens on the windows. The house had electricity, so I didn't have to worry about putting out any fires. After the administration of the ether, I started pulling on the fetus. I pulled and tugged for over two hours. As I was doing this, the flies were crawling all over my face, and I wasn't able to brush them off.

I was exhausted but finally delivered the fetus. The patient was sleeping peacefully. It was about 5:30 a.m. when we finally left.

On our way back to town, I said to my receptionist, "Mrs. Beaman, I'm going to have to build that damn hospital right away. I can't stand much more of this."

"I'm glad to hear you say that because I can't stand much more either," she agreed.

As I thought more and more about the matter, it occurred to me that I would have to get some information regarding the whole set-up of a hospital before I went in too deeply. What I needed to do was find someone who had already successfully taken on the task of building a hospital from scratch.

The only person I could think of at that time was Dr. Vaughn D. Mizell of Fort Lauderdale, Florida. I got on the phone with him and explained the situation. We decided that I should go to Florida to visit him. Helen, Jr., was about a year old at that time and had just started walking well. Desegregation had hit the railroads, and I decided that traveling with my wife and baby on the long train trip to Florida would be too much for us in the day coach. I went to the station in Rocky Mount and told the stationmaster that I wanted a drawing room on a Pullman car to Fort Lauderdale.

There were two types of passenger service. One was called a "day coach," which was a passenger car with seats only. You got on the car and selected a vacant seat and remained there until you got to your destination. Now this is all right for a trip of three or four hours, but a rail trip that might last as long as eighteen or twenty hours would be too long for most people, especially with children.

There were Pullman cars on the same train. These were constructed so that the seats could be pulled together and made into beds, and the compartment above the seats could also be opened into a comfortable bed. Those were the accommodations found in the open sections of the sleeping cars. In addition to the open sections, the car usually had compartments, or small rooms, partitioned off from the rest of the car. In the small room you had an upper and lower berth. Then there were drawing rooms, which contained an upper and lower berth and a couch that could be made into a third bed, along with toilet facilities.

I requested a compartment because I did not want to create an embarrassing situation that might develop when passengers awoke and found that they were sleeping in a Pullman car with Blacks or "colored people," as we were called then. The station-master consulted his records and found that no compartments were available. However, I insisted that he get me a compartment. He tried to explain that conditions had changed to such an extent that the people in the Pullmans did not object to colored passengers. I continued insisting on a compartment. Finally, he said, "Okay, all right, I'll get you a compartment."

After boarding the train, I found that he had still been unable to get a compartment and had to give me a section that had upper and lower berths in the middle of the car. I had to accept that section. The Black porter was glad to see me. He was glad to see any colored person take advantage of the accommodations that were open to them.

"Now, Doctor," the porter explained the following morning, "we will soon be getting into Jacksonville for a ten-minute stop. They make the first call for breakfast after we leave Jacksonville. I'll tell you what would be better for you to do. When we make the stop, you and your family get off the train and go to the car next to the dining car, and when they say, 'All aboard,' you get on the dining car and be seated. They are going to pull the curtains around your table, so you won't be eating with the white folks."

"I know," I said. "I'm accustomed to that sort of thing."

Florida, as a part of the South, had the same segregated customs as North Carolina—when a colored person boarded a train and attempted to go into the dining car, they wouldn't keep him out, but they had a way of seating him in a corner and pulling a curtain around him so that nobody would be able to see him. I knew that was coming, so we were prepared for it.

When the train stopped, we did just what the porter told us to do. When the conductor said, "All aboard!" we boarded the train and went to the dining car. The steward did not have to direct us to a corner table. I knew where to go. He was flabbergasted when he didn't have to direct me in the presence of all the white diners. We had a nice breakfast. The colored waiters were very glad to see us and happy to see the baby. The waiter took Helen, Jr., all over the train and kept her entertained until we finished our breakfast. We were still on the train when lunchtime came around. When we went to the dining car for lunch, the steward did not pull the curtain around us.

I had first met Dr. Vaughn D. Mizell when we were students at Meharry. He was short and stocky, very light-brown-complexioned with fairly good hair. In fact, he could have passed as a Latino, especially in that portion of Florida where he lived. He had been considered one of the best students in his class and sailed through his freshman and sophomore years.

The situation in Florida at that time was about the same as it was in Tarboro. There was a county hospital, Broward County Hospital, with a few beds reserved for Black patients. If those beds were filled and a Black patient was unable to be sent to Miami for treatment, or if he had no money, he had to content himself with whatever treatment he could obtain from Black doctors in his home. If a Black patient required hospitalization but was unable to get in, he most probably would die from lack of proper treatment.

Dr. Mizell had been back in Florida three or four years by the time I went to see him. He had the blessings, goodwill, and the assistance of the community's Black people and was able to build a twenty-five-bed hospital, which, he named Provident Hospital of Fort Lauderdale, Florida. At the outset, he was the only doctor at the hospital. However, he was soon joined by other Black doctors of the community so that in a few short years the hospital increased in size to over fifty beds.

When we got off the train, we were met by Dr. Mizell, who escorted us to the place he had reserved for us to stay for a couple weeks. At that time, there were no hotel facilities available for colored people. While visiting the hospital there, I observed the layout, assisted in operations, and got answers to the questions that came to mind. My wife was busy getting acquainted with management of the financial end of operating a hospital. I found a staff of very dedicated nurses on duty at all times. All kinds of questions arose in my mind: How to operate such a place on a small budget? What about laboratory work? Where would I get the supervisor of personnel to staff the hospital? And a dozen others!

Dr. Mizell was a wealth of information and shared it all with me. I was particularly interested in how he had such qualified staff. He had to seek out registered nurses who had recently finished their training. In addition to their nursing duties, some were given special laboratory training. One was dispatched to the hospital in Miami where she was given training as an x-ray technician. A third was sent to the dietary department of a hospital where she was given special instructions in the dietary management of a hospital. In other words, he saw to it that each RN was given some type of special training, enabling her to do two jobs.

When I returned to Tarboro, I set to work laying the groundwork for building my hospital. First of all, I had to brush up on my surgical techniques. A friend of mine from school, Dr. W.F.

Clark, was general surgeon at a well-established hospital, St. Agnes Hospital in Raleigh. I visited him and explained my situation.

"Quig, I think you have a great idea and can make it," he encouraged me. "I will be glad to do whatever you need to help."

I said, "First of all, I've got to catch up on my surgical techniques."

"Fine. Suppose you come over every Monday, Wednesday, and Friday, and assist in the operations over here?"

I took him up on that, dividing my time between Tarboro and Raleigh.

Helen and I put our heads together and started planning our venture. It was 1945. We decided to try to build a twenty-five-bed hospital. I took our ideas to Henderson Lumber Company and received assistance from Mr. Moore, the manager, who drew up the plans. World War II was still in progress at that time, which made it hard to get any type of steel to use in the building—the Army and Navy had priority status for that.

We needed steel and a cast iron pipe for our sewage system. It was in short supply, and we had to get permission from the federal government in Washington, D.C., to buy it. We had to make an application to a bureau handling these affairs at the regional office in Greensboro. We came back to Tarboro, waited two months, but heard nothing. We went back to Greensboro and asked why. The manager advised us that all applications had to be sent to Washington, D.C., for approval or disapproval by the bureau.

"How much longer will it take before we can get the material?" I asked impatiently.

"I don't know," the manager said. "You know, when it comes to those bureaucrats, they take their time, sit on their butts, and do nothing."

"How in the world can I speed up the process?" I asked.

"It may be possible for you to go to Washington and walk the application through in three hours. I bet when you get there, you find your application on somebody's desk who hasn't even looked at it. You may have to talk to the guards because security is tight."

Helen's father lived in Washington, D.C., and worked in government service. He knew many people who worked in the different offices, including the one to which I had to go for implementation of my application. "If you know anybody," he informed me, "even any of the guards, you can get by the front door and will be home free to get your application through."

Sure enough, we went and found one guard who knew Helen's father. He let us in the building, and I found the office I was looking for. When I went in, I found about thirty men sitting around, some with their feet on their desks, some smoking, and some just whiling away the time sipping coffee. One asked, "What can I do for you?" I told him I had come to get my application approved, a requisition for some steel. Four men jumped up and almost knocked each other down trying to help me.

"Let me do it."

"No, I'll do it."

"Let me do it."

"I can handle this."

They must have been very bored, sitting there waiting for something to do. I got my application approved in about half an hour.

When I came back to Tarboro, our next order of business was to get financing. We only had about ten thousand dollars in cash to use for the project. I went to Edgecombe Bank & Trust Company, the local bank in the area, and applied for a thirty-five-thousand-dollar loan. Someone on the Board of Directors told me that when the application was presented, the president of the bank said, "How in the world does he think he can run a hospital? Hospitals don't ever make any money, so how does he think he's going to pay back this loan? I move that we disapprove this loan."

I then went to the other bank in town. At that time, it was the Security & Trust Company with headquarters in Greensboro. The vice president in charge of this branch, Mr. W. J. Ausbon, took my application and forwarded it to Greensboro. In about ten days, he called me back to his office. He had a long answer to my application. It went something like this: "We appreciate your efforts. We think it is a fine thing that you are attempting to do. However, since we are in war time and money is scarce, we don't feel we could advance this loan unless certain criteria could be met." He kept reading all the things I would have to do.

I stopped him about halfway down the letter. "Wait a minute, Mr. Ausbon. That means they're not going to be able to let me have the money, doesn't it?"

"Well, it looks that way, Doc."

"I guess I'll just have to give up on my idea of building a hospital," I said sadly.

Mr. Ausbon looked me straight in the eye and said, "How much money do you have?"

"About ten thousand in cash that I could put into this venture."

"I'll tell you what to do," he said. "You start the foundation."

I explained to him that that was a big job because I was building the hospital on a hillside. Further, I was building it on a riverbank, and in order to have a stable structure, it would be necessary to dig about twenty feet below the ground surface on the side nearest the river.

He said again, "You go on, take your ten thousand and go as far as you can with the foundation. Then start on your masonry. By the time your money runs out, I'll see to it that you have enough to finish your hospital."

I replied, "Wait a minute, Mr. Ausbon. All I have is ten thousand dollars, and I have been turned down by two banks, and now you're telling me that you'll be able to help me borrow thirty-five thousand?"

"Now, if you want to build that hospital," he replied, "you do what I say and don't worry about the money. I'm on the board of a Building and Loan association in Rocky Mount, and when I present this proposition to the board members, I'm quite sure they will help you. I have faith in you and your ability. I will see to it that you get the money if I have to go on the note myself."

With his assurance, we started the building. I made an application to the Builders Federal Loan Association in Rocky Mount for thirty-five thousand dollars. After the board of directors went over my plans, I guess they saw that the building would easily be worth that in the event it was finished. They advanced me seventeen thousand dollars and advised that the balance would be forthcoming whenever this money ran out in the building process. The building was well underway when the first portion of the loan ran out.

I went back to Mr. Ausbon and the board, and he asked, "How much do you need this time?"

I said, "I believe I'll need all of the original amount we set out to get in the beginning."

"Suppose we let you have fifteen thousand dollars now, and if you need any more when that is exhausted, we'll see about advancing you more money," he offered.

I went ahead and took the fifteen thousand.

It was just about that time that the war was ending, and the *Journal of the American Medical Association* listed surplus military and naval equipment available for sale. I needed everything! Equipment was available in Norfolk at the naval yard where some ships had been damaged in combat and were being decommissioned. At Newport News, I was able to obtain a used operating table and operating room lights. I was advised that I could possibly obtain an autoclave, a sterilizer for instruments and supplies that would be used in operations. Luckily, there were several new uncrated autoclaves that had been declared surplus. What would have cost me about three thousand dollars if I'd bought it through regular channels cost me just seven hundred fifty. I was able to get twenty-five hospital beds on a deferred payment plan from the BETZ Company in Indiana, a medical supply firm. I finally had enough equipment to go into business.

There was one hitch. The contractor we were using had several jobs going at the same time. My hospital was supposed to be finished by September 1. In mid-November, there was still a lot to do on the building. I was in a jam. I had employed three young RNs and was having to pay them to keep them from accepting other jobs. I pleaded with the contractor, the plumber, the electricians, and everyone involved, but I was being put off each day. I finally got a lawyer to call all three gentlemen in for a conference. He stated that since the building had been promised by the first of September and it was now mid-November and the building was still incomplete, they would be sued for damages unless the building was finished. My building was then finished in two weeks. The plumbing was in, the lights were on, and I began moving equipment in. I was finally able to announce the opening.

December 1, 1946, opening day of my hospital, was such a happy day for me, Helen, and our children. Helen, Jr., was about two years old, and Milton, Jr., was six months old. I had an open house on Sunday so people could come and see it. The local paper even gave us a full-page spread. Every Black person in Tarboro was overjoyed except the members of "Uncle Tom's Cabinet," who came to look us over but made no comment.

One of my doctor friends said, "Well, Quig, I hope your building doesn't fall into the river."

"With the Lord's help, it'll stay put where it is," I replied.

Another friend said, "I hope you don't need a new car soon because I don't see how you would be able to buy one and keep up the payments on this building."

I smiled and went about my business.

I received no gifts nor any funds other than the money I borrowed from Builders Federal except for a desk and twenty-five bedsheets that were donated by the St. Stephens Baptist Church. I believe that the Elks Lodge made a donation of fifty dollars.

One lady in the community, whom I had treated for syphilis over a long period of years, was a seamstress and had made the curtains for the windows of the office I had been using. She asked me if there was something she could do to help with the hospital. When I told her I needed surgical gowns, she asked, "How many do you need?"

"I will need about two dozen to start off with."

She said, "I'll tell you what I will do. You buy the material, and I'll make the gowns. I'll also make your patients' gowns and won't charge you a penny. You have been nice to me, and I will never forget it. I'm glad that I can do something to help." In treating her syphilis, I had been able to give her free medication from the health department and only charged her one dollar per a visit, enabling her to get proper treatment in the privacy so dear to her. Her gift to the hospital made me happy because I didn't have the money to buy any gowns.

Before I opened the Quigless Clinic-Hospital, an elderly lady asked me to her home to check her grandchild who had been having severe stomach pains over a period of seven to eight days. She had been seen by the pediatrician in the area, who told the grandmother that the child was suffering from a disease known as pneumococcal salpingitis. The child had an infection of the fallopian tubes caused by a germ usually associated with pneumonia. I called the doctor in question, and he informed me that he had begun treating the child by giving her Coca-Cola and popsicles. I could not control my astonishment.

When I examined the child and found her vomiting and complaining of abdominal pain, her abdomen was distended and very tender to the touch. I believed she had all the symptoms and signs of a ruptured appendix. The grandmother had no money at all, and I knew it would be impossible to get the child into the hospital in Tarboro. I called Dr. Clark at St. Agnes Hospital in Raleigh and explained the situation. Even though she had no money, the grandmother had assured me that if the patient lived, the doctor would be paid. Dr. Clark agreed to do the operation, and I took her to Raleigh for the surgery. Sure enough, during the operation he found a ruptured appendix with dense adhesions. The child was in such critical condition that the only thing that could be done was to insert a drain into the abdomen and fight the virulent infection. With drainage established, the child got better.

Later, Dr. Clark was able to operate a second time and found the adhesions so dense that he had to remove part of her intestines. Following this operation, the child continued to develop symptoms of intestinal obstruction, and Dr. Clark found it necessary to operate a third time to remove more of her intestine. The child recovered following the third operation. In total, she was hospitalized for over five months, but she had no further trouble with intestinal obstruction.

As a result of three operations, she had post-operative scars all over her abdomen. She laughed about her experiences later, but it was not a laughing matter at that time. Her ruptured appendix, misdiagnosed as pneumococcal salpingitis, could have been fatal. During her long stay in the hospital, the entire staff became greatly attached to her. She never forgot her experiences at St. Agnes Hospital, so much so that after finishing high school in Tarboro, she returned to St. Agnes and completed nurse's training!

The operation of the Quigless Clinic-Hospital was quite a challenge. I would not be able to handle the workload relative to the operation of the hospital and handle my practice at the same time without some help. I knew of several graduates, even some who had passed the NC Board but who didn't have the funds necessary to start their own practices. I knew they would be available for me to hire as associates in my hospital. Graduate physicians from Class B medical schools could not be certified to practice in the State of North Carolina on their own, but at that day and time, it was acceptable to hire them to assist in the hospital practice as long as they didn't go into general practice.

I was able to hire a Class A medical school graduate who had taken the exam of the NC Board of Medical Examiners. That took care of my physician's associate.

The next challenge was finding nurses to operate the hospital on a twenty-four-hour basis. I talked with my friend Dr. Clark in Raleigh and asked about the availability of graduate nurses for my hospital. He recommended three young ladies who had nursing training and had recently obtained their certificates as registered nurses. I hired one who had completed her training at Good Samaritan Hospital. It was easy for me to recruit two high school graduates as nurse's aides from this area.

I was able to obtain a cook and a young man who was glad to serve as an orderly. Dr. Clark agreed to take on the position of chief surgeon since I had been under his tutelage for six months prior to opening my hospital. And I took Dr. Mizell's good advice as to giving special training in different fields to my registered nurses so they could take on more than one job.

My surgical team consisted of the in-hospital physician as my surgical assistant and nurses as my second surgical assistant and scrub nurse. One of my nurses had been trained to take care of the anesthesia.

At that time, ether was the only general anesthesia that I used. It was comparatively safe; the four stages of anesthesia were easily demarcated, and the surgeon in charge could coach the anesthetist along as to how much to use, when to apply the anesthetic, and when to ease up on it. This allowed the patient to be kept in the third stage of surgical anesthesia without fear of his going into the dangerous post stage which could lead to his death if not corrected in time. I had no anesthesia deaths.

However, I did have occasional deaths from severe cardiovascular accidents and one from strangulated hernia. The hernia strangulation had been done several days before the patient came to the hospital. As to obstetrics, we were extremely lucky and, except for premature deliveries where infants weighed less than four pounds, were able to salvage 90 percent of those infants.

As I tried to establish the hospital rules with my nursing staff, I had to deal with a disturbing test of my authority, which happened about six months after I began taking patients into the hospital. I happened to come by the hospital one night about midnight, and as I entered the building, I smelled food being cooked. I went to the kitchen and found three nurses cooking their breakfast. The meals we gave our nurses were well-balanced, and there should be no reason for them to be cooking any food at night. I remonstrated them and told them that if this was repeated, I would discharge any who were caught. About three months later, the cook informed me that someone had been cooking food—steaks, pork chops, bacon, and eggs—when she came in the mornings. I wrote letters to the three previously caught, telling them that I was giving them thirty days in which to find employment, after which time they would be discharged.

Three nights later, one of the nurse's aides called to tell me that all three of the nurses had collected their belongings and had left the building about midnight. That left only one registered nurse to care for twenty patients plus three post-operative patients. I got on the phone with the administrators of three Black hospitals and explained my plight to them. Each let me have one of their nurses. My nursing staff had been replenished within a period of twenty-four hours. I had no further trouble with nurses taking over my kitchen from that time until I closed the hospital.

I asked Dr. Clark to come from Raleigh to do surgeries for the first eight months after opening the hospital. He then assisted me for another six months, and after that, I was on my own. After my first month of operations, I was able to repay my loan at five hundred dollars per month and did not miss one single payment. It goes without saying that the Board of Directors of Builders Federal in Rocky Mount was very pleased with the good deed they had done, and I must say that without their help, I never would have been able to build the Quigless Clinic-Hospital.

My first patient was a transfer patient whom Dr. Clark sent from Raleigh for a convalescence period. He had been injured attempting to change a flat tire on the highway. A passing motorist ran over him, causing a compound fracture of his leg. Dr. Clark had to amputate his injured extremity, and because the patient was recovering without complications and was a resident of Tarboro, he suggested to the patient and his family that he be moved to my facility.

At that time, the elevator was not in operation, and we had to carry him upstairs on a stretcher. It so happened, however, that the man's family did not like the idea of him coming to my hospital and had him removed the very next day so he could be attended by a white physician. The incident did not discourage me in any way because it was entirely expected. I had known the family's attitude from the beginning. They were the type of people who believed that a Black doctor could in no way equal a white doctor in competence. I recognized this when I saw it and was not in the least bit disturbed by the outcome.

Within the first week, I had admitted patients with pneumonia, chronic inflammatory disease, asthma, and diabetes. Business was picking up and going smoothly. Along came acute appendicitis, simple and compound fractures, tubal ligations, and hysterectomies. I had patients for normal deliveries and children for tonsillectomies. About two months after opening, I admitted a four-year-old child with a fractured thigh. I had already obtained equipment for converting ordinary hospital beds into fracture beds. That made it easy for me to take care of that type of injury. In less than a year, my patient occupancy was around 75 to 90 percent.

Shortly after I opened the Quigless Clinic-Hospital, I realized that my most important challenge would be keeping proper nursing personnel. I realized that there was a large reservoir of talent around—raw talent that, with the proper encouragement, could be converted into efficient nursing personnel.

One of my nurse challenges was Barbara Ann, who I had known since she was four years old, when her family lived across the street from me. She was a vivacious little girl. One day she fell, cut her arm, and was taken up to my hospital for treatment. During the time we were treating her, she became fascinated with the hospital, especially the nurses, and expressed a desire to become a nurse when she was older.

As the years passed, her enthusiasm remained high, and she expressed her desire to become a nurse every time I had a chance to talk with her. When the time came for her to finish high school, she asked me for help because her parents were poor and could not afford to pay for her nurse's training. I contacted my friends at St. Agnes Hospital in Raleigh, a hospital established and maintained under the auspices of the Episcopal church. We were able to get Barbara Ann enrolled in the nurse's training program at that hospital. The tuition was very reasonable, and her parents were able to handle the expenses through most of her training. However, when graduation time came, Barbara Ann owed just under two hundred dollars, which had to be paid before graduation. I was glad to advance her the money, and she graduated on time.

We had an understanding that after graduation she would come work for me at the Quigless Clinic-Hospital. We were very happy to receive her, but it soon became apparent that she did not have the proper attitude to serve on our staff. For instance, one of her first acts upon taking up nursing duties was to stand in the middle of the ward and announce very loudly, "My name is Barbara Ann, and I am in charge of this ward. I am the only person who gives orders here. Do you see this white cap on my head? I have worked very hard to be able to wear it, and I'm going to be the boss as long as I'm here. Don't ask me to come after bedpans or straighten up your beds. That's the duty of the nurse's aides and LPNs. Now get that in your heads and act accordingly."

There was a post-operative patient on the ward at the time that Barbara Ann began work. She had only been working with us for three days when I began to get complaints. I was making rounds and came to this patient's bed. She said to me, "Dr. Quigless, I like everybody up here, and everybody has been treating me very nicely. But that new nurse doesn't do anything but run off at the mouth every time I ask her anything. Now, Dr. Quigless, I'm going to tell you straight. If that woman comes in here bothering me again, I'm strong enough, and I'll throw her out this second-story window. I will stand for no such foolishness."

I was very much upset, so I talked to the other patients in the ward who also expressed the fact that my "new nurse" made them all feel uncomfortable. I had to call Barbara Ann to my office and inform her of all the complaints I had received.

"After all, Doctor," she replied, "I'm a registered nurse now, and it is my place to give orders. If they don't like the way I'm doing things, then I guess I'll just have to quit."

"I'm sorry things have turned out this way," I said. "However, under the circumstances, I guess it would be better if you discontinued working for me. As to the money you owe me, it would be perfectly all right for you to pay it back at your convenience whenever you get a job at another institution."

"I promised to work it out in your hospital," she said. "If you don't want it like that, then I don't see how you're gonna get your money back." She then turned and walked out.

Barbara Ann and her family moved to Washington, D.C. I often wondered if she worked as an RN there and if she went into another hospital with the same attitude she had when she left us. That's the last I heard of Barbara Ann. I just had to kiss that money goodbye. She's the only person who I helped who showed their appreciation in that manner.

***

One patient's case I remember knocked every bit of egotism out of me. A young lady under my care became pregnant. This was her first pregnancy, and after about the third month, it was diagnosed that she was expecting twins. I followed the patient through her entire pregnancy, and along about her eighth month when I examined her, she asked, "Doctor, do you think I'll be all right? Do you think anything might happen that would cause me to be in trouble, serious trouble?"

I turned to her and said, "Mrs. Smith, your pregnancy is normal so far. I can't foresee any complications that we won't be able to handle. No matter what should occur, I'll be ready. Your babies seem to be in very good condition now, and in the event that anything should happen at the time of delivery, I'll be ready to do a Caesarean section. I guarantee that you'll have two beautiful babies."

In due time, she went into labor and seemed to be progressing normally. The delivery of the infants was eminent. I encouraged the patient to bear down and assured her that labor would soon be over. Shortly after I made that statement, my patient went into deep shock. She became very pale, her respiration became rapid and shallow, her pulse increased to 150, and her blood pressure dropped precipitously. We were in serious trouble. I hastily delivered the first twin, which was followed shortly by the delivery of the second. Both infants were dead. Her bleeding was somewhat profuse, and the only thing I could think of was a ruptured uterus.

We then directed our efforts toward getting the patient out of shock, but the low blood pressure, elevated pulse rate, and all other symptoms of shock persisted. I hastily called my friend at one of the medical centers. I explained the situation and was advised to get the patient to his hospital as soon as possible. She made the ninety-mile trip to the hospital still in shock but conscious and very apprehensive.

At 4 a.m. the next morning, I was called by one of the hospital's residents, who asked that I go over the details of the delivery from beginning to end. The resident stated that she was still in shock, and he could not do anything to reverse the condition. The patient died at the medical center, and her family refused to have an autopsy performed. I was so depressed by the entire incident that I felt like giving up, throwing in the sponge, and closing my hospital.

However, reality hit me, and I knew that I could not give up at that point. All twenty-five beds of the Quigless Clinic-Hospital were filled. The physicians at the medical center were as confused about the situation as I was. They could offer me no explanations for the series of events that culminated in the patient's death. However, the question kept recurring in my mind: Why? Why? Why? Now here was a case in which the delivery was progressing normally, then all of a sudden, the patient went into irreversible shock which culminated in her death. There were two beautiful babies delivered—both dead. The whole community was shocked.

Shortly thereafter, I returned to St. Louis, Missouri, for my annual interns' alumni meeting and talked with gynecologists from St. Louis University and the Barnes Hospital. They were unable to give me any explanations as to why the incident happened. About six months later, one of the gynecologists from St. Louis called me with an explanation for the disastrous incident. He related the story of a patient he had attended. He stated that things were progressing normally, and suddenly she went into shock and died within a few minutes.

An autopsy revealed that the placenta had partially pulled away from the wall of the uterus, opening the veins that connected the uterus to the placenta. During contractions, amniotic fluid surrounding the developing fetus was squeezed into the circulation of the patient. The fluid, consisting mostly of water, brought on the symptoms of shock. The patient died before they could do anything about it. He stated that a few days following that incident, they had another case where the patient went into shock. They opened the abdomen and removed the entire uterus. However, the shock was so profound that the patient died, but at least they had found the cause of the problem.

By the time I returned to St. Louis a year later, the gynecologists told me that they had seen two more patients with the same problem. The first patient died, but the second survived when the hysterectomy was done immediately after the developing symptoms of shock. I was able to explain the situation to the husband of the young lady who had died as a result of the condition that developed in my hospital. My explanation came just in time because the young man was preparing to sue me for malpractice.

So, everything did not always go smoothly with the passing of years. We were successful in most cases, but we didn't learn very much from the successful ones. However, we learned a hell of a lot from those unfortunate cases that went wrong.

Another difficulty I encountered while practicing medicine involved another gynecological case. I had done a hysterectomy on a patient who was suffering from uterine fibroids. She had lost a great deal of blood, so I gave her two units following the surgery. Her hemoglobin, however, remained low, so I started looking for blood donors to speed her recovery. There was no blood bank at that time, so we were under pressure to reach out and find our own volunteers. Their blood had to be typed, cross-matched, and then given to the patient. We found a young man who volunteered to give blood for this patient. His blood type was okay and cross-matched okay, so we drew two units of his blood and gave it to the patient.

About six hours after receiving this transfusion, she developed chills and fever, and her temperature elevated. A few hours later, her temperature returned to normal, and her chills subsided. I called the young man donating the blood and asked if he had ever been in the military service. He said he had served in the Pacific area for a time. I immediately took a blood smear from the patient, and what did I find? I found malaria parasites in all stages of development. I had infested the patient with malaria. Intra-muscular injections of quinine resulted in a lessening of the chills and fever. The patient, feeling fine, was discharged from the hospital six days later. I had learned a valuable lesson—never use a blood donor who has done service in the Pacific area.

Another challenging incident happened about four or five years after I started practicing in Tarboro. A certain lady, who worked as a cook for some of the good white folks in town, had syphilis and came to me for treatment. Like many with this condition, she was too embarrassed to obtain treatment at the public health department because she felt everyone would know what was wrong with her. Several years after finishing her treatments, she came to my office complaining of pain in the upper portion of her abdomen. The pain intensified whenever she ate greasy food. She became nauseated and had to be given morphine and atropine for pain relief.

My diagnosis was clear. She was suffering from gall bladder disease. After two or three painful attacks, I informed her that she needed an operation to remove her gall bladder. She kept putting off the surgery. Periodically, I gave her injections for pain whenever she ate greasy food. I repeatedly informed her that she needed the surgery and would not get any better until she had it. But instead of the surgery, she would call every time she had an attack.

One day she had an attack in her employer's kitchen. Her employer called in another doctor who said she needed a gall bladder operation. Although I had repeatedly told her she needed surgery, she said nothing about my advice to the other doctor. Her employer was very loud in condemning me for my "ignorance." The patient even began condemning me when talking about it with her friends and kin. Surgery revealed that her gall bladder was full of stones.

She was also allergic to nearly forty different substances. She developed eczematoid dermatitis whenever she worked in her garden, inhaled dust or cigarette smoke, or ate tomatoes. About four years after her gall bladder surgery, she developed an upper-respiratory infection.

The same doctor who advised gall bladder surgery was called in to see her at home. He gave her an intra-muscular injection of penicillin. Immediately after the injection, the patient developed respiratory difficulties. The doctor was confronted with a very serious situation and had nothing in his bag to counteract the penicillin reaction. He advised the family that he was going back to the hospital to get her some medication. He left the house and did not return, and the lady died within thirty minutes of his departure.

Although the family was very much upset, no blame was ever put on the physician. Instead, they just said, "It was the Lord's will." Now if I had been the doctor administering that lethal dose of penicillin, I bet instead of saying "it was the Lord's will," they would have said, "that nigger doctor didn't know what he was doing." I had to put up with a lot whenever an untoward reaction occurred after my treatment of ailments or whenever one of my patients died. Even many of my good Black brothers and sisters still had the ingrained opinion or notion that Black doctors did not know as much as white doctors.

***

During the early years of the Quigless Clinic-Hospital, my wife Helen served as my secretary. She kept track of correspondence, typed insurance reports, and checked my finances, including charges made for treating patients, payments, deposits, disbursements, and everything that had to do with my financial affairs. With young children to look after, it became increasingly difficult, if not impossible, for her to look after both my office and the children. We felt that the children were more important than anything else.

We looked for someone else to be my secretary and found a young lady from Tarboro named Elaine (which is not her true name). After some training from Helen, Elaine took over the job of secretary. I felt that she could be trusted to handle my affairs without much scrutiny. Everything went along nicely for about two years. My collections were coming in nicely, and I was never in a financial bind.

Until then, I had handled my income tax returns without any outside help. Then one day, I received a letter from the Internal Revenue Service stating that an investigator was being sent to audit my income tax records. I knew that I had been honest and had declared everything to the IRS. The investigator came and went over my returns. He questioned some of the items, and we disagreed. He stated that in all fairness to me and the IRS, I should call in a third party to help settle our partial differences. I contacted Mr. Gassaway, a CPA from Rocky Mount. Instead of agreeing with me, the CPA agreed with the IRS investigator. At that juncture and without further deliberation, I asked Mr. Gassaway to take over my income tax reports and returns.

About two years later, my CPA informed me that there was a problem with my financial records. He stated that my deposits did not agree with my income, as evidenced when the duplicate receipts were checked. He put it this way: "Dr. Quigless, you've got to go back and dig up some of that money you're hiding. You're taking it in, but your deposits are not agreeing with your receipts. You are either hiding it, or someone else is hiding it from you."

I did not know what to think! After carefully checking my deposits against my receipts, I found that there was a deficit of several thousand dollars over a period of three years. I called Helen in to see if she could help me find out what was going on. It did not take her long to discover that some of the checks submitted in payment for treatments were not being deposited into my account.

The next thing we did was check with the bank. In short, we found that some checks were being cashed but not recorded in my deposits. We asked the bank for copies of all the checks issued to me or the Quigless Clinic-Hospital. When we reviewed the copies, we found that my signature had been forged on the backs of some checks.

Next in the investigation was an interrogation of the tellers. One of the tellers quickly admitted that some of the checks had been brought in by my secretary who requested that they be cashed. Those checks had not been included on my deposit slips. In other words, Elaine had forged my name to the checks, had them cashed, and kept the money.

When faced with the evidence, Elaine readily admitted to having diverted the funds. She begged me not to prosecute her. Her mother joined the pleadings, realizing that this would have a serious effect on the family's standing in the area. Of course, if I had gone through with the prosecution for embezzlement, it probably would have resulted in a prison term for her. The bank would have had to reimburse me, and I would have been able to recover the missing funds.

However, I listened to the pleas of Elaine and her family, and we agreed that Elaine would take out an insurance policy and a twenty-year endowment policy so that at the end of that time, I could be reimbursed for the money she had taken. That way they could repay this money and protect the family's name. The policy was bought, and Elaine and her family agreed to make monthly payments on the policy. I dropped the matter at that point. But the premiums on the policy were kept up for only about two years, and then the policy was allowed to lapse. The result was that the family's good name had been saved, but I was out of thousands of dollars.

***

For several days during visiting hours, I noticed a gentleman, Reverend Lewis, standing in the hall wearing a white barber's coat. One day I asked how he was doing. He replied, "I'm doing all right, Doctor. I came in to visit one or two of your patients who are members of my church."

"Go right ahead, Reverend." He was visiting the hospital regularly.

One day, a patient called me over to her bed and said, "Doctor, why don't you stop that man from coming in this hospital and worrying your patients?"

"He's a minister," I said, "and he's supposed to come and see the members of his church as often as necessary."

"But, Doctor, that isn't what he's coming in here to do. That man came up to me and said, 'Lady, the best thing for you to do is get out of this hospital and let me pray over you. That doctor doesn't know what he's doing. He doesn't know what's wrong with you. I know what's wrong with you. You've got cancer, and I can cure it. All you have to do is just come and let me pray over you.'"

Well, that sort of steamed me, but I didn't say anything. I just waited until the good reverend came in again. Then I went up to him and said, "Now, look here, Lewis. I don't mind you coming in and seeing your members, but I'll be damned if I'm gonna have you coming in here telling my patients that I don't know what's wrong with them. And I'll be damned if I'm gonna have you coming in here telling them that you can cure them by praying over them. You get your butt out of this place and don't ever let me see you coming up these stairs again."

I have very little faith in these so-called "faith healers." I feel that prayer and a good pep talk may do something for a person who is suffering from a psychosomatic condition. However, I have yet to observe a patient who has obtained any relief from the incantations of a faith healer.

I believe in prayer. I know prayer can move mountains and do a lot of things, but I don't feel that God has endowed every Tom, Dick, and Harry who can sing loud with the ability to perform miracles. I feel that God is performing miracles every day through dedicated individuals who look to Him for guidance, administering to ailments of man, and who spend their entire lives in laboratories trying to present the facts that are revealed to them as a result of profound dedication through the art and science of medicine.

***

About two years before opening the Quigless Hospital-Clinic I had a call from a white dentist. "Dr. Quigless," he began, "I have a good colored dentist here in my office who is thinking about starting a practice in Tarboro. I understand that he finished dentistry at Howard University Dental School. He took the examination of the Dental Board here in North Carolina, and I understand from the Chairman of the Board of Examiners that he had the highest mark of any taking the examination. You know we need a good colored dentist in this town more than we need anything else right now."

I lost no time in going to the dentist's office to meet the new dentist, Dr. Moses Ray. Dr. Ray informed me that he had finished dentistry in the same class with my brother-in-law, Dr. Frederick Gordon, who later went to Albany, New York to practice. Dr. Ray said that he and Fred had served together in the Dental Corps of the U.S. Army during World War II. I welcomed Dr. Ray to town and assured him that I would do everything possible to help him get established.

Dr. Ray began his practice in two rooms of his home. I offered him space in my building, so he could have an operating room, and the use of all my facilities, including utilities, telephone, and the rest. I told him that I would charge him thirty dollars per month for the first six months and sixty dollars per month after that. He thought the arrangement was satisfactory and agreed to my offer. I went ahead and roughed in the necessary water and drainage connections he would need along with the necessary power cables to his dental unit. As I got farther along in my plans, I saw the need for more space for myself. However, I had made the offer to Dr. Ray and was resigned to stand by my commitment.

I was not the only person welcoming Dr. Ray to Tarboro. Some of the older citizens welcomed him as well. Dr. Ray joined one of the local churches and began taking part in our people's civic activities. When we were well along with roughing in the necessary changes the dental unit required, Dr. Ray called me to say that he had thought over our agreement and felt it was all right for me to charge him thirty dollars per month for the first six months, but it would be asking too much for him to pay sixty dollars per month after that.

For the life of me, I could not understand why he wouldn't accept the offer, so in our phone conversation I went over every step of the agreement, including the fact that he wouldn't have to pay for any utilities or a receptionist. He still insisted that it was too much to pay. I explained that I had promised to give him every assistance I could when he came to Tarboro, and I stood by my commitment. He insisted that he could not come into my building with these financial arrangements.

By that time, I could plainly understand that some of the older residents of Tarboro had warned Dr. Ray to steer clear of me, saying that I would probably do him more harm than good. I had no ulterior motives in mind, and while I regretted his decision to turn my offer down, I looked at his refusal as a way for me to get out of my commitment.

A few years later, a two-story building was constructed in East Tarboro, in which Dr. Ray was able to obtain facilities more suitable for his dental office. It is to be remembered that I gave up trying to help the people in this community when the older citizens went out of their way to counteract every proposal I made to the Town Council. Dr. Ray, however, joined the Civic League and began advancing his ideas. The people of the community witnessed my troubles and assumed that without leadership they were unable to make any advances. When Dr. Ray came along, he was quickly elevated to a position of leadership. Under his leadership, the organization became known as the East Tarboro Citizens League. He received better cooperation from the people than I had ever achieved and was able to mold the East Tarboro Citizens League into a very effective organization, which was able to improve the lot of the Black people to a great extent.

CHAPTER 20

LAST ADDITION TO MY FAMILY

When Milton was about four years of age, my wife, Helen, became pregnant with our third child. We already had a boy and a girl, so the gender of this new child was immaterial to us. Helen had the usual pregnancy symptoms—nausea, vomiting, and abhorrence of smelling cooking food. Some symptoms developed, however, that indicated a probable ectopic pregnancy—a pregnancy in the fallopian tubes.

One Saturday morning, I contacted my good friend, Dr. Clark, in Raleigh. An immediate operation was indicated. Because no active symptoms were present, we decided to operate on Monday morning, two days later. But the next morning about 10 a.m., Helen developed severe lower abdominal pain, became dizzy, and fainted. I knew right away just what was happening—the ectopic pregnancy had ruptured. This was very serious. The first thing I did was call an ambulance and had her transported to my hospital. I tried to contact two other surgeons in Tarboro, Dr. Ed Roberson and Dr. Green. Neither could be found.

To add to my dilemma, I had recently employed a nurse who had previously assisted in an ectopic pregnancy surgery at St. Agnes Hospital. However, in that case, the patient lost too much blood and died on the operating table, which left quite a memory with my new nurse. As soon as she heard what was happening, she started screaming, "Oh, Dr. Quigless, please do something right away."

I called Mrs. Beaman, my anesthetist, who was preparing to go to church. I told her, "Come right now. I need you right away. Come as you are."

Since as I could not contact any doctor in Tarboro, I called and roused Dr. L.H. Webb out of bed. He had been my assistant in the hospital two years before going into practice on his own in Rich Square, North Carolina. I said, "Come now. You can come in your damn pajamas, but I need you right now."

In the meantime. Helen's blood pressure was 80 over 40. My nurse monitored the blood pressure, and Mrs. Beaman began administering ether. Because Helen was already in shock, I knew how important it was to get into her abdomen without delay. I had operated on three other ectopics, and all three of the patients had been saved. Immediately after entering the abdomen, I located the ruptured tube by touch, and a clamp was applied, stopping the hemorrhage. As I was taught in St. Louis, the free blood in the abdomen was aspirated, drawn out, and placed in a sterile container. The ruptured tube was removed, and in the meantime her blood pressure started reviving.

While in St. Louis, I was taught that in cases of ectopic pregnancies, where the abdomen was entered and no blood donor was present, the blood taken from the cavity could be strained through sterile gauze and reintroduced into the patient's bloodstream. In other words, the blood could be returned by auto-transfusion. In order to make blood available for auto-transfusion, the blood had to be strained through at least six thicknesses of gauze which had been washed eight or ten times so the blood could be strained through a sterile funnel and reintroduced into the circulatory system of the surgical patient. I had used this procedure with my previous ectopic pregnancies with no untoward results.

In checking Helen's hemoglobin the night following the operation, I found it was 9.5, which was still on the low side. I decided to play it safe and find a suitable donor for at least one unit of blood. The donor was Sylvester Brown, a Black teacher in the community. Helen was duly transfused and back home after a stay of five days in the hospital. Her recovery was uneventful.

Helen became pregnant again about eighteen months after the ectopic pregnancy. This pregnancy was followed closely and had no emergencies. However, I thought it would be better if she had a Caesarean section since she already had a midline incision, and I didn't want to take the chance of a rupture with a second abdominal incision. I called my friend, Dr. Mizell of Fort Lauderdale and asked if he'd come and do Helen's Caesarean section when we determined her nine months had passed. Dr. Mizell came and delivered our baby girl, Carol Marie. It so happened that during the Caesarean delivery we made a tape recording. I kept that recording and could relive the moment when I heard Carol's first cry.

Up until that time, Mary Cherry had been helping Helen with the two children at home. At eighteen years old, she was the eldest of a very large family. When we brought Carol home from the hospital, Mary took one look at her and said, "Well, I'm sorry, Dr. and Mrs. Quigless, but I'm going to have to quit now. After taking care of nine babies, I swore to my Lord that I'd never take care of another. I love all of you, and I love that child, but I'm telling you right here and now that I ain't going to be taking care of no more babies. I'm quitting."

When Mary decided to quit, we looked for someone to take her place. About one year before Carol's birth, I began treating Ms. Lena Mayo for chronic arthritis. I immediately thought of her because I knew that she had worked for many years as cook for one of the white families in the county, which would help us out. She had expressed a desire to move to town, so we contacted her.

Ms. Lena's arthritis symptoms had subsided considerably under my treatment. She weighed about one hundred eighty pounds, was very dark-complexioned, had a disarming smile, a deep mellow voice, and when she laughed, you somehow felt compelled to smile with her. She was a very fine lady who had come up the hard way. She married early in life, and she and her husband had been sharecroppers. She told me of the many years she had labored alongside her husband from sunup to sundown in the tobacco fields to eke out a meager existence. They had one child who had left the area for New York. After Mr. Mayo's death, she had been left on her own. She did not have the benefit of an education but had a remarkable memory. She was an excellent cook, a wonderful housekeeper, and had a way with children that could not be touched by anyone.

When my son Milton had just entered school, he learned that Ms. Lena could neither read nor write, and he took it upon himself to teach her. They had some wonderful times together. In most instances, the teaching would end with Ms. Lena challenging Milton to a checkers match. After the game, he would scratch his head and look puzzled, and Ms. Lena would laugh. He would then make this promise: "I'll get you next time."

Ms. Lena had some misgivings about taking the job because she was arthritic. I said, "Ms. Lena, I think the best thing in the world for you to do is work for a doctor, at least a doctor who is giving you some relief from your symptoms. And remember, Ms. Lena, if you are working for us, it would be to our advantage to keep you healthy so that you could look after our little girl."

I took Ms. Lena around the house. She took one look at Carol and fell in love with her. When I think about it, falling in love was mutual between Carol and Ms. Lena. Carol soon became devoted to Ms. Lena and looked to her for everything instead of looking to her mother.

When Carol was about six months old, she developed a severe case of diarrhea which lasted for about a week. At the end of that time, she had lost a lot of weight and was greatly dehydrated. Her appetite was very poor, and we couldn't get her to eat anything. However, Ms. Lena had a solution. She said, "Give her here." She then sat Carol in her lap at the dinner table and started eating the food from her plate using her hands. Carol watched Ms. Lena's hands go to the plate, pick up the food, and put the food in her mouth. She watched the procedure about half a minute, grabbed the food off Ms. Lena's plate, and put it in her mouth. Soon, she was eating everything on her plate. In no time flat she had regained her strength, and her appetite continued to be ravenous. In about six months' time, Carol looked just like Ms. Lena—fat.

The two became inseparable. At the end of the day, Ms. Lena would have to slip away from the house to keep Carol from following her. If Carol caught her leaving, she would grab her by one leg and have to be forcibly removed. Most of the time, however, Carol knew just about the time Ms. Lena would be ready to leave for home. She would grab her bottle, tuck it under her arm, and say, "Ms. Lena, let's go home now."

Ms. Lena attended the Few in Number Baptist Church in the country. She would always go to church with Carol following closely behind. Carol even walked like Ms. Lena by that time. When Ms. Lena would take a vacation, Carol insisted that she go along. Carol was the happiest child. Because she was the third child, she was often getting into fights with her siblings, Helen and Milton. She seemed to win every time, or at least they would let her win. So, she began bossing everyone around. If she couldn't have her way, she would run to Ms. Lena, knowing full well that she would take her side. Ms. Lena had become part of our family.

Later, Ms. Lena began suffering from shortness of breath, her ankles swelled, and she had all the symptoms of a failing heart. The many years of laboring hard under adverse conditions had taken their toll. When Carol was about six years old, Ms. Lena decided to leave our employment. I pleaded with her, Carol pleaded with her—we all pleaded with her, promising to lighten her load and do everything possible to keep her with us and contented. However, she insisted upon leaving us. She took a job with a very fine lady in Tarboro where she remained for several years.

Ms. Lena had saved her money and was able to buy a small, comfortable home—quite a feat for a person in her circumstances. She was extremely happy, and Carol took advantage of every chance that came along to keep in touch with Ms. Lena as the years passed. I found it necessary to put her in the hospital on several occasions due to her heart condition. After bed rest and medication, she was always able to return to full employment.

However, the time finally arrived when she became so disabled that she had to be admitted to the hospital because of increased breathing difficulties. The night following her admission, Ms. Lena called me to her room and said, "Doctor, you have put me in this hospital many times, and I've gotten out feeling much better. However, this is the last time. I'll not be able to get out of here alive."

I scoffed, "Oh, no, Ms. Lena, we'll be able to do something for you this time, too. In four or five days, you'll be out and going about your confounded business."

But she was right. In spite of everything that could be done, her condition worsened, and she died. Carol had finished grade school and was enrolled in a private boarding school—The Putney School in Putney, Vermont—with our other two children when this happened. Because she was so far away, she was unable to attend Ms. Lena's funeral. As a friend of the family and her former employer, I was asked to say a few words at the funeral. I spoke of her devotion to the church, her friends and relatives, and our close relationship. I spoke of the adverse circumstances under which she lived. She was a very fine person, and I thought of all the good things she had done for everyone. I thought of her stage of semi-retirement and her great sense of satisfaction when she was able to buy her home. That was the only brief period of happiness I believe the lady ever had. It was a sad occasion, and as a rule I'm not given to a great show of emotion. However, I could not keep the tears from flowing as I saw the funeral procession leave the church, knowing full well that her body would be placed in a lonely grave to be forgotten by most, except for a few. Carol was one of those few.

Helen, Jr., and Milton, Jr., grew up so fast. There was no such thing as kindergarten in this area at that time. When they became four and three years old respectively, we enrolled them in a little private school run by Mrs. Weston, the wife of the Black priest at the colored Episcopal Church. Mrs. Weston's father had served as priest of that church for many years. When he died, Mrs. Weston's husband succeeded him as priest. Mrs. Weston had been a teacher all her life and continued teaching in the Perry School, a private school. All who could afford it sent their children to Mrs. Weston's school for early training. She gave kindergarten and elementary school instruction to students in second and third grade.

Under her influence, students were very well prepared when they made the transition to the public school. In fact, our children were enrolled in the second grade of the public school when they left Mrs. Weston's tutelage. I remember that Milton, Jr., was enrolled in the third grade and was much younger than his classmates. One child, two years older than he, had a habit of jumping on his back, throwing him to the ground, and engaging him in a tussle. Of course, being older than Milton, he would win every time. Milton confided in me one day that he was getting tired of having to tussle every time he left the classroom. I told him, "Bro, you will have to take care of that situation yourself."

He said, "Daddy, he's bigger, older, and stronger than me. I can't do a thing but fall over on the ground."

I said, "I'll tell you what to do, Bro. Tomorrow, when you go to school, get a stick, lean it against the door, and when he jumps on you and throws you to the ground, just do the best you can. But when you get up, reach over, grab that stick, and hit him over the head."

"But Daddy, if I hit him, he is going to whip me."

I said, "Bro, if you hit him hard enough across his head, he's not going to do a thing but grin and walk off."

He said, "Well, Daddy, you told me to do it, and I'm going to."

About three days later, he came right down to my office after school and said, "Daddy, I want to talk to you for a minute."

"What's happening?"

He said, "I did just what you told me to do. I hit that boy right across his head, and he didn't do a thing but get up, rub his head, and grin."

I said, "Well, Bro, that's the way it's going to be. You're going to have to look after yourself. If you find that someone is too strong for you, you've got to have a way to circumvent that strength and come out on top. That's what I've always had to do!"

CHAPTER 21

THE FARM

After being in Tarboro about four years, I had treated many farmers and their families, and, of course, had learned a lot about their problems. I felt I would like to identify more closely with the farmers. I noted a small farm advertised for sale. It was the same farm on which I had conducted maternity, prenatal, and infant welfare clinics, so I was quite familiar with it. The farm buildings were not in such good shape. However, the land was very fertile, and the crop allotments were satisfactorily proportioned to the amount of crop land on the farm. The asking price was not considered exorbitant, and because I could purchase the land by making a down payment and borrow the remainder from the Farmers' Loan Cooperative at a reasonable rate, I decided to buy the farm.

I informed Mrs. Sue Pender, who had shared her folk wisdom at the previously mentioned maternity clinics, that I had purchased the farm, and she said, "Doctor, I'm so glad you bought this place. I hope you'll let me stay on here. But there is one thing I want you to do, and I want you to do it right away."

"What is that, Mrs. Pender?"

"I want you to dig a well out here," she said. "That well in the backyard is in bad shape. It has caved in on all sides, leaving a big hole. Chickens fall in sometimes, and there are three or four frogs in there. I stay afraid that some of my grandchildren might fall in. I've been trying to get the other owner to dig one for fifteen years. I want you to dig a new well, and I want it right away."

I turned to her and said, "Mrs. Pender, am I to understand that you were after the owner to dig a well for fifteen years, and he hadn't done it in all this time?"

"Yea, that's the truth."

"Well now, as soon as I say I'm buying this farm," I said, "you tell me that I've got to dig you a well right away."

She said, "That's right. I want it right away."

"Mrs. Pender, I'm going to take my time in digging that well," I said to her surprise. "If you want to stay on this farm, I will be glad to have you. But if you insist on my digging a well right away, and you let the former owner go for fifteen years, it'll be all right if you move."

She said, "Doctor, I don't mean that. I don't want to move, but I would like for you to dig a well because I don't want my grandchildren falling in the old one."

"Don't worry, Mrs. Pender, I will do it as soon as I can get around to it."

The farm was situated on a paved highway. There was a scuppernong grapevine, at least fifty years old, situated close to the house. The vine was supported by a substantial trellis covering an area of about thirty to fifty feet. It produced an abundant crop of greenish-brown scuppernong grapes, excellent for eating and better still for making wine.

I secured a tenant to farm the land and bought the necessary farm equipment. My agreement with the tenant was half and half. I would furnish the equipment, and we'd jointly furnish the fertilizer, seeds, and plants. The tenant would furnish the labor. When the crop was harvested, I would deduct one-half the costs of the farm supplies, the tenant would pay the other half, and we'd split the profits from the sale. I wouldn't pay the tenant a salary but would advance him money to take care of his living expenses until the crop was harvested and not charge any interest during the year.

Everything went along well. I had a new well dug adjacent to the back porch of the house, so Mrs. Pender would not be exposed to the weather whenever she wanted to draw water. After the well was in working order, I told her to have her son-in-law fill in the old well. She said, "Wait a minute, Doctor. I don't want to fill that well up right now."

"Why?"

"I can still use that water to wash my clothes in."

"Mrs. Pender," I said, "you've been after me time and again to dig that well, insisting that I dig it because it was a menace to your health and your grandchildren's safety. You said the water was unfit for drinking. I feel that if it is unfit for drinking purposes, then it's unfit for anything. What about the frogs and chickens that were falling into the well? What about the danger to your grandchildren? Now, Mrs. Pender, I insist you have your son-in-law fill in that well right away. If anything should happen to you or your family, you would be the first one to sue me."

The old well was filled in soon after that encounter.

When the hospital was in operation, and I was using a lot of both white and sweet potatoes to feed my patients, I decided to grow some on my farm to cut down on my food expenses. I made a deal with the tenant, saying I would buy potato vines and seedlings if he would raise them.

When harvest time came, I would take half and give him half. I asked him if he would be satisfied with that arrangement, and he said he would. Accordingly, I bought the vines and seedlings, and they were planted.

The potatoes grew, and, in the early fall, I checked their growth and found them ready for harvest. The tenant agreed to do the harvesting. I rode out one day to take a look, and he stated that he was just about finished. I noticed that I had about twelve bushels of sweet potatoes and about twelve or fourteen bushels of white potatoes. I asked him if that was the yield, and he said, "Yes." I was a little suspicious because I was expecting much more. However, I took my half and went back to town.

I then decided to go back out to the farm. When I did, I found him plowing the potatoes again. I discovered that he had harvested the first time by plowing very shallowly. The second plowing was much deeper and yielded more potatoes than the first. I decided to wait until he finished plowing, and then we divided the potatoes again. After that incident I found I couldn't trust him. After all the crops had been harvested and we settled up, I advised him that I would no longer need him on my farm.

I knew another farmer who had been a sharecropper all his life, and he'd told me he would like to work for me. We came to terms regarding division of the crop at the end of the year, and I also agreed to advance him money for living expenses, month by month, until the end of the year. I further advised him that I would not charge interest. Everything went along smoothly except this man had no mechanical ability. He was unable to make any repairs or adjustments to the farm machinery. I'd have to call a mechanic whenever any of the equipment wasn't working properly.

A few years later, I had more trouble with him. A friend and I drove out to the farm and were looking around when I saw a column of smoke rising from the woods. "Something is wrong down there," I said. "See the smoke? It looks like the woods are on fire. Let's go see what's happening."

We started toward the smoke. When we got halfway there, the smoke suddenly stopped. At that time there were moonshiners in the region, and I knew that someone had a still down there. I found the man and said, "Look here, what in hell is going on in the woods? I saw smoke rising, and when I started down, it stopped."

He said, "Don't go down in those woods."

"I'm not going down there, but you tell whoever is down there making moonshine that he'd better get out today because I'm going to call the law."

I went back to my office and started treating patients. Not too long afterward, a man came in. "Okay, what's your trouble?" I asked.

He said, "I know you saw smoke in the woods today and started down to see what was wrong. I had a still down there and was running off a batch of liquor. Now, if you'll let me finish that batch, I'll pay you fifty dollars. After that, I'll move my still."

"Look here, man," I said angrily, "let me tell you one damn thing right now. You'd better get that still out of there this afternoon because I'm going to notify the sheriff at five p.m. If he goes out and finds the still, I'm going to tell him who owns it."

"Okay, Doc, I'll get out," he said. And he did.

Later, I received a call from the sheriff's office, and one of the deputies stated that my tenant was in jail for making whiskey.

"Hell, that guy hasn't got sense enough to build a still. There's something wrong here," I said. "I know he isn't making whiskey." I went down to the jail, and there was my tenant sitting behind bars.

I said, "What in the hell is going on here, fellow? The sheriff said he found a still down on my land and that you were the operator. Now, you know damn well you wouldn't even know how to build a still. What happened?"

"Well, Doc," he said, "I'll tell you the truth. A man agreed to give me fifty dollars to let him put the still down there. I know I did wrong, but that's what happened. When the sheriff caught me, I was afraid to tell who owned the still because I thought the man might do something to me if I told on him. So, I took the responsibility, and here I am."

I posted his bond. He was tried and convicted of operating a still and fined six hundred dollars. I paid it so he could carry on my farming operation that year. Needless to say, I needed to get rid of that fellow after that. It was the early 1960s, and Peyton Beery had started recruiting workers for a textile firm that was moving to Tarboro—Glenoit Mills. I asked Mr. Beery to put my tenant's name down as a potential worker for this plant. Mr. Beery agreed to do so, and that took care of that.

I had quite a problem trying to find someone to look after my farm. But at last, I found a good tenant. For about eight months I had been treating Mrs. Knight, a nice lady suffering from hypertension. I checked her kidney function, monitored her blood pressure, and prescribed medication. I was unable to pinpoint the cause for her hypertension.

One day I said, "Mrs. Knight, I can't understand why the devil your blood pressure doesn't come down. Are you having any trouble at home? Is there anybody who causes you to worry all the time?"

"Well, Doc, I'll tell you," she answered. "I've been having some trouble. It's not trouble with my husband, Travis, but it's connected with our financing and farming. We bought a farm out on Dicken's Hill and had been getting along pretty well with it, but something happened that caused us to lose our farm, our entire savings, and all the work we have done. All we were left with was our pickup truck. Travis had nowhere to turn and no one to help him out."

Now here was Travis Knight with a wife with high blood pressure, a child with diabetes, and three other minor children.

I asked Mrs. Knight where they were living, and she said that after being evicted from the farm, Travis found a job with another farmer as a day laborer. As well as doing farm work, he was required to take care of all the farming equipment. I knew Travis, and I knew his ability as a farmer. He was mechanically inclined and able to take care of the farming equipment. That was the man I needed for my farm.

I asked directions to their house near Palmyra. I knew better than to go to another man's farm during the day to talk with his tenant about hiring him for my farm, so I waited until about ten o'clock one night and drove out. I talked with Travis about two hours. I made a deal with him to come and look after my farm, but I made a different deal with Travis than I had with the others. I agreed to pay him one hundred dollars each month plus half the proceeds from the farm products which he grew, less the cost of the fertilizer, seed, and such.

It was about that time that I decided to go into the hog-raising business. I agreed to give him five percent of the proceeds from the sale of the hogs raised on the farm. I knew that under that arrangement I would not make much money. However, my medical practice was taking care of my needs, and I was very glad to help this man out, especially because I knew I would not lose in the end. Accordingly, Travis moved his family to my farm.

At that juncture, I was also able to acquire another parcel of land near my farm. A farmer who had moved here from the Midwest to buy a five-hundred-acre parcel of farmland had brought with him the farming methods which he had used in the Midwest. Instead of raising cotton, corn, and peanuts, he confined his operation to raising small grain, like wheat, oats, and barley. When I talked with him, he stated that he had come here with the idea of teaching these people how to farm. However, after about five years, he got so deeply in debt that he had to sell out. Since his farm was near mine, I decided to buy one-third of his acreage. With Travis looking after everything, I thought it would be a worthwhile investment. I hired another tenant to help Travis. With the acquisition of more farmland, I needed and found more tenants to work the farm under Travis's supervision. That's when my real tenant trouble started.

The first tenant I hired was quite elderly but had several teen-age children. I felt he could take care of a section of the farm, so I decided to employ him. Everything was going along fine through planting time. However, it soon got to the place where he was too old to do his part and couldn't control his children. At the end of the year, I had to let him go.

I was determined to get the proper type of tenant to look after my land. Instead of getting the proper type, I got the worst type possible. A man was referred to me by a person I thought was a good friend. He was able to do the work he was assigned, but I found out he was known as a troublemaker and very hard to get along with. After he'd been on the farm about four months, Travis started having difficulty because of the man's bad temper.

In those days, while harvesting peanuts, a farmer would first plow them up, then put them in stacks where they would stay until they were dry, and the vines could be hauled away. At this juncture, a peanut thrashing machine would be brought in to separate the peanuts from the vines. They would then be sold.

After the peanuts had been stacked, the cows got out and into this particular man's peanut field. The cows ate one of the peanut stacks and knocked over two others. This bad-tempered man came to me and said, "The cows have eaten up three stacks of peanuts, and I've got to be paid for them."

"Let's go down and check it out," I said.

Travis and I went to the farm to see what the damage was. I knew the man had a bad temper, and I didn't intend to get into trouble with him, so when I went to check on things, I put a little pistol in my pocket. Sure enough, we got out, checked the stacks of peanuts, and found that the cows had really only eaten one stack. The two other stacks had been knocked over but not eaten.

I said, "You told me that the cows had destroyed three stacks, when in truth only one stack has been eaten."

He got very agitated and angry. He came up with an ax handle, attempting to attack Travis. Travis weighed about two-hundred-forty pounds, and I weighed about one hundred thirty-five. Travis attempted to evade the fellow and tried crouching behind me. "Wait a minute here, fellow," I said. "You're not going to do anything to Travis or to me because I'll blow your damn brains out."

He backed off, and we had no further trouble with him until we started harvesting tobacco.

This tenant cured his tobacco very well. He called me to the farm when he took out his first tobacco. He said, "Doc, when we take the tobacco from the barn, we'll divide your part and my part at the barn door, and that's the way we'll sell it."

"No," I said, "we won't do it that way. We'll sell the tobacco, figure up all the returns, and you'll get your share of the money. We'll pay off the expenses first, then divide what's left."

"Now that isn't the way I'm going to do it. We're going to do it like this. We'll divide the tobacco at the barn."

"We're not going to do it like that," I said firmly. "We're going to do it my way." He finally reluctantly agreed.

I thought to myself, "I'm going to have to figure out a way of getting this damn man off my farm." About the middle of October, I informed him that I would not be able to keep him on the farm any longer. I gave him one month to get off the farm.

"I'm going to stay on this damn farm as long as I want to, and I ain't leaving here before January," he informed me.

I told him two or three more times. I didn't want to get him riled up because I knew he had a bad temper. I finally said, "Okay, I'll give you one month to get off the farm, and if you don't, I'll have you evicted."

He didn't get off. He stayed right there, so I had him evicted.

It was about that time that Travis decided he was through farming. During the last three or four years on the farm, Travis had developed hypertension, and old age had hold of him. His hypertension got worse, and he had developed heart disease. In the meantime, his wife's parents had died and left them a home in the little town of Speed. He died about three years after leaving our farm. Mrs. Knight lived about three years longer before hypertension finally carried her away, too.

When Travis left my farm, I decided it was a little too much for me to handle on my own. That's when I began looking around for someone to manage my farm, and I engaged the services of a white farmer who had been very successful in his own farming operations.

About this time, everyone was noticing my rise from being a penniless physician who had come here under adverse circumstances to a successful man who could buy farmland and turn around and buy more. Not everyone was in my corner. There was a man living in Tarboro who had other interests. The farming bug had also bitten him. Watching my progress, this particular man was extremely jealous, although I didn't know it at the time.

In those days, during the process of harvesting tobacco, after the tobacco leaves became ripe and ready for harvesting, they would be put into what we called "slides," pulled by mules between the tobacco rows. The tenants harvesting the tobacco would pull the ripe leaves, place them on the slide until they got to the end of a row, then the leaves would be transferred to a table and prepared to be placed in the tobacco barns. In the barns, the tobacco would be heated until properly cured.

There was a farmer going out of business who had several mules for sale. I went to the auction and picked out the mule I thought would best serve my needs and decided to bid on it. When the mule came up for auction, I bid twenty-five dollars.

Everyone laughed. I wasn't thinking about putting much money into a mule that probably wouldn't last but a couple of years.

Someone said, "Thirty-five dollars."

The auctioneer said, "Thirty-five, thirty-five, thirty-five. The mule is going for thirty-five dollars. Who'll bid forty?"

I said, "Forty dollars."

"Forty dollars, once, twice. Who'll bid forty-five?"

Someone said, "Forty-five."

"Who'll bid fifty dollars? Fifty dollars."

"Fifty."

"Fifty dollars. Going once, twice. Who'll bid fifty-five?"

I said to myself, "What in the hell is going on here? Somebody is trying to get that old mule. He isn't worth that much, but I'm going to have myself some fun." I bid sixty-five dollars.

"We have a bid for sixty-five dollars. Who'll bid seventy?"

After a while the auctioneer said, "Seventy dollars. Sold to this man right over here." He pointed in my direction.

I said, "Wait a minute now. I didn't bid seventy dollars. I'm not going to pay seventy dollars for that old mule."

The auctioneer said, "I wasn't pointing at you, Doc. I was pointing at the gentleman standing behind you."

I looked around, and there was this old guy, the one jealous of my farming operation, standing right behind me. The funny thing about it though was that John Freeman, Sr., the Black man who looked after his farm, was standing in front of me. When the bid started going up, John started looking uncomfortable. I didn't know what the hell was going on.

After the auction was over, John came over to me and said, "Doc, I thought there was something fishy going on. I don't know how come my boss paid all that money for that mule."

I knew what was going on. I said, "After all, John, that was a good mule, and that farmer knows what he's doing. I guess he did what was right."

I was doing fairly well with my farming operation and was making a little money—however, not much. I was spending far too much due to my ignorance of farming operations in general. Anyway, I knew another white man who was interested in timber and real estate. He'd buy a farm with a lot of timber on it, sell the timber at a profit, then sell the farm and make a little more profit. He had several farms for sale at all times. He was having medical problems and had gone to various area physicians. He didn't improve under their treatments. He came to me as a last resort. I checked his history, examined him, and found he had far-advanced diabetes. He stated that the other physicians had not recognized his symptoms as being diabetes. The man was in so much trouble that I referred him to Duke Hospital for treatment. His diabetic symptoms improved, and he came back, expressing his gratitude.

This gentleman was so grateful that he said, "Now, Doc, I have a good farm for sale, and I want you to buy it. I ain't going to sell you nothing bad."

About a year later he came to me again and quoted me a good price, so I went out to look at it. With Travis taking care of my regular farm operation, I decided to take it on. My jealous neighboring farmer became even more jealous. There was a tenant living on the farm I bought.

I asked the man I bought the farm from, "What about this fellow?" He replied, "Oh, he's all right. Cephus is a good farmer."

I decided to keep him on the farm. It turned out that he wasn't the man for me. He couldn't take proper care of my farming equipment and was extremely dishonest. Once I had him cutting some wood which I was selling. During the first winter, when the farming operation was slow, I had him cutting the wood and stacking it in cords. I went out with a friend of mine to inspect the work Cephus had done. Cephus had several cords of wood cut and stacked. However, when I examined the wood, I found that each piece was only three feet in length. My friend reminded me that the standard length for cord wood was four feet. I pointed this out to Cephus, and he admitted he had cheated me. When I paid him, I took into consideration that each piece of wood was one foot shorter. Cephus reluctantly agreed to my payment terms. However, he told my friend that he didn't have any damn business coming out there reminding me of anything. That ended my wood cutting with Cephus.

***

I had gone into the hog business. I took some out to Cephus for him to raise with the understanding that he'd receive five percent of the gross sale. The hogs were coming along nicely. About the middle of May, the corn I'd raised to feed the hogs gave out, and I was obliged to buy enough feed to last until the hogs matured enough for sale. Here is where the trouble occurred.

One day, I went out to the farm to find two of my hogs, which were about ready for sale, butchered and hanging up. Cephus was not at home, so I asked his wife why he had butchered the hogs. She said the hogs had choked to death on the feed. The hogs were not discolored as they should have been by choking to death. There was someone with me, so we took the hogs down and took them to town to the freezer plant to be examined by the Department of Agriculture inspector. He stated that if the hogs had choked to death, they would have been discolored from a lack of oxygen in the bloodstream. I immediately sold the hogs to the processing plant.

Cephus came in all upset about it. He asked what I had done with the hogs, and I told him. He insisted that they had choked to death. I told him that they had not and proceeded to give him five percent of the money I received from the processing plant. After paying him, I asked him to get off my farm right away. He was a very belligerent fellow and went around threatening me and everyone else involved with the affair. I was not afraid, however.

I soon found another tenant for that farm. Everything was going along fine. I increased my hog operation by buying some Hampshire gilts (young female pigs). From time to time, hog breeders replaced their brood sows with gilts to keep up the production. I used purebred Hampshire gilts with a Duroc boar (male hog). I found that crossbreeding Hampshires with Durocs produced a better, leaner hog than the purebred types.

About five years into the breeding process I felt my existing boar was getting too old for breeding, so I decided to replace him with a younger Duroc boar. Hog cholera was prevalent in the area at the time. It was necessary to vaccinate the new boar with a live virus vaccine before turning him loose with my breeding sows. Using the live virus vaccine to immunize the boar made it necessary to keep him apart from the rest of the herd for a time so the vaccine could get in his system. Otherwise, he would infect the remainder of the herd.

I kept him apart for a time but guess what happened? The old boar broke in on the new one, and they fought. Before we knew it, the new boar was in with the rest of the herd and had infected the entire herd with cholera. My hogs started dropping off—eight or ten a day. I called the County Extension Agent who notified the State Health Department. They sent an inspector to check, and I was told that I would have to slaughter and deeply bury the entire herd.

All the land walked on by the hogs would have to be plowed deeply and left free of any living creatures for at least two years. The State Department of Agriculture did reimburse me fifty percent of the value of the hog herd. That put a temporary stop to my hog operation.

After a two-year hiatus, I went back into business. I bought a group of Hampshire gilts and a purebred Duroc boar, since it appeared that that crossbreed of animal raised for meat developed faster than any others. From then on, my hog-raising project progressed without further setbacks until terminating the program after Travis left my farm.

One day I had the entire family in the car, traveling along Granville Street. There was a truck going along ahead of us fully loaded with hogs bound for the market. Suddenly, a pig had fell from the truck. I was unable to alert the truck driver, and he didn't return to the scene. I yelled to Bro, "Bro, jump out, grab that pig, and bring it here." He brought the pig to the car. That thing was stinking. We took him out to the farm. One of my sows had delivered a litter of ten pigs, and I didn't know whether she would accept this new one.

However, I cautiously eased the pig down among the others. With one or two grunts, the new pig was accepted. He saw a teat and started feeding. The newborn pig, whom we called "Granville," was male. As he developed, we did not have him castrated as we had all the other male pigs. Consequently, Granville matured into a well-developed boar hog. We kept him on the farm, and when he grew older, I could not bring myself to sell him for lard. About ten years later he died of old age on the farm.

**

Whenever we planted a crop with proper fertilization and cultivation, the crops were fine through May and June. However, beginning the first part of July, the crops began wilting in the field despite anything we tried. In the end, the yield was depressed. It was at that juncture that I called Rad Bailey, the Soil Conservation Agent. I explained the situation, and he agreed to come and take a look. We walked all over the farm. He had an augur with him, and at intervals he would stop and bore a hole in the ground for a soil sample. He'd rub the soil in his hands, walk a little farther along, stop, and do the same thing again, taking samples from several depths. After walking over the farm, we sat under a tree, and I asked, "Mr. Bailey, what do you think about this farm?"

He said, "Doc, you want me to tell you the truth?"

"That's what I asked you for."

He said, "This farm isn't worth a damn. The subsoil is pure sand. There's about six inches of topsoil on top of it. When you planted the crops, you used fertilizer and tilled as you should have, and everything went along fine until about the first of July when the weather became very dry. All the moisture evaporated or was drawn up from the soil by the plants. Consequently, the crops withered in the field from lack of nutrients."

"That sounds pretty bad to me. Now, what should I do?"

He said, "Plant another crop next year. Till it properly, put on plenty of fertilizer, then sell this damn farm about the middle of June."

I said, "I know you know what you're talking about, and that's exactly what I'm going to do."

I told no one about this incident and followed Rad Bailey's advice the next year. I had very good stands of corn, peanuts, and tobacco. I let the word out that I was going to sell the farm because it was too far removed from my other farming operation. I wanted my good, jealous fellow farmer to hear it. Sure enough, he came to me right away. He said, "I understand you're going to sell that farm."

"I'm thinking about it."

My heart was pounding in my chest when I told that lie.

He said, "I have land next to this farm, and I'd like us to swap land because my other farming operation is close to this farm."

"No, I've decided not to sell the farm. I'm going to keep it."

He said, "Now, Doc, think about this thing."

The land he had adjacent to mine was very low. In fact, it badly needed drainage. The crops planted there never did very well. The only thing the land needed was better drainage. I knew that if I acquired it and put in proper drainage ditches, I would have better crops than I had before.

He came to me again. "Doc, I understand that you're still thinking of selling that land."

"No, I've thought better of it. I'm not selling the land." My heart was jumping, and I thought, "I'm going to get this sucker right here."

It was mid-June when he finally came again. He said, "This is the last time I'm going to ask you about this, but are you still saying that you're not going to sell the land?"

I said, "Well, I'll tell you what we'll do. There's about the same acreage in my land that there is in the land you've got out there that stays wet all the time. Suppose we swap?"

He was elated but tried to appear calm and said, "Well, that's good. We'll swap that land."

"Wait a minute now," I said. "The land I want to get from you requires a lot of drainage. I just couldn't swap farm for farm because it's going to cost me to put the drainage in. I'll swap the land if you'll give me five thousand dollars in addition to the farm."

He hemmed and hawed but finally agreed to it. The transaction was made the next day because time was short, and I knew what was going to happen to the farm he was getting. He was satisfied that everything was going along fine. I was happy, knowing I had made the trade.

I had another state man come to survey the new property and determine the sites for the required ditches. When the drainage crew pulled in their bulldozer, there was so much moisture in the ground that the bulldozer sank to the top of the caterpillar treads. We had to wait two months for the land to dry out so the stalled caterpillar could be moved. In the meantime, the crops deteriorated on the farm I sold. After establishment of proper drainage on the farm I acquired, the crops came out beautifully.

***

My wife Helen had gone through all the ups and downs with me in my farming projects. To tell the truth, she knew more about it than I did. When I hired a farmer to take over management of my farm, she took over management of the finances. Everything went along smoothly for a while. The farm manager saw to it that everything was planted. When time came to harvest tobacco, the process was not going fast enough to suit me. Ripe tobacco was remaining in the field too long. I went out one day to check on things. I saw my tenant with my tractor and a load of tobacco, taking it to the barn. I stopped him. "Hey, fellow, you're getting my tobacco after all, aren't you?"

He said, "No, sir. This is not your tobacco. This is the boss man's tobacco." "Who in the hell are you talking about? I own the farm."

He said, "The boss man is the man you got running the farm."

My manager was using my tobacco barns to cure his tobacco and leaving mine to burn up in the field. I looked that sucker up right away and said, "Look here, Bro. You've got to change your way of doing. You're using my tractor and my barns to house your tobacco and leaving my tobacco in the field to burn up."

After that exchange, I checked on him every day and looked after my tobacco to make sure it was being cured on time. From that time on, I saw that he was a little crooked. He was taking care of his farming operations and leaving mine until after finishing his. We checked on him daily until the end of the year. Helen recorded all the transactions during the year. When time came to settle up, he began questioning her figures. However, we were able to prove him wrong.

He finally said, "Well, Doc, I've enjoyed working with you. I'll work your farm again next year but not if your wife is going to handle the finances." I thanked him but told him I'd decided to turn management of my farm over to one of the banks specializing in that type of service. I went through another year with the bank managing the farm, and that arrangement also proved unsatisfactory. The farm manager did not check on the tenants to see if they had done the work properly.

I decided to sell my farm equipment, hogs, and cattle and rent the farm out on a yearly basis. I leased my property to Russell Harris, a Black farmer who was very successful in his farming activities. In addition to his own farm, he leased about five hundred acres of my land. He had heavy equipment and was able to make money even with the high cost of production. He produced hogs and used what we call hog parlors, where a large number of sows are kept in production.

By that time, my grandchildren who lived in Raleigh were being city-raised, so I took them out to see Mr. Harris's farm setup and hog parlors. Although it's a very smelly operation, they were able to see about fourteen sows with young pigs in all stages of growth. I was very proud of the progress Mr. Harris was making and assured him that I'd be glad to cooperate with him as long as he wanted to use my farm.

In addition to my farming operation, I had an on-going project of raising timber. The timber buyers bought the standing timber and removed it from the property. I then replanted the harvested areas with seedling pine trees. I was very happy to let things go on as they did and finally just rent it out. After all, I found out that I was a much better physician than I was a farmer. And everything turned out all right.

CHAPTER 22

OUR SWIMMING POOL

One day I was driving along with my daughter, Helen, who was young at the time. We passed by the municipal swimming pool and saw the white kids swimming and having a big time. "Oh, Daddy," she said, "look at those children swimming. Can we please watch them for a little while?"

"Okay." We sat and watched the children swimming for about fifteen minutes, then drove on.

About two or three days later, Helen said, "Daddy, I'd like for you to take me back to see the children swimming again."

I took her, and again we sat and watched them swimming for a while.

Helen turned to me this time and said, "I want to swim. Can I go over there and swim?"

"Helen, I'm going to have to tell you the facts of life," I began. "White children and colored children are not allowed to swim together."

"Why?"

"You'll understand why when you are older, but you're just not allowed to swim together. You will never be able to come up here and swim in this pool."

"Well, I want to swim, and if I can't swim here, I want you to build me a swimming pool," she said.

I thought, "Uh oh! I'm in trouble now!"

"Okay, if you want a swimming pool, then I will have to build you one," I agreed.

"Hooray, hooray! Daddy's going to build me a pool." Helen was so happy.

I didn't have the money to build a pool at that time. However, it occurred to me that I could build a pool at our big farm in the country. So, I went home, talked it over with my wife, and we drove out to the farm to decide where to build the pool. The area we chose was undeveloped, full of trees, bushes, and weeds. I hired a bulldozer driver to clean up an area of about five acres.

I decided to build the pool myself. I knew I would need lumber for the forms and would need concrete to pour into them. We outlined a section sixteen feet wide and thirty-two feet long. I used a tractor and an earth-moving scoop to excavate the site. We looked at the excavation and decided that because we were building the pool ourselves, we shouldn't settle for such a short one. We ended up building our pool about thirty feet wide and sixty feet long.

I traded some of my big pine trees to a lumber company for enough lumber to build the forms for the sides of the pool. Because I knew nothing about building a pool, I hired the services of a bricklayer and a plasterer.

We poured concrete for the sides before pouring the floor. That was a big mistake. The floor and sides should have been poured at the same time. Since they were poured at different times, a seam was left between the sides and bottom which gave us some trouble later on. I had one of the local men dig three shallow wells in order to be able to fill the pool. To my dismay, I found that the water was contaminated and discolored.

So, I had to get a certified well-digger to come and dig a well one hundred thirteen feet deep. The water from the deep well was very clear. Sometime after we began using the water, white sand and bits of shell were pumped with the water to the surface. The sand and shell fragments settled to the bottom of the pool. At that point, I decided to build two settling partitions in the pool before allowing the water to run in. That arrangement appeared satisfactory. From that time on the water in the pool was clear.

Our daughter, Carol, was about one year old when the pool was finished. One day, she was walking around the shallow end when she missed her footing and fell into the water. I pulled her out, wiped her face, and put her back into the pool. I knew full well that if I didn't put her back in, she might develop a fear of the water, which would defeat my purposes for building the pool.

I built a shelter at one end of the pool so we could have a place to escape the rain whenever a storm occurred. During the first summer after the pool was finished, there was a severe storm while we were swimming. The first thing I did was get everyone out of the water and under the shelter. We were standing under the shelter when lightning struck a tree near the pool area. Those of us standing under the shelter felt a shock run through our feet. Helen, Jr., was sitting near an electrical outlet and felt a shock run through her back. We decided then and there that we needed more of a shelter.

The next step was building a cottage for protection from the storms and to facilitate our enjoyment of the pool itself. We began planning the building. From a shelter it evolved into a patio with broken tile flooring, a large kitchen that could serve as a dining area, and a recreation room along with showers and storage facilities. We added a fireplace, and a built-in bar to keep refreshments for friends who enjoyed something stronger than water or Coca-Cola.

The year after finishing the cottage, we came up with the idea of having a Fourth of July celebration with a barbecue. We invited about fifty of our friends. I had hogs and cattle on the farm at that time, so it was easy for me to arrange for barbecued pork and T-bone steaks without putting a strain on my wallet. Everyone enjoyed the outing and begged us to repeat the event the following year.

The next year we had another barbecue and invited a hundred of our friends and had a really good time. The third year we invited more than one hundred fifty friends. Everyone seemed to enjoy themselves—that is, everyone except us. It worked the heck out of us, so we enjoyed entertaining less and less.

One of our guests got carried away on one occasion, imbibing a whole fifth of Scotch. He became very loquacious and asked if I was going to put any bedrooms in my cottage. I told him I'd been thinking about it. He said, "Good. When you do, just let me know, and I'll come and spend a few weeks." That ended my thoughts on adding bedrooms. We did, however, buy sleeping bags for the children and a roll-away bed for us so that our family could spend a few nights out there. I bought a hammock and hung it between two trees so I could snooze after eating dinner at the cottage. Everything went along merrily. The children learned to swim, and we all enjoyed our outings at the pool and cottage.

Some of my friends began sending their children off in the summer to Camp Atwater in Pennsylvania. Helen and Milton stated that they would like to go to camp also. We decided to send them for two weeks. The children were ready to go until the time came for them to leave. Milton then decided he wanted to stay home, but I made him go anyway. Before they left for camp, their mother gave them some paper and stamped envelopes addressed to us so they could write home whenever they wanted to tell us anything.

Milton was most unhappy at camp. He wrote us a letter saying, "Dear Mother and Daddy, I don't like this place. Come and get me. Don't send nothing. Just come and get me." We made up our minds to let him stay until the end of the two-week period. On the day they were supposed to return home, I sent someone to meet the train and bring them out to the pool. When they arrived, Milton gave me some angry glances, threw some blue ribbons at me, pulled off his clothes, and jumped into the pool. After swimming all he wanted, he got out of the water.

I said, "Bro, what was it that you didn't like about Camp Atwater?"

"Daddy, they didn't have a swimming pool like this. We had to swim in the lake where the leeches were, and they almost ate me up. The nights were cold, and we didn't have enough cover," he continued. "The food was bad. All we had was peanut butter at bedtime. I don't want to ever go to another camp. Never, no more."

We used the pool every summer until the children left to go to their boarding school in Putney, Vermont. With the children gone, our interest in the pool waned. The seam in the bottom of the pool began giving us some trouble about that time. Groundwater seeped into the pool through the seam when it was empty, and when it was full, pool water seeped into the ground. We decided to abandon the pool. My wife Helen then had a pool built in our backyard behind our home in Tarboro.

CHAPTER 23

SUCCESS STORIES

My brother, John, was living and operating a small grocery store in Newellton, Louisiana. He and his wife, Ruby, had one child named Charles Richard Quigless. At that time, the school situation in Louisiana was just about the same as it was in Mississippi and North Carolina—separate but unequal. Charles had reached the fourth-grade level when his parents decided to send him to Natchez, Mississippi, because the schools were a little better. He attended school in Natchez until he finished the eighth grade.

Ruby and John discussed the matter of bringing Charles to North Carolina to be admitted to high school. I had been in North Carolina about twelve years and knew the state school situation well. My wife Helen was able to use her connections in D.C. to arrange for Charles to attend a high school there, and to reside with Helen's parents. Charles was a teenager, and I felt that this would be an opportune time for him to get out and get some experience in relationships with people. If he should get a job which would place him in contact with the public, it would teach him how to relate to people and at the same time help him make some extra money during the summer months.

Charlie Brown was a local young man who worked at a restaurant in Virginia Beach for the summer to make enough money to help him through college. Tarboro is not so far removed from that portion of Virginia Beach where a lot of recreational facilities and vacation spots are located on the Atlantic coast. Several teenage boys and young men in this area usually went there for the summer and worked in restaurants as waiters, cooks, busboys, and the like.

I contacted Charlie and asked him to take Charles to Virginia Beach. He agreed to do so. Charlie had been working at the same resort for several years and had become an excellent waiter. He took Charles along with him. The lady who operated the facility was very much interested in the students and did all she could to help them along. She insisted that he familiarize himself not only with the food service, but with food preparation procedures as well. Accordingly, she started Charles in the kitchen as a kitchen helper. His duties were to peel potatoes, prepare fish, and generally assist the cooks in whatever they wanted him to do.

After four weeks, Charles was upgraded to the status of waiter. He did not make much money that year. However, he gained a lot of valuable experience. The next summer, he went to Virginia Beach and worked full-time as a waiter. From the second summer on, he continued to fill that position. Charles told me that he wouldn't take anything for the experience he gained during his summers at Virginia Beach. He learned to get along with and please people. I don't care what you go into—that public relations thing is something to be desired.

After finishing high school in Washington, D.C., he enrolled at the University of Illinois as a pre-dental student. He formed a lasting relationship with a pre-med student named Leslie Bond. Leslie was the son of the physician, Dr. Bond, who had encouraged me to study medicine at Alcorn College.

Charles was later drafted into the Army and served in the combat area of the South Pacific. He did not return to the University of Illinois following his army stint. Instead, he went to Southern

University in Baton Rouge, Louisiana, where he finished his pre-dental training and then went to Howard University for his dental training. Following his graduation from dental school, he was able to obtain an internship at the Guggenheim dental facility in New York City.

That same year, I attended my interns' alumni meeting at Homer G. Phillips Hospital in Missouri where I met my old friend, Dr. Brooks, who was the head of the dental department at that hospital. Dr. Brooks trained two dental interns each year. When I informed him that Charles was going to Guggenheim, he insisted that Charles become one of his dental interns. That was a very lucky move for Charles because he served his internship at Homer G. Phillips and went into a residency for three years.

At the end of that time, Dr. Brooks was about ready to retire and was able to recommend Charles as his replacement. Charles remained as head of the dental clinic in St. Louis and also had a private practice until his retirement.

***

In 1938, a Black teacher living about twenty miles from Tarboro noted the development of a firm enlargement in her lower abdomen. She went to a physician who examined her, and then informed her that she had a large fibroid tumor of the uterus and advised surgery. The lady continued teaching for several months and suddenly developed vaginal bleeding. The poor, misguided doctor examined her and told her that the vaginal bleeding was coming from the tumor and advised her to go to the hospital for removal of her uterus.

She was being transported to Chapel Hill by ambulance when, of all things, she developed labor pains. A male child was delivered in the ambulance. The teacher was not married and was very embarrassed by the incident. She didn't know what to do but had the presence of mind to have the driver stop the ambulance and gave the newborn baby to the first woman she saw. The ambulance then proceeded to Rocky Mount, where she was taken to the hospital.

The woman to whom she had given the baby was married to a wino. The foster mother did what she could for the child, whom she had named Elijah. However, she and her husband were share-croppers and had very meager means. When Elijah turned six years old, he was enrolled in school. He loved to go to school, but when he turned ten, the wino and his wife took him out and made him pick cotton. Elijah resented being removed from school, but what could he do? At that time the colored county schools closed for about two months during cotton-picking time (more separate but unequal rights). By the time Elijah was twelve, he was taken out of school and given a full-time farm job.

I met Elijah when he was about sixteen years old. His parents had moved to town, and he was looking around for odd jobs. That's when Elijah came to me. I needed someone to run errands during the afternoon and do a little cleaning up around the hospital, so I hired him. Piece by piece, I learned his story.

Elijah was very bitter toward his foster father. He realized, however, that his foster mother had done all she could to help him along, even to the extent that she would be beaten by her wino husband whenever she remonstrated with him and begged him to let Elijah go back to school. I encouraged him to go back and re-enter school. Here he was, now seventeen, and he had only finished the fifth grade, just as I had done in Mississippi. He hated the idea of going back to school and being in classes with kids much younger than he was. However, he swallowed his pride and did it. During the year he re-entered school, his foster parents' house burned to the ground. He had to withdraw from school and help his foster mother because his wino father had deserted them. Elijah finally gave up the idea of ever going back to school.

When Elijah was around nineteen, he got a job with an electrical company, repairing power lines. He remained with the company for several years and learned the craft very well. He was soon upgraded to a crew that installed and maintained high voltage power lines. His job carried him away from Tarboro.

When I saw Elijah again it was about twelve years later. He had married a teacher in one of the nearby towns and had a fine family. Despite his upbringing, he developed into a fine, upstanding citizen. He said, "Dr. Quigless, you did everything you could to help me. I shall be eternally grateful to you. I'll see to it that my children have the opportunities that I missed." What a tragic story, but what a nice, happy ending.

***

Black physicians had no chance to study the advances in medical techniques except through their own scientific societies, such as the Old North State Medical Society and the National Medical Association. We realized that medicine was changing from day to day, and we further realized that some changes were on the way, such as Medicare and Medicaid, and that if we were not affiliated with organized medicine, we would be unable to participate and practice medicine as it would be practiced in the foreseeable future. What I mean by "organized medicine" is that we had to be members of the NC Medical Society. I had once attended a NC Medical Society meeting in Wilson and had to wait outside the hotel until the white doctors finished their meal. That method of obtaining information was entirely unacceptable to me.

Those problems were discussed in the Old North State Medical Society meetings, and we were determined to change the conditions, whatever price it might entail. We decided to apply for membership in the all-white NC Medical Society. Our applications were answered by the secretary of the Society who spelled out the rules and regulations concerning membership: The applicants had to be graduates of a Class A medical school; must be licensed by the NC Board of Medical Examiners; and thirdly, there was a "white only" clause.

All of us were graduates of Class A medical schools, all licensed by the NC Board of Medical Examiners, but none of us could get by with the "white only" clause. We all had white physicians and surgeons as friends, but this group of white physicians was resistant to change.

Our first order of business was to try and have that "white only" clause eliminated. In order to accomplish this, we enlisted the aid of our white friends who stood before the annual meeting of the NC Medical Society and insisted that the clause be eliminated. We then requested a meeting with a committee from the Society. We had a frank discussion with the Society's committee whom we questioned, "Why is it that we cannot be admitted to the NC Medical Society?"

Their answers were vague, enlightening, and somewhat frivolous. One committee member stated that he had no idea where we could meet as a desegregated group. Another said that there were social events, and he did not know what would happen if a Black doctor sat beside his wife to eat dinner. He said he knew quite well that he couldn't stand it if a Black doctor asked his wife or daughter to dance. Another related an experience of attending a meeting in a northern state. He said that Black doctors were included in the membership of the Society, and at one of the dances, one of the Black doctors brought his wife, children, and a big picnic basket. In between dances, he said they sat at the table and munched cake, barbecue, and collard greens. We knew that was a lie.

Finally, we were offered a "scientific membership." That is, we would be allowed to attend the scientific meetings. We would not, however, be allowed to participate in the social activities. Just about all of us felt that scientific stipulation represented a humiliating, stigmatizing, stinking, repulsive insult inasmuch as we felt our wives, sisters, and children were due the same respect and consideration as any other doctors' wives, children, and relatives should have.

Believe it or not, two Black physicians in another part of the state accepted the scientific membership! When we learned of it, we did everything except kick their tails all over North Carolina. We sent word to the NC Medical Society that we could not accept that type of membership. This fight went on for two more years. In fact, the fight was on until the Hill-Burton Bill was passed, allocating monies to build and upgrade the hospitals in this country. One stipulation was that any physician in good standing would be allowed to practice in the hospitals. It was then that the barriers fell, and we were admitted full membership in the NC Medical Society.

We were grateful to our white colleagues who had exposed themselves to vilification and ridicule because of their efforts to help us obtain the recognition that we so badly needed.

CHAPTER 24

INTEGRATION

It was just about that time when Blacks throughout the nation were voicing their discontent with the status quo. Martin Luther King, Jr., had come forward with his non-violent stand for complete and total integration. He had been jailed, kicked, beaten, and shot, but had not yet been murdered. The fever for total integration had enveloped the entire land. The students from AT&T had sat down in a drug store in Greensboro and demanded service. The exponents of non-violence had made their point. However, some of the demonstrators were not so non-violent.

We did not seem to be making much headway in Tarboro at that time. There were marches and demonstrations in surrounding towns, however. The demonstrations in Williamston, North Carolina, brought violent reactions on both sides. Everyone was wondering just what was going to happen in Tarboro.

Although interracial committees were being formed throughout the southern states, no such step had been taken in Tarboro. One summer, when our Black college students returned to Tarboro, they decided to take things into their own hands and conduct a sit-in demonstration in one of the restaurants on Main Street. They were instructed to be non-violent and to make their demands known to the proprietor but to leave when they were threatened with arrest or jail. My son, Milton, Jr., was one of the demonstrators. After sitting down in the restaurant, the waitress demanded, "What are you doing in here? What do you want?"

They said, "We came here to be served."

"Do you know that it is against the law to serve colored people in here?" she asked. "You can't eat here."

One of the young fellows, Dr. Ray's son, reached over to pick up a glass of water that had been placed on the counter. The waitress snatched the glass out of his hand. They all laughed. There was some give-and-take between the students, the waitress, and the proprietor. They were finally told that if they didn't leave, they would be arrested.

The proprietor called Harry Alderman, Tarboro's Chief of Police. Harry came in and talked to the students. He said, "You know we can't let you eat in here, and you know it's against the law."

Bro spoke up, saying, "The law is wrong."

Chief Alderman did not know Bro because he had been to school out of town. He turned to Bro and said, "Who are you anyway? What are you doing in here? Are you one of those outside agitators?"

Bro said, "No sir, I live here. I was born and raised in Tarboro."

"Who are your people?" he questioned.

"It doesn't make any difference who my people are," Bro said. "My daddy pays taxes, is a law-abiding citizen, and I don't see any reason why I can't be allowed to eat here."

Chief Alderman repeated, "It's against the law."

"The law is wrong," Bro said again.

They all—Chief Alderman, the students, the waitress, and the proprietor—argued back and forth in a friendly manner. The students were finally told that if they didn't leave, they would be arrested. At that juncture, they got up and started walking out.

Chief Alderman asked Bro again, "Who are you anyway?"

Bro then told him who he was. You know one thing? Bro and

Harry Alderman are now the best of friends. Nobody wanted a confrontation like they were having in places such as Williamston, Greenville, and surrounding towns. After the sit-in demonstration, an interracial committee was formed, chaired by Dr. Howard S. Hussey. I don't remember the other white members of the committee, but Dr. Ray, Nat Gray, Mrs. Beatrice Garrett, Mrs. Pearl Bennett, and I were designated as the Black members. We discussed our grievances during the first meeting.

First of all, they had segregated tax-listing books, movies, and eating establishments. Whenever a tent show came to town, it, too, was segregated. Even at the courthouse, all the Blacks sat on the left side of the aisle and the whites, on the right. These and other segregated policies were related to the committee. There were, of course, segregated schools—separate but unequal. We did have a bus line in Tarboro, but, true to form, the Black riders had to be seated at the back. There were no toilet facilities in any public places for Blacks.

In one of our leading department stores, a colored lady and her little daughter were in the store making some purchases when the little girl told her mother that she had to use the restroom. Her mother asked the clerk the way to the restroom facilities. The clerk stated that they did not have restroom facilities for coloreds. "My little girl has to go, and she has to go right now," the mother pleaded.

"I am sorry," the clerk said, "but we don't have any place for you."

The mother turned around and said to her little girl, "Put it right down there in the aisle." The little girl did her "number two" in the middle of the aisle. The mother was threatened with arrest, but nothing came of it.

Blacks were not allowed to try on merchandise in the stores to see if the clothes would fit. However, they were welcome to buy the merchandise in the stores.

Another incident happened in Scotland Neck when a Black man was on the street and felt the urge to urinate. There were no toilet facilities anywhere around, so he had to go into an alley to relieve himself. A white woman saw him and screamed. He was arrested and given a jail term for indecent exposure!

It goes without saying that the hospitals were segregated. There were white wards and colored wards. The linen was marked "colored ward," and most of it was patched.

At the second meeting of Tarboro's interracial committee, the owner of the restaurant singled out for the demonstration spoke to us, saying that he did not mind serving colored people. However, he knew that if he ever did serve the colored people in his restaurant, he would be boycotted by the whites. At that time the Civil Rights Bill was being debated in Congress. The white merchants gave us their solemn promise that "the day the Civil Rights Law passes, we will desegregate everything."

On the day that the law passed, it was broadcast on the radio at 10 a.m. When I left my office and drove up Main Street, I passed the movie theater. Heretofore, if a Black person wanted to see a movie, he had to climb the stairs to the balcony. There was a side door with a sign that read, "Colored Balcony." In fact, a Black person could not buy a ticket for the movie in the foyer of the theater. He had to buy his ticket in a little cubbyhole at the steps to the colored balcony.

The idea of ascending to the colored balcony was so repulsive to me that I had only seen about six movies in that theater, and those six were movies in which colored stars performed. On that day, I noticed that a piece of tape had been placed over the "Colored" portion of the sign at the side door.

Signs of segregation vanished in Tarboro. When I had first arrived in Tarboro, I found that there was a nucleus of good people in this town. The good white people knew that the Black man was being treated unfairly. However, because of peer pressure, they did not have the courage to stand up for the Black man. After passage of the law, the early compliance of the white citizenry verified my first impressions of white people in this area. Now I must say that I do not mean that everybody complied. We had rebels, rednecks, turkey necks, or whatever you call them, back then, and we still have some of them left today. The only thing that will change their minds is a funeral at which a redneck is the guest of honor.

There was a die-hard rebel, a segregationist, or whatever you want to call him, who took advantage of Blacks at every turn. But when the old so-and-so died, he had a standing request that Black pallbearers carry him to his grave. I wondered why in hell he thought he could fool the Almighty God by making that acquiescence, and only making it after he was dead. I think Fats Waller had that type of person in mind when he was singing the song, "I'll be Glad When You're Dead, You Rascal, You."

I was told of another incident that happened not too many years ago. One white man of considerable means lived in this area and was advised that he would have to have a major operation. He was further advised that he would probably need three or four blood donors. By that time, a blood bank had been set up by the Red Cross, and blood donors, regardless of race, were welcome to donate blood. This particular man wanted to be sure that he would not be infused with any Negro blood, so when he went to

Richmond for his operation, he took along several white "gentle-men" who had the same blood type, thereby making sure that he would not be given any Negro blood. You know, many white people felt that Negro blood was more powerful than white blood. It was the usual conception that one drop of Negro blood would make a white man Black. However, on the other hand, there was never the thought that even ten gallons of a white man's blood would make a Black man white!

Yes, times changed in Tarboro, and that is the one main reason I am writing this book in such detail. Kids growing up in our community should know these things. Blacks should know just what it took to get them to the place where they can hold their heads up and walk like men and women. Whites should know the hardships that Blacks suffered to get to where we are at this time. When I talk to white kids, they are amazed to hear these details.

I am reminded here of a verse in the Negro national hymn composed by J. Rosman Johnson and James Weldon Johnson:

Stony the road we trod, Bitter the chast'ning rod
Felt in the days when hope unborn had died.
Yet with a steady beat, Have not our weary feet
Come to the place for which our fathers sighed.
We have come over a way that with tears have been watered.
We have come, treading our path thro'
the blood of the slaughtered.
Out of the gloomy past, Till now we stand at last
Where the white gleam of our bright star is cast.

CHAPTER 25

FAMILY LIFE

My children were growing up during all this furor. Milton, Jr., was my constant companion. At an early age, he loved fishing as much as I did. Bro was also interested in farming and was on the farm, running around every chance he had. He was always a sleepyhead, fast asleep in bed every night by 8 p.m., except for the nights before we made a trip to the coast. We would leave Tarboro between 2 and 3 a.m., drive to Morehead City or Sneed's Ferry where we chartered a boat, and troll for King Mackerel or go deep sea fishing at the continental shelf for Red Snapper.

On one trip, we chartered a fishing boat for a day of trolling in an effort to bring in some King Mackerel. My brother-in-law and his wife were visiting us from Buffalo, New York, and went with us. After we had been trolling for about three hours, his wife became tired and decided to take a short nap. She turned her fishing rod over to Bro, who was about eight years of age at that time. In about five minutes, he began yelling, "I got him. I got him. I don't know whether I can hold him, but I got him. I got him."

We rushed over to assist Bro, but we let him reel the fish in. When it was finally brought on board, it was about thirty-two inches long. Bro was out of his mind with joy. All of us were very proud that he was able to land the fish with a minimum of assistance. I had the King Mackerel mounted, and that fish was one of his proudest possessions.

As with Bro, Helen, Jr., also grew up very nicely. She took piano lessons, although she was more interested in dance than anything else. I enjoyed their presence. However, I knew the time would come when they would leave us in order to get the education we wanted for them.

My wife Helen's mother died when she was quite young, leaving her, a sister, and two brothers to be raised by her father, Mr. Gordon. Mrs. Leona Boyd, a neighbor who lived adjacent to the Gordons came over and assisted him in preparing his children for school. She made sure they were properly dressed, fed, and everything else. Mrs. Boyd was not married and had a position in Government Services. She had adopted a little girl named Denise, who was very smart. Mrs. Boyd sent Denise to The Putney School in Putney, Vermont, where she was able to get a scholarship. Denise had done very well there and had also studied in France. In fact, she had done so well that she was awarded a Fulbright Scholarship.

So, when it came time for Helen and me to decide where to send our children to school, Mrs. Boyd recommended Helen, Jr., and Milton, Jr., for scholarships at The Putney School. They were interviewed and accepted. It was up to me to pay the balance left that was not covered by scholarships. Neither Helen nor Bro was very pleased with our decision to send them to Vermont. In fact, on our way up to the school, Bro kept saying, "Well, Dad and Mother dear, I thought you loved me, but I see you are shipping me off to Siberia. Putney School is so far up north that I am going to freeze to death."

A month after being admitted to Putney, they liked it a little better. Putney is a highly rated prep school, drawing students from New England states as well as New York and all over, including some foreign countries.

As a child, Helen was very much interested in music, and from the time she was about six years old until she left Tarboro for Putney, she was given music lessons by Mrs. Boddie. Mrs. Boddie found her to be a very adept pupil, and by the time she left Tarboro, she was well along in the study of classical music and continued music training at Putney. She was also very much interested in dance and maintained good grades at school.

I had a conference with her school advisor prior to her graduation, and that dear lady summed up her impression of Helen briefly by stating, "I consider Helen a very fine person. She is an adorable girl. However, I don't think she will ever become a serious student. You know, the best thing that she could possibly do after leaving here would be to get married, settle down, and have some children. I feel that she would make a lovely wife and mother, but I don't see much of a future for her as a serious student."

I thanked her profusely but had no doubt in my mind that Helen would become a serious student. When the time came for us to choose a college for the continuation of her education, we considered several schools in the New England area. We finally settled on Bard College, a small institution rated very highly, located at Annandale-on-the-Hudson. Helen was very happy there, selecting modern dance as a major and English as a minor.

While a senior at Putney, she began being plagued with joint pains that continued to increase in severity. She was examined by the school physician at Bard regarding her joint pains. After a brief period of hospitalization, he advised us that Helen was suffering from rheumatoid arthritis. That was a very depressing revelation since I knew that the disease was very hard to treat with any measure of success. During her second year at Bard, her bouts of joint pain became more frequent and her disability more pronounced. At the end of her sophomore year, we decided to transfer her from Bard, where the winters were so severe, to Fisk University in Nashville, where the climate was more suitable to a person suffering from arthritis. I wanted her to continue treatments at Meharry Medical College under the care of some of my classmates who had remained there at a financial sacrifice in order to train future Black physicians and surgeons.

Fisk University was founded by the American Missionary Association shortly after the Civil War. Those pioneers in education, who came from northern states to teach the Black youths, were not interested in just teaching the rudiments of reading, writing, and arithmetic. They were full of the spirit of confidence and knowledge that would enable them to further enlighten Blacks as to the arts and sciences.

Helen, Jr., continued to be plagued by arthritis through her two years at Fisk, where she graduated on the dean's list. She became more interested in literature and decided to further her education by working toward a master's degree in library science at Atlanta University in Atlanta, Georgia. She was elected president of her class shortly after enrolling and held the post until graduating. After earning her master's degree, she was able to obtain a position in Washington, D.C., at Federal City College, where she made her mark as a member of the library staff.

However, arthritis continued to plague her until she became totally disabled and had to withdraw from teaching and return home to Tarboro.

During my years of practice in Tarboro, I treated hundreds of arthritic patients with some success in the relief of their symptoms. However, Helen's arthritis was a type that could only be slowed but not completely halted. With her arthritis is an associated syndrome, which involves the atrophy and drying up of tear glands which furnish lubrication for the eyes. The result of this syndrome is that Helen had to undergo more than twenty corneal transplants to retain partial vision in both of her eyes.

Despite her suffering, pain, and disability, she maintained interest in literature and, I must say, had more spunk than any person I know. She was looking ahead to further horizons. I cannot help but recall the conversation I had with her doubtful advisor at The Putney School when I see how far she has come—and is still going.

As for Milton, I hated to see the day come when he would leave Tarboro. I recall several incidents during his early childhood that are outstanding even to this day. When he was about five years old, I bought him a Boxer puppy. That boy really enjoyed that puppy—they played together day in and day out. However, the dog got so strong that he was able to rough Bro up to the extent that he sometimes had to call for help, so I decided to confine Boxer in the pen. That was a sad day for Bro and Boxer. The dog was never vicious, but his playful antics were so overpowering that Bro and Boxer could only be together for a short while at a time.

The night before he left for Putney for the first time, Bro brought Boxer inside to share his room and bed. At Putney, Bro became interested in sculpture. His art teacher had a very definite influence on him, and as a result, he produced outstanding pieces under his tutelage. For one of his first projects, he fashioned Boxer in rosewood. He has kept this sculpture and featured it in his office many years later.

I never did try to talk Bro into studying medicine; it was something he decided on his own. He heard the phone ring one morning about 3 a.m., and I had to rush out on a labor case. He fell back to sleep soon after that. The next morning at breakfast, out of the clear blue sky, he said, "Daddy, I heard you go out last night, but I never heard you come back. You know, I want to be a doctor. But I don't think that I would like the idea of having to get up and go out any time of night, though."

"Well, Bro," I said, "let me tell you one thing. It doesn't make any difference. There are bound to be some distasteful elements involved in whatever you set out to do. For instance, you know Ms. Lena cooks and cleans house. She loves to cook but hates doing the dishes. In most anything you do, there will be parts of it you'll like and parts of it you won't. But just like dishwashing goes along with cooking, if you want to be a doctor, you'll enjoy helping people, and there'll be certain times when distasteful elements will be involved. You have got to take the bad along with the good. What do you think?"

"I guess I'll have to take the bad along with the good because I want to be a doctor just like you," he said.

I felt good inside, but I tried not to show it to him. From that time on, we both knew he would become a doctor if he ever got grown. Thanks to Mrs. Weston at Perry School and the dedicated teachers at the colored Tarboro Elementary, Bro was well prepared to continue his studies at Putney. While a student there, I encouraged him in all his interests, including sculpture. However, way down deep in my soul I said to myself, "Lord, I hope he doesn't become a sculptor!"

CHAPTER 26

ON TO EDGECOMBE GENERAL

J ust about that same time, my rate of occupancy in the Quigless Clinic- Hospital was nearly 90 percent. In the early spring, a representative of the NC Medical Care Commission inspected my facility and suggested some alterations and physical changes they felt should be made to the facility. The Commission was responsible for pointing out hazardous and/or unsafe conditions.

My hospital, built in 1946, had undergone a lot of changes in specifications aimed at ensuring the safety of patients. I had adequate exits and fire escapes on both floors, however, the inspector pointed out that I did not have a sprinkler system, that my second-floor halls were not wide enough to allow two stretchers to pass one another going in opposite directions, and that the doors to the second-floor rooms were not wide enough. I had to agree with the inspector on all those counts. To tell the truth, I had been reading accounts in newspapers of deaths occurring in hospitals and nursing homes because of inadequate fire safety measures.

I remember having two nightmares; in both, my hospital caught fire during the night and patients died. I awoke in a cold sweat and called the hospital to be assured that everything was secure and that I was just dreaming. After receiving the Commission's report, I thought about the cost that would be involved and decided I would not be able to comply with their suggestions. The Quigless Clinic-Hospital had served its purpose, putting me into the mainstream. It did not take long to decide that it would be better to close my facility and take a staff appointment at Edgecombe General Hospital. I could carry on my surgical activities at Edgecombe General and continue seeing patients in Tarboro. So, I wrote a letter to the Chief of Staff, advising him of my decision. Dr. Ed Roberson had championed my cause for years, and when he read the letter, he called, complimenting me, and saying that I should have been working at the hospital years ago.

As soon as I discharged the last hospital patient from my hospital, I went to the office of Lewis Ridgeway, administrator of Edgecombe General Hospital, who was my good friend. Lewis greeted me warmly, giving me keys to the doctors' private entrance and a plastic card used for opening the physicians' private parking lot, then took me on a tour of all the hospital departments, introducing me to the persons in charge as a full-time staff member with surgical, obstetrical, gynecological, and medical privileges. When he passed the callboard in the lobby, he insisted that I push the button that illuminated my name.

My first patient was a lady admitted to surgery for an appendectomy the very next day. I had no trouble at all. Patient number two was a lady with enlarged fibroids. This is when trouble began.

In my own hospital, I had my own operating team whom I had trained. They knew me so well that I wouldn't have to ask for the next instrument because they would know what I needed. The only general anesthetic we used was ether. I could tell from the reaction of the patient what stage of anesthesia he or she was under. As a rule, whenever things were proceeding properly, I would either be discussing the case or talking about anything else that came to mind—in other words, just talking. Whenever I found myself in trouble, I would stop talking. My scrub nurse was Mrs. Rebecca Rogers, who had retired from the Halifax County Health

Department. She would always start a little prayer that went like this: "Lord Jesus, come down and help this man, I pray..." You know, I came to depend on that little prayer. Whenever I got into trouble, Mrs. Rogers would say that prayer, and I would get to feeling better.

Well, here I was, about to perform surgery, and I did not know any of this surgery team. I had never seen them before, and they did not know me at all. I was performing a major operation and had to give directions to nurses whose names I did not know nor had time to learn. The operating room supervisor, Mrs. Duncan, assigned the surgery team. When she looked at me, I felt she was making an appraisal, comparing me with the other surgeons with whom she had worked. I may be wrong, but somehow, I thought she felt uncertain as to my ability.

I was not satisfied with my performance as a surgeon until I had been at Edgecombe General for about three months—until I had done a dozen hernias, three appendectomies, five or six uterine fibroids, and three Caesarean sections. I hope Mrs. Duncan will forgive my early appraisal of her because she turned out to be one of my best friends. After about six months at the hospital, I felt that all the surgical nurses had a warm spot for me. They all seemed eager to work with me. The entire time I did surgery at Edgecombe General I only had one fatality. I am sorry, but I must place the blame where it belongs.

The patient was a thirty-six-year-old Black female with a small fibroid tumor that caused profuse bleeding at each menstrual period. She had three little girls. The oldest child was waiting in the lobby when her mother was admitted for the operation. The child remembered me, and when I entered the lobby, she ran up to me, saying, "Dr. Quig, I know you are going to make my Mommy well."

"You bet I will," I assured her.

I proceeded to the operating room where the team was scrubbing up, waiting for the anesthetist to give us the word that the patient was ready. When word came, we draped the patient and took our places around the operating table. I asked the anesthetist again if the patient was ready, and she stated she was. I made a primary incision. To my horror, the blood that escaped was black, not red as it should have been. This indicated a complete lack of oxygen.

The entire operating team gasped. We immediately set about trying to revive the patient. However, in spite of our resuscitation efforts, the patient did not respond.

Why did it happen? In all probability, the anesthetist was thrown off guard by the patient's complexion. Her face was very dark, so the anesthetist was unable to notice skin changes, which are discernible with patients of lighter skin. It was clearly an anesthetic accident, but I had to face the patient's family. That was the most difficult task I have ever faced. Fortunately for me, the patient's children had left the hospital before surgery started, but I had to face the patient's husband and mother. The death of that patient was the only unpleasant experience I encountered during the time I was on staff at Edgecombe General Hospital.

Along about 1965, the Black physicians of Rocky Mount applied for privileges in the Rocky Mount hospitals. They sent a committee of two to the governing bodies of both hospitals in the city. The hospital boards recognized that changes were coming with the times and agreed to grant limited privileges to the two committee members representing the Black physicians. Privileges were granted in the fields of general medicine and obstetrics.

About a year-and-a-half after granting these privileges, the Rocky Mount hospitals saw fit to limit participation of the two

Black physicians by refusing, point-blank, to admit Black patients into the hospitals under the care of the Black physicians. I was greatly relieved, after passage of the Hill Burton Bill and the construction of the new Nash General Hospital, when the Black physicians were admitted and allowed to treat patients at the new hospital. But there was no Black physician in the area who had been trained in surgery.

It so happened that I met a native North Carolinian, Dr. Porter, who was a surgery resident of Homer G. Phillips Hospital. In the year prior to the opening of Nash General Hospital, I talked to Dr. Porter and learned that he was interested in returning to North Carolina to enter the practice of surgery. He was thinking of setting up practice in Dunn where a small general hospital was located. I immediately got in touch with Dr. F. Burnett Bryant, a Black general practitioner whose area of practice included Nash General and Rocky Mount and inquired as to whether they had any Black surgeons in mind to work at Nash General. He stated that he knew of no Black surgeons who were under consideration. I told him about Dr. Porter.

Dr. Bryant said, "Send him on to us. We need that man."

It didn't take me long to change Dr. Porter's mind about Dunn. He came to Rocky Mount, and with the support and encouragement of the Black physicians of the area, his surgical practice grew to the extent that he was busy at all times. I spoke to the governing board of Edgecombe General Hospital about Dr. Porter, and upon reviewing his application, he was extended privileges to practice surgery in that hospital as well. That was a good break for me as well as for Dr. Porter.

There were some types of surgery cases that I turned down and referred to others because the particular operation would require participation of one or more surgeons. Dr. Porter began assisting me, and I assisted him on patients admitted to Edgecombe General Hospital. We worked this way, not because I had anything against operating in conjunction with the area's white physicians, but because they were overworked already.

Now here was Dr. Porter in Rocky Mount with a full surgical practice while at the same time operating at Edgecombe General on his own and also assisting me there. In other words, within six months he was a very busy man. I happened to be in Rocky Mount one day about 6 p.m. and was passing by Dr. Porter's and three other Black physicians' offices. I walked in to see what was going on and found the waiting room full of patients. Dr. Porter was the only doctor present.

I said, "Who's going to see all of these patients?"

"I am," he said. "They are all my patients."

"Look here, bro," I said. "I know you have a full-time surgical schedule, doing two or three surgical procedures every day, so when in hell do you have time to see patients at this time of day? And more importantly, why do you do it?"

He said, "Well, Quig, these are Medicare/Medicaid patients. The other doctors are too busy and don't have time to see them. So, I just took it upon myself to take care of them. I feel it's my duty to see that everyone in Rocky Mount who has need of a physician will be seen."

About ten years after joining the Edgecombe General staff, I developed a cataract in my left eye and began having cloudy vision. During one operation, I had trouble controlling the bleeding from a severed artery. I applied three clamps before the bleeding was controlled. My decision was made then and there—my career as a surgeon had come to an end. I continued treating medical patients for five more years until I grew tired of having to travel across town to the hospital. It was then that I gave up my medical privileges at Edgecombe General Hospital and confined my activities to treating out-patients in my own clinic.

EPILOGUE

November 22, 1997

I t was a mild fall day. It had rained the night before, so the air was clear and crisp; the wind pushed a few gray-laced clouds against the Carolina blue sky. The sunlight caught the glint of the brass trimming on his black coffin as it was being carried into the school auditorium for the funeral service. Even until the very end, life and the heavens showed my father, Milton Douglas Quigless, grace.

The minister scheduled to officiate over the service never showed up; yet Reverend Doctor Frank Weaver, who was to present the eulogy, stepped in at the request of my brother, and all went well. It turned out to be a service my father would have loved. The Tarboro Jubilee Singers sang with unmatched passion, led by Walter Plemmer, a man whose life my father saved. My father's funeral was attended by many, and his treasured friends and colleagues were the floral bearers, active pallbearers, and honorary pallbearers. Black and gold, colors of nobility for a noble man.

My sister (my parents' oldest child) Helen caught his essence in the obituary: "After years of frustration with segregation laws which prevented Dr. Quigless from performing surgery and admitting seriously ill patients to Edgecombe General Hospital, he opened the Quigless Clinic-Hospital on December 3, 1946. His wife, Helen, was his partner in this enterprise, serving as administrator, bookkeeper, and personnel manager. At that time, patients came from a radius of two hundred miles, but at the end of his career, they came from as far away as Connecticut, Massachusetts, and even Italy. He became well known for his work in dermatology, arthritis, weight control, asthma, and allergies. He treated patients for their entire lifespan and usually whole families. He is famous for his hypodermic shots and would tell patients, 'I'm going to shoot the hell out of you!' as he gathered up the weapons of choice.

"He was a whiz at diagnosis and creative in the application of his science. He has used a God-given talent to do amazing things in his time. He performed difficult operations in country homes on kitchen tables; he sewed on a severed fingertip; he found a treatment for hemophilia, which has kept the patient alive and free of blood transfusions for over fifty years. He has relieved so many people of the pain of arthritis from which there is not yet a cure. Even in the last weeks of his life patients were seeking his help."

My sister Helen adored her father, in spite of his inability to ease her pain or retard the advancement of her arthritis. She delighted in our dad's company and no doubt garnered inspiration from him to persevere. Hers was an extremely difficult plight for someone who wanted to be a professional dancer. She dropped her dance dreams in college with the onset of arthritis, graduated from Fisk University and went on to get her master's degree in library science from Atlanta University, earning induction into the national library science honor society. She worked at Federal City College in Washington, D.C., before returning home to Tarboro as her illness progressed rapidly. She remained there until her death from complications of arthritis on January 17, 2004.

She made a definite imprint on life—her poetry was published in several critically acclaimed Black poetry anthologies (even one posthumously in 2006), she started a summer art camp for underprivileged children, ran for city council, and maintained a network of many friends that included people from all over the world. Helen was also the founder of the Phoenix Historical Society, which researches and honors the accomplishments of African Americans in Edgecombe County, of both local and national influence. It was Helen who introduced our family to the venerable Congressman John Lewis and his wife Lillian. She had the vision for the current exhibit regarding our father down at the Quigless Clinic-Hospital building and was the one who urged him to write his autobiography.

She and our mother organized Doctor Quigless Day in Tarboro with Glennie Matthewson, celebrating his fifty years of service. Our dad introduced Helen to Doris Stith, who, with Patricia Mabry, would take Helen to the Newport Jazz Festival. Even after Helen could no longer get around, just thinking about their good times at the Festival always brought a broad grin to her face. Helen was a jazz buff and never missed listening to the Tom "The Jazz Man" radio show every Sunday night. She was also the honored guest in the early 1990s at the Martin Luther King, Jr., banquet dinner for her leadership in the African American community. Helen did not shed a tear about our dad's death until months later when she was brought to the clinic to see what things had to be sorted and sifted through.

She told me that she was in his treatment room, standing in a shaft of sunlight through the window, and she felt his vibe, as if his spirit was there. No doubt, he was there.

The years from the 1980s to my dad's death mirrored his previous years. He worked hard, loved his work, and loved and cared for friends and patients alike. I remember him always studying, reading up on medical things, keeping current. He was at peace, particularly because he lived long enough to see the effects of integration and become respected and beloved at Edgecombe General Hospital. So many colleagues and friends from Edgecombe General were at his funeral as well as people from way back when, when he started up the Quigless Clinic-Hospital. Some of the early nurses were there, including Miss Shirley Mays and Miss Dozier.

His wife, my mother Helen, brought her strength to bear, particularly during the last few months of my dad's life. Their relationship was one of the strangest ones I've seen. Although they separated in the late 1960s, they never divorced. They could not live with each other, nor without each other as their lives remained profoundly intertwined. If family company came to town, it was understood that my dad would preside at the head of the dining room table, telling the stories from his stage, as if he had never been gone. Amidst fussing and fighting, they remained confidantes. In fact, for the last five years of his life, my dad came to my mother's house for dinner every evening, sometimes contributing a pan of raisin-laced brownies or Jiffy Mix corn muffins that were crunchy because he proudly added extra corn meal. He was famous for his brandied figs, you know.

When my mother became ill with heart disease, my dad was there, attentive to all treatments she received. She was told in 1988 that she probably would only have two more years to live. She persevered and thrived for an additional sixteen years, which prompted her Duke doctors to call her their "miracle patient." But I know that it was not only the medicine or their expertise keeping her alive—we all know that it was her amazing will power and sense of purpose. That was the mettle she was made of. That was the woman that had my dad's back through all the years. She was every bit his match because she was raised to be a strong woman.

She succumbed to her disease September 16, 2005.

Eight years before that, it became apparent that my dad's emphysema was getting much worse. My dad had been famous for lighting up a cigarette while another still lay burning in an ashtray. But once he got emphysema, he had no trouble quitting smoking. Months before his death, my mother had him come back home so that he could be well cared for. He stayed in what used to be Brother's bedroom when we were growing up.

My dad was often very, very proud of my brother, Milton, Jr. ("Brother" or "Bro," as we called him). He became a fine general surgeon. As you can tell from the prologue, Brother shared a special relationship with our dad, which often was one of mutual admiration. Brother graduated from our dad's alma mater, Meharry Medical College, in 1971. He followed in our dad's foot-steps as he was inducted into the Alpha Omega Medical Society during his third year at Meharry. This society is reserved for only the top 10 percent of each class. Brother did his internship and residency at George H. Hubbard Hospital at Meharry and was chief resident during his last year. He was also Doctor of the Year for the Old North State Medical Society in 1984 and president of the medical staff at Wake Medical Center in 1987. He is certified by the American Board of Surgery and is a fellow of the American College of Surgeons. He lived in Japan as a contracted civilian surgeon for the armed forces for a time, and he is now retired. After two previous marriages, Brother has remarried and lives in Columbus, Georgia. He has five beautiful, brilliant adult children living currently in all parts of the USA and the world.

As for me, Carol, I returned to Tarboro in 2003 to help out with my sister and my mother who, by that time, were both very ill. I had spent twenty-six years in Los Angeles learning about alternative treatments and working as a nutritional chef, sometimes to Hollywood luminaries. My sister Helen died six months after my return, and my mother died a year and a half later. After their deaths, I decided to stay in Tarboro, a place I consider to be the quintessential southern small town. I opened the Quigless Natural Health Center of Tarboro, which, you can see from its name, used natural, holistic methods of healing. Today, I live in Charlottesville, Virginia where I have an essential oil business, Flourish Essential Oils LLC.

My dad would not have agreed with the natural approach. Because he formulated some of his own medicines, ointments, and injections, there is a misunderstanding that he employed natural means and herbology in his practice. In fact, he had nothing but scorn for such practices.

However, he would be very proud of the results I have been getting through Russian medical massage, clinical aromatherapy, Reiki, herbology, and energy medicine. One of his old patients came in to see me about a skin problem she had that I helped clear up. She said my dad had been the only one able to help her out. She looked at me and said, "When your dad was getting up in age, I asked him who was going to help me out when he was gone. He said, 'There will be somebody around to help you out.' And it seems like it's you!" That gave me a chill up my spine, and I thank God the lady is doing fine!

I do not know why my dad stopped working on his autobiography in the 1980s. I know that there were so many more stories he had to tell. There were stories about his kindness, such as the time when an older man rode a bicycle over twenty miles with a huge, open painful sore on his leg. My dad treated him, and the man could have been sent home. But instead, my dad allowed him to stay ten days in the hospital at no charge because he needed some rest and good nourishment. My dad also talked about lots of people he intended to include in the book whenever he got back around to working on it, including me, his youngest child! For whatever the reasons, he just never got back into continuing the book. Perhaps the recent years were too fresh—he was very comfortable with the past. You also have to understand that my dad never thought of himself as old or elderly and thought he had lots of time left.

At the graveside, after his funeral and interment, I happened to look back at the grave and saw the funeral director, Jesse Baker, fidgeting with the lid of the vault. He looked up and said, "I'm just making sure that it's sealed tight." It was a caring, loving gesture as if he was caring for my father the way he cared for so many others. The body was sealed, but my dad's spirit and legacy have lived on well past that funeral service.

In 1998, the NC Museum of History opened an exhibit dealing with the healing arts in North Carolina in which my dad's operating room was reproduced and his story told. It was an exhibit that was to close in 2003, but, due to its popularity, it ran until 2008. I was assured that my dad's place in the exhibit had a lot to do with its popularity. My dad was posthumously inducted into the Hall of Fame in Rocky Mount in 2004, which was a great honor. Other posthumous honorees are Thomas H. Battle, Dr. Casey Chavis, Spencer Case Fountain, James Kern "Kay" Kyser, Walter "Buck" Leonard, and living honorees are Harold Denton, General Hugh Shelton, and Joseph Daniel "Danny" Talbott. As you can see, he was in great company, and General Shelton spoke very highly of my dad.

His spirit lives on in the impact of his brilliance at treating people and his nerve and courage to persevere through all barriers—economic, racial, and social. But especially I see that his spirit lives on in the faces of people—some total strangers to me—that light up with joy, gratitude, and laughter as they tell me a story about their encounter with my dad.

They often end the story with, "Yes, Doc was a mess! I went everywhere, but he was the only one who could help me out." Sometimes it's his old patients' children or grandchildren who carry on the stories. I also hear many stories of how he encouraged those wanting to go into the medical field but who got discouraged by the odds against them. He told them to never give up, that if he could do it, they could, too.

That there is still such a buzz about my dad so many years after his death is amazing. I see the impact of his practice and his indomitable spirit every day of my life here in Tarboro, Edgecombe County, North Carolina. My father lives on because his impact transcends space and time.

– Carol M. Quigless

DR. QUIGLESS'S SPEECHES

I completed my internship at City Hospital No. 2 in St. Louis, Missouri, which later became known as Homer G. Phillips Hospital. This hospital's alumni association was organized in 1936. Although I missed the first two meetings, I found it to be very advantageous to attend them regularly once I began going. For many years before the time that many medical journals were published, my attendance at the annual alumni association and the Old North State Medical Society meetings were the only way I could halfway attempt to keep up with the rapid pace of advancing medicine.

I was elected President of the Homer G. Phillips Hospital Alumni Association in 1958. The following is the address I gave at the annual meeting that year. It gives some insight into the development of the hospital and mentions some of the men who contributed much to advance medicine for the Black people.

Presidential Address of the 13th Annual Meeting of the Homer G. Phillips Hospital Interns Alumni Association

Mr. Chairman and members of the Homer G. Phillips Hospital Interns Alumni Association, I feel that I have been awarded a single honor in being elected to serve as your president, especially when one remembers that only a selected few may hope to attain such an honor with the passing of the years. Indeed, through the past year I have attempted to search myself and discover whatever traits I possess that would lead this august and learned body to select me as president. I can't get it. I just arrive at the same conclusion—that is, an organization, as well as an individual, can make a mistake.

Believe me when I say that I have never made a speech in my life, and I don't think you fellows are in the mood for me to practice speech-making now. In my vain efforts to keep up with the trends of medicine from day to day, the words of the philosophers of old have been so crowded out of my mind that my memory seems to be blank when I try to recall the writing of the immortal bards and sages of old.

Although I interned at City Hospital No. 2 and have returned here for about ten of the twelve meetings, I did not know much about the origin and development of City Hospital No. 2 and Homer G. Phillips Hospital. I wrote several former interns who had been in St. Louis for many years, seeking sources of information concerning the origin of our institution, but, as usual, only one or two answered my letters. Dr. Thomas was one of those, and he advised me to write to Dr. Haskell. Dr. Haskell, I found, was one who could and did give me the information I needed inasmuch as he was one of the original group of stalwarts responsible for the establishment of City Hospital No. 2.

According to Dr. Haskell, years ago, our professional group in St. Louis realized that if they were expected to reach the highest development in the science of medicine, they must have opportunities and advantages of training afforded only in large institutions like municipal hospitals where there is an abundance of clinical material. There, opportunities were denied our group, although our taxes were used to help train the members of the other group.

This small group of men in St. Louis realized that taxation without representation was unjust. They felt their group should demand that they share in the training of interns and doctors, at that time underway. In 1916, a group of men met in the office of Mr. C. K. Robinson, editor of a weekly paper known as *The Palladium*, for the purpose of forming an organization to prevail upon the city authorities to appoint physicians, interns, and nurses of our group to the staff of the municipal hospital. The group consisted of Mrs. John T. Clark, Charles Turpin, A. W. Lloyd, I. H. Bradbury, Frank Field, C. K. Robinson, and A. E. Malone; the following clergy: B. G. Shaw, Noah Williams, and P. W. Dunavon; Attorney Homer G. Phillips; and Drs. S. P. Stafford, J. T. Caston, G. B. Key, C. H. Phillips, and R. C. Haskell. All are now deceased except A. W. Lloyd and Drs. G. B. Key and R. C. Haskell.

The group met in the office of Mayor Henry Keil, who was then up for re-election as mayor, and presented their claim. The mayor listened attentively, said there was merit in their claims, and gave his personal approval. As might have been expected, the Board of Aldermen and some of the other authorities disapproved of the mixing of the races under the same roof (remember that was back in 1916). The matter became a campaign issue.

The two medical schools at that time were opposed to the appointment of colored professional personnel to the municipal hospital. So, rather than give up their plight, the colored group accepted a compromise in the form of a separate institution. The city fathers offered to purchase the old vacant Barnes Hospital and Medical College building. They agreed to remodel the property and make it suitable for general hospital purposes. In December 1918, Dr. Haskell was appointed superintendent and was sent to the white hospital for training. Several graduate nurses and interns were appointed and were also sent to the white hospital for training. Contrary to predictions even at that time, no race riot developed as a result of their presence in the white hospitals.

In November 1919, City Hospital No. 2 was opened with twelve junior interns, one resident on medicine, one resident on surgery, a staff of graduate nurses, and twelve student nurses. A visiting staff composed of physicians from Washington University and an associated visiting staff composed of local colored physicians were appointed. The patients were transferred from the white hospitals. City Hospital No. 2 was, in the words of our great philosopher, Dr. C. V. Roman, "born of the exigencies of American environment." Within two years, the hospital was so crowded that patients had to be placed in the halls.

In 1922, a bond issue was voted on and passed for the erection of new hospitals in the city of St. Louis. City Hospital No. 2 was included. Another fight developed at that time as a group within the city wanted to build an annex to the white hospital for colored patients instead of a separate institution. This fight lasted about ten years before a new hospital was assured for colored patients. The building was started. In 1936, the new building was completed and named for the militant leader, Attorney Homer G. Phillips. Thus ends the first chapter of our story. A group of determined men has presented to us, you and I, our heritage. The dictionary defines the word "heritage" as "an estate that passes from an ancestor to a descendent," and that is what every alumnus of Homer G. Phillips should consider this hospital—ours by the right of inheritance—with all of the obligations that go along with any heritage.

The Homer G. Phillips Interns Alumni Association is not an organization that has just materialized out of nowhere. Our present organization has developed over a period of years by steps—sometimes uncertain and sometimes faltering, but always forward—from the humble beginning more than thirteen years ago. This organization is the brainchild, to a great extent, of the men who carried the load back in the days of City Hospital No. 2 with its dilapidated building, outmoded equipment, overcrowded wards, overworked and undermanned staff. These were the days when the pioneers of No. 2 toiled, and without monetary reward, to ease the suffering of "Black St. Louis." They toiled with the hope of a better tomorrow. They longed to see the day come when our group would have adequate buildings, funds, equipment, and personnel to make a worthwhile contribution to the health of St. Louis and to the sum total of medical knowledge.

As a member of the last group of interns to be trained at City Hospital No. 2, I can speak with firsthand knowledge of the conditions that existed in that day and time. I was attracted to St. Louis and City Hospital No. 2 by the type of men I met coming from that hospital. Their energy and resourcefulness, their self-sufficiency without ostentation, their willingness to reach down and help the neophytes, their utter lack of selfishness and greed, instilled in me a desire to become one of them. On arriving in St. Louis and taking my first look at No. 2, I felt shaky (if I may use that word) when I reported to Drs. McClelland and Hampton in that rambling structure with creaking floors, fat cockroaches, and one elevator for six floors. And do you remember the OB ward up on the sixth floor with one elevator, and that elevator being tied up most of the time? Or the TB wards in July with beds a foot apart, and the air conditioning—or I should say, the oscillating fans—blowing the acid-fast-laden air hither and yon, creating a noise that drowned out the sepulcher-coughs of the wretched patients who lay there exhausted, awaiting the touch of the "Grim Reaper?"

There were the operating rooms—small, tight, overcrowded, and with one team anxiously awaiting the completion of a cholecystectomy so that they could get started on a hysterectomy. Dr. Vaughn had me over a barrel one day in a minor operating room. Everything was tied up, so he demonstrated how easy it was to do a herniotomy under local anesthesia on an elderly patient who had an incarcerated hernia with threatening gangrene. Those were raw times for indigent patients of our group in St. Louis. They were also raw times for the staff because of inadequate equipment and quarters, which took their toll on the interns as well as the patients. But those were the days when men worked, and dreamed, and planned. Those were the days when Homer G. Phillips Hospital was conceived and born to alter, spawn, this great organization which we represent today. As we look back over the years, we would like to pause a moment to salute those martyrs who gave their lives in the development of our present hospital. I mean the patients who died because of inadequate facilities and the interns whose lives were sacrificed because of overwork, overcrowding, and equipment that became booby traps.

I have painted a dark picture—dark, but true, however. This picture, among other things, serves to furnish a background revealing, in all of its splendor, the institution that we have at our disposal today. Those veterans among us today who have survived to see the fulfillment of their dreams should feel proud of their handiwork. Those whom I have been privileged to know and learned to revere include Drs. Taylor, Thomas, Curtis, Hampton, McClelland, Vaughn, Sherrod, Blanche, and Sinkler. You may add to the list. Let's not forget those who have answered the last roll call. Many of us remember Drs. Breedlove, Cheatum, Gaykins, Mormon, Weathers, and others. You may be able to add to that list also. Those were the men who pioneered in the development of Homer G. Phillips as we know it today. They should be hailed as heroes by every member of our association.

I have already mentioned the fact that I was attracted to St. Louis by the type of men that our hospital produced and sent out into the world. Doubtless, many of you have been anxiously asked by nurses and other hospitals for staff assignments, "Doctor, where did you intern?" When you answered, "Homer G. Phillips," you could see an expression of relief cross the countenance of your interrogator. He or she knew at that instant that the doctor reporting was ready for his job; knew, too, that he was competent, skilled, and ready to cope with whatever situation might arise. In short, Homer G. Phillips has the reputation for turning out doctors who are well-rounded and ready. That is a well-deserved reputation, and it has not been attained without determined effort on the part of the staff.

For many years now, we have been blessed with the sympathy, understanding, and cooperation of the heads of two outstanding medical schools and many hospitals. It is a great achievement to become a physician, to be able to complete the requirements outlined in order to be awarded the degree of Doctor of Medicine. One has to be a real man or woman, one who is able to take it without complaint, and ready to come back for more. Maybe I am biased by having been trained here. However, I do sincerely feel that being accepted for internship at Homer G. Phillips Hospital is an achievement second only to the completion of a person's medical studies. Where else could you find better facilities for the application of the precepts you have mastered during your four-year grind? Where else would you find such a wealth of clinical material? Where else would you find a more unselfish house staff ? Where else would you find a more concerned governing body than we have here at Homer G. Phillips?

A few years ago, Dr. Evarts A. Graham was presented a plaque at the Keil Auditorium for the part he played in the development of Homer G. Phillips Hospital as a training center. He commented that he could not understand why he was being so honored. He could not recall having done anything that should have merited such an honor. But most of us here know that he opened many doors for us that had been heretofore closed to our group. But, through his insistence, he made them realize that man could not be classified as inferior, incompetent, or unworthy until after he had been given a trial and found wanting. We all know that Dr. Graham was a great man. His greatness was accentuated by his humility.

A few years ago, in Washington at the Park Plaza Hotel, we heard Dr. Elman's comments in response to an introduction in which he was presented as a most important benefactor to the physicians of our group in St. Louis. He said he "had worked with the men of Homer G. Phillips and had learned a lot about mankind." He also stated that he had shown no favors to the men of our group. Wherever he found a man capable of doing a job, he let the man do it regardless of race. We all know Dr. Elman as a man who has made invaluable contributions to the science of medicine—one of America's greats in the field of medicine.

A few years ago, we were present when Dr. Walter E. Henneric, Hospital Commissioner for the city of St. Louis, was presented a plaque by this organization on behalf of the important part he played in helping to obtain this great hospital for us and for his continuous battle for equalization of hospital facilities for all. When the eventful program of integration of patients was inaugurated in St. Louis, he was at the helm, guiding the destinies of Homer G. Phillips through one of the most critical periods of its existence.

Drs. Graham, Elman, and Henneric have all departed this life, but not before they made "footprints on the sands of time" that will long remain to guide our faltering steps to greater heights on the medical horizon—heights that are yet beyond our field of vision. When I think of those three great men and what they have meant to this hospital, teaching institution, research center, and to the Homer G. Phillips Interns Alumni Association, I am reminded of the words of William Cullen Bryant in the "Ode to a Waterfall": *Thou are gone, the abyss of heaven hath swallowed up thy form; yet, on my heart, deeply hath sunk the lesson thou hast given, and shall not soon depart.*

You may ask why I am devoting so much time to these men. They have been acclaimed and honored for their research in the field of surgery. They were elevated to the highest offices and positions in scientific societies in America and abroad. But I feel that enough can never be said of the part they have played in calling the attention of the medical world to the fact that, given a chance to demonstrate his ability, the Negro physician and surgeon could and would add to the sum total of medical knowledge as well as physicians and surgeons of any group.

As a result of their insistence for a fair chance for everyone, we find members of the Homer G. Phillips' staff holding important teaching assignments in the two top-flight medical schools in St. Louis. Fearless in the face of biased criticism of their fellows, they insisted that our men be given fair treatment and started us on our way to the full realization of our dreams of becoming contrib-utors to the march of medical progress. At the present time, the incumbent staff of Homer G. Phillips is writing history, day by day. I am happy to repeat that statement here. The work being done here is recognized not only in St. Louis, but throughout America. If you were not thrilled by reading Dr. Sinkler's letter of March 12, 1958, you have no right to be a member of this Homer G. Phillips Hospital Interns Alumni Association. Our hospital, under the present leadership, is developing a place for itself in the world of medicine of which we should be proud. This is commendable since some institutions much like ours have been scrapped or have lost their identity by other means as a result of change inci-dent to integration.

Homer G. Phillips has taken integration in stride and has retained its identity as a contributing unit in the health set-up of St. Louis. That fact speaks well for our staff. That fact speaks well for the city of St. Louis. In spite of the political changes that have occurred from the time of the establishment of City Hospital No. 2 to this day, our institution has been able to find friends among the incumbent administrations in the political circles of the city, thus making for continuous progress here at our hospital. The very existence of this hospital in its present state speaks well for St. Louis politics, regardless of the party in power at any given time. In other words, the people of St. Louis have seen to it that their regard for the welfare of less fortunate individuals should transcend all party lines. For this fine spirit to be found only in St. Louis, we salute the people of St. Louis.

At the present time, there are some clouds on the horizon. Early in my address, the statement was made that I was impressed by the type of doctors developed at City Hospital No. 2. Back in the days when many of us finished medicine, opportunities for internship were limited. Graduates of Negro medical schools were happy to be accepted in St. Louis and five or six other cities as interns. The pay was almost nothing. The work was hard, but the number of worthwhile internships was so limited that a mad scramble developed in our senior year to get an appointment to one of the more important hospitals. The Intern Committee has an easy time selecting the cream of the crop.

Today integration has changed the picture. Negro medical school graduates are welcomed in many of our larger American hospitals. They are welcomed because our graduates and the graduates of other Negro-staffed hospitals have demonstrated that they are as well trained as any interns in America, and their medical training has prepared them, as to make them worthy of the chances afforded in any hospital anywhere. The men who have been trained in the specialties here are to be found in teaching positions in many large medical centers and are doing such good jobs that the way has been opened for other Negroes. With all the hospitals now bidding for services of graduates of Howard and Meharry, we are finding it more difficult to satisfy our needs for junior house staff members. The hospital staff has worked hard to establish residences in different fields. Now we are experiencing difficulty in finding men prepared to accept the residences.

The alumni of City Hospital No. 2 and Homer G. Phillips Hospital make up a good-sized segment of the graduates of Howard and Meharry. We have been trained here and have gone out into our respective communities to practice and reap the rewards of the training we received in St. Louis. We have returned to our alma mater where we observe the superior advantages afforded by our hospital—the house staff, second to none in training and experience; a visiting staff made up of some of the best minds to be found in America; clinical material in abundance; facilities for research; and the same spirit of helpfulness and encouragement that we found here years ago.

All great institutions have their traditions. One of our most outstanding traditions is that of encouraging the fellows who show ability. Greed and selfishness do not exist in the members of the house staff of Homer G. Phillips.

We ask only a few favors of our alumni. First of all, we ask your active support in attending conventions. You will probably be asked for financial support in order to improve the recreational and living facilities of our resident staff. But most importantly, we are asking your support in recruiting interns of the caliber that would be worthy of our institution. We are insisting that you exert your influence as fathers, uncles, brothers, sisters, and/or advisors of fellows graduating from your medical schools today to see that our quota of interns is filled to overflowing.

Questions may arise concerning interns' pay, housing, recreation, etc. You may answer positively that steps are now being taken to bring our institution in line with the best hospitals in America in every respect. Our medical director has informed us that we now hold an enviable position as a hospital and training center. But we cannot hold our position without a full complement of top-flight interns. We have the responsibility of seeing to it that our hospital is adequately staffed before consideration can be given to the institutions which are just now beginning to open their doors to Negroes.

So, let us all roll up our sleeves and go to work to make sure that our institution maintains its enviable place in the world of medicine today. Let us instill ourselves to see that Homer G.

Phillips' interns' quota is filled. Let us set about to justify the faith and trust that those who have gone before have placed in us, to maintain this institution in the place of pre-eminence that it has attained by the hard work of many men who fought our battles while we were helpless to lend aid. Ours is a great heritage. Let us pray to the Almighty God that we may be able to live up to the responsibilities that go along with membership in the Homer G. Phillips Intern Alumni Association.

***

I attended just about every meeting of the Black state and national medical organizations each year. I became the recording secretary of the Old North State Medical Association and held that position for about four years. I then became vice president and, subsequently, president of the Old North State Medical Association. The following is my address to that association at the time I was inaugurated as president.

Inaugural Address to Old North State Medical Association

I feel that I have been highly honored in having been elected president of this venerable organization. I have always thought that the office of president should be reserved for the man who had exhibited outstanding characteristics that would set him apart as a shining example to be followed and admired by the membership of the organization. I have attended meetings regularly and have done all that I could to keep the Old North State Medical Society going strong.

I am reminded here of a true story that happened in Mississippi. There was a teacher at Alcorn who saved every penny he could and invested his money in real estate in a nearby city. The real estate increased in value. He collected lots of rent and, in short, became very wealthy. He retired, his wife died, and after a few months he began showing some interest in a young chick. Some of his former students became alarmed as he began to go more and more steady with the young lady.

One man got up the courage to speak to the old professor about it. He said, "Professor Jones, I have always admired you and followed your advice, but I am somewhat disturbed by the interest you are showing in Miss Smith. After all, you are old enough to be her father, and anybody can see that all she is after is what you have got."

The old professor replied, "Well, son, the only thing I am after is what she's got."

I worked in this organization for what I could get out of it, and I assure you that my labors have been rewarded long before I was elected president. The Society owes me nothing, but I feel that I owe it everything. There is the prestige of belonging to an organized medical group with the authority to speak for all Negro doctors. There is the undisputed privilege of joining in discussions of policy, and, if you have something on the ball, seeing your ideas influence the thought and action commensurate with the responsibilities. There are priceless ties of fellowships that are developed that bind friends together as long as life lasts. There is a chance to join in for the fight for complete emancipation of our race. The Old North State Medical Society is a great organization. I feel that most of us have taken this organization for granted and have either forgotten, or have never known, the part that it played in the forward march of the Negro physician in North Carolina and in America.

There is one sure way to make me speechless, and that is to put me in a position in which I have to make a speech. I don't seem to be able to find the words. In seeking material for this address, I asked Dr. Donnell for help, and he sent me a souvenir program of the Old North State Medical, Dental, and Pharmaceutical Society that was published for the fiftieth annual session, which incidentally, was held in Durham at this same time in 1937, just one year after I unloaded my trunk in Tarboro. I read that booklet from cover to cover several times and was astonished at the amount of interesting information it contained. It should be common knowledge to all of us that the Old North State Medical, Dental, and Pharmaceutical Society was the first state medical society established by Negroes in America. In the words of Dr. C. V. Romans, "It was born of the exigencies of our American environment."

In the year 1887, the following physicians came together to establish this organization: Drs. M. T. Pope, A. M. Moore, J. T. Williams, L. A. Scruggs, and Marcus A. Alston. Back seventy-one years ago, when this organization was looked upon as something yet untried and, accordingly, looked upon with mingled feelings of distrust and hope by millions of their neglected, suffering fellowmen, these five young Negro doctors, fresh out of Leonard Medical College, saw the need to develop a statewide organization with the purpose of working together for the advancement of the Negro in medicine. That was the prime reason for the establishment of the Old North State Medical, Dental, and Pharmaceutical Society. Thus, we see our society as a pioneer in the field of professional relationships to be followed soon by groups in other states who could readily see the wisdom of the concerned efforts initiated by fine men from Leonard Medical College in the Old North State.

Later, the medical men were joined by the dentists and pharmacists of our state to form a strong organization, which thrived and served to enhance the stature of professional men in our state for many years. Diversity of interest later brought about divisions of the parent organization, but the Old North State Medical Society is still the father of them all, and a cordial relationship still remains with our dental and pharmaceutical brothers. We are happy that we are all meeting concurrently in Durham and enjoying the fellowship that should exist among men and women with very similar problems, interests, and ambitions.

You know, at times I am disturbed by the attitude some of the medics appear to take relative to their relationship to the manifold problems that confront us as a group. Instead of joining the society, working with us, and joining community organizations and taking an active part in guiding the destinies of the group, they are showing a tendency to isolate themselves from the masses, joining only long enough to extract as much cash as the traffic will bear. Apparently, the fact has never dawned on them that we, as a race, are in a fight for first-class citizenship, and we of the Old North State Medical Society are in a fight for full recognition as American physicians.

I am reminded here of a young classmate that I knew when I was a kid. We were studying the verb "to go." The teacher asked him to use the word "went" in a sentence. The boy said, "I have went." The teacher said it was wrong. The boy said, "I know it's wrong." The teacher asked why it was wrong. The boy answered, "Because I ain't went yet." In other words, we have only made a start toward reaching our objective.

What is our objective? Our objective is to hasten the day when Negro physicians will be accepted as just another physician in North Carolina and throughout the length and breadth of America. Many years ago, Sir William Osler, often called the father of modern medicine, spoke these words: "Distinctions of race, nationality, color, and creed are unknown within the portals of the Temple of Aesculapius. Dare we dream that this harmony and cohesion so rapidly developing in medicine, obliterating the strongest lines of division, knowing no tie of loyalty, but loyalty to truth; dare we hope, I say, that in the wider range of human affairs a similar solidarity may be reached?"

When we ponder the words of Sir William Osler, a few factors crystallize themselves clearly, ever so clearly. First of all, he envisioned a day when men of medicine, regardless of race, color, and creed, would stand together as brothers. Secondly, he charged, or at least expected the medical profession to lead the way to a universal state of brotherhood by their examples of fellowship and mutual esteem. I wonder what Sir William Osler would say were he alive today, if he could see America's largest minority fighting for first-class citizenship in this, the greatest country of the world, this great country that they carved out of the wilderness, sweating blood and bathed in tears. I wonder what he would think of that stubborn minority of physicians engaged today in a life-and-death struggle for our rightful place in organized medicine, blinded by raw, irrational, and indefensible prejudice—a minority that aids and abets the efforts of agitators to undermine the good name and exalted position of the United States throughout the world by their insistence that the Negro should be subordinated and maintained in an inferior status in organized medicine.

The entire world has its eyes on America and its management of the racial problems. The entire world, its population predominantly colored, is watching while a minority of the physicians in organized medicine play into the hands of the agitators abroad who seize every opportunity to expose our country's faults and fallacies. Our international status as a truly democratic nation suffers as a minority of short-sighted individuals influence the masses to hate and discriminate, while one of the most influential groups in our country ignores the challenge of Sir William Osler.

I would not like to be misunderstood. I have said, and I repeat, that a minority of physicians in our state and our country are responsible for the lack of leadership of the profession in matters relative to the full fruition of the ideal state of national brotherhood. The vast majority of the physicians with whom I have come in contact in two score years have exemplified everything that is stated or implied in the Hippocratic Oath. In my own community, I could hope for no better cooperation, but there is always a fly in the ointment.

With Sir William Osler, those of us gathered here tonight are looking forward to the day when, to paraphrase Osler, we can look around us and truthfully say, "Distinctions of race, color, and creed are unknown within these portals." And we may be able to look about us and see that the harmony and cohesion developed within the medical profession, obliterating the strongest lines of division, and knowing no ties or loyalty but loyalty to truth, has helped to develop those virtues in the wider range of human affairs, so that a similar solidarity has developed throughout America.

As for me and many other members of the Old North State Medical Society, we shall not be satisfied with half a loaf. We have faith in the majority of the medical profession. We believe that they will ultimately bring themselves around so that they may be numbered among the members of this noble profession who live up to the letter and the spirit of the Hippocratic Oath.

In the meantime, what are we, the members of the Old North State Medical Society, going to do? What should we do? We should, first of all, strive to live up to the high standards prescribed by Hippocrates as a code of ethics for our profession. We should keep ourselves abreast of the most recent trends of thought and action with our profession. We should assume our parts in the civic life of our communities. We should be good, loyal Americans all, and, as true Americans, work aggressively to achieve the same status that other men of medicine enjoy in the United States. We should look forward to the day when we will no longer be offered half a loaf. The Old North State Medical Society has been in existence for seventy-one years. Although individuals tend to degenerate with age and finally pass off the stage of life, organizations such as ours are expected to show improvement with the passing of years and justify their existence with worthwhile contributions to society.

***

TRANSCRIPTS FROM DR. MILTON D. QUILGLESS'S DIARY BEGINNING JULY 1, 1933

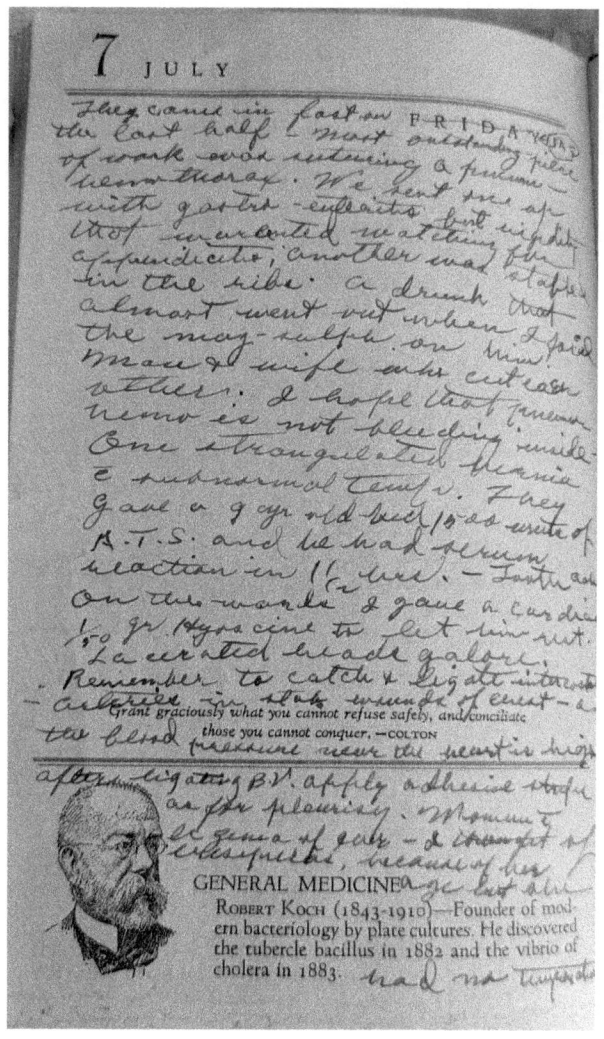

Excerpt from Dr. Milton's Diary

Dr. George Bryan to Dr. M. D. Quigless

1933

July 4, 1934

JANUARY

SUN	MON	TUE	WED	THU	FRI	SAT
1	2	3	4	5	6	7
8	9	10	11	12	13	14
15	16	17	18	19	20	21
22	23	24	25	26	27	28
29	30	31	-	-	-	-

FEBRUARY

SUN	MON	TUE	WED	THU	FRI	SAT
-	-	1	2	3	4
5	6	7	8	9	10	11
12	13	14	15	16	17	18
19	20	21	22	23	24	25
26	27	28	-	-	-	-

MARCH

SUN	MON	TUE	WED	THU	FRI	SAT
-	-	-	1	2	3	4
5	6	7	8	9	10	11
12	13	14	15	16	17	18
19	20	21	22	23	24	25
26	27	28	29	30	31	-

APRIL

SUN	MON	TUE	WED	THU	FRI	SAT
-	-	-	-	-	-	1
2	3	4	5	6	7	8
9	10	11	12	13	14	15
16	17	18	19	20	21	22
23/30	24	25	26	27	28	29

MAY

SUN	MON	TUE	WED	THU	FRI	SAT
-	1	2	3	4	5	6
7	8	9	10	11	12	13
14	15	16	17	18	19	20
21	22	23	24	25	26	27
28	29	30	31	-	-	-

JUNE

SUN	MON	TUE	WED	THU	FRI	SAT
-	-	-	-	1	2	3
4	5	6	7	8	9	10
11	12	13	14	15	16	17
18	19	20	21	22	23	24
25	26	27	28	29	30	-

JULY

SUN	MON	TUE	WED	THU	FRI	SAT
-	-	-	-	-	-	1
2	3	4	5	6	7	8
9	10	11	12	13	14	15
16	17	18	19	20	21	22
23/30	24/31	25	26	27	28	29

AUGUST

SUN	MON	TUE	WED	THU	FRI	SAT
-	-	1	2	3	4	5
6	7	8	9	10	11	12
13	14	15	16	17	18	19
20	21	22	23	24	25	26
27	28	29	30	31	-	-

SEPTEMBER

SUN	MON	TUE	WED	THU	FRI	SAT
-	-	-	-	-	1	2
3	4	5	6	7	8	9
10	11	12	13	14	15	16
17	18	19	20	21	22	23
24	25	26	27	28	29	30

OCTOBER

SUN	MON	TUE	WED	THU	FRI	SAT
1	2	3	4	5	6	7
8	9	10	11	12	13	14
15	16	17	18	19	20	21
22	23	24	25	26	27	28
29	30	31	-	-	-	-

NOVEMBER

SUN	MON	TUE	WED	THU	FRI	SAT
-	-	-	1	2	3	4
5	6	7	8	9	10	11
12	13	14	15	16	17	18
19	20	21	22	23	24	25
26	27	28	29	30	-	-

DECEMBER

SUN	MON	TUE	WED	THU	FRI	SAT
-	-	-	-	-	1	2
3	4	5	6	7	8	9
10	11	12	13	14	15	16
17	18	19	20	21	22	23
24/31	25	26	27	28	29	30

Excerpt from Dr. Milton's Diary

Dr. Quigless's handwriting was nearly impossible to read – not only did he have the famed scratchy handwriting of a doctor, he also was left-handed which made it worse! With hours of work and diligence on the parts of Carol Quigless, Lynn Murray and Dr. Richard Pantalone, we were able to provide the following transcripts. Blank spaces indicate handwriting that was indecipherable.

Sunday – just waiting for tonight when I begin on the receiving door of the hospital. The hospital is old and decrepit but gee – the clinical material – I slipped down to watch Dr.Hale work – he sewed on one man 2 hours – and the man died today - what a loss of suture material. It's a revolting sight – so much blood lost – the operating table all red. I sickened but I'll become accustomed to it.

Monday July 2. Drunk women – it is revolting! Blood – it makes me sick and faint but this is life – the other side of life in St Louis – however I think I shall like it when I get broken in. Tis quite a helpless feeling that and experiences on this first at "Day Watch" at the receiving door.
Knife wounds – sick kids (too much sour kraut) pregnant women and gyn cases – a salmagard/"salamagundi"(good play on words) that I must learn to relish. Dr. Hale Pee Wee's cousin is a fine fellow and we'll make make it o.k.

July 3 Day watch. This is bloody business, cuts, broken bones – powder burns and hematomas.
One woman – Doctor I've been bitten. "Where" - "I've been bitten" Physical exam revealed a lacerated vulva. Shocking but true!!!

July 4. Wed. Day Watch – She had never seen a man – she had menorrhagia (we thought) and sent her off but she expelled a 2 month fetus in bed – ... bleeding as an ectopic (pregnancy)_____.
Women are funny indeed.
I suture now without a needle holder and like it – sewed on the tip of a guy's nose – also closed a hole in a woman's mouth – through and through.

July 5. Doggonit Will I ever learn how to fill out those entrance folders? Sewed up lots of heads last night. About six I guess. Powder burns galore with A.T.S. (anti-tetanus serum)
One poor sap trying to be a burglar_got plugged above the 7th rib, on the right seemed to have missed his heart.
But did that guy scuffle to keep off the table when Dr. Hale said he did not care anything about him. More pelvic inflammation
The chief hated t o spoil his hand with stitches. That drunk and his head cut (cant read the rest)..and handsome.
Hale is letting me hold the rein now –I do fairly well but one woman returned with a secondary hemorrhage showing that I don't know it all.

July 6. Friday. Another steadily busy night is gone. My finger is sore and tender from putting sutures in heads limbs backs side, etc.
Gee but I had a time stopping the hemorrhage on "Corine." Her arm gashed with a knife, she came with blood spurting. , weak from whisky and loss of fluid. Got in and promptly fainted. The blood spurted I clamped and missed and clamped again. Dr. Hale left her to me and I sweated. When finally finished the new janitor complimented me or working fast and accurately – if he only

knew how I I messed up!!!! Young couple with a baby who fell out of bed, old stuff with lye (..his eyes)

Pleursey;the girl with "rheumatism"had keloid cellulitis(?) Bite on the cheek>. Continuing cleaning blood from finger nails with H2O2

July 7 Saturday They came in fast and the last half – most outstanding piece of work was suturing a pneumo hemothorax. We sent one after over with gastric enteritis but rigidity that warranted watching for appendicitis, another was stabbed in the ribs. A drunk that almost went out when I injected the mag sulphate in him. Man and wife who cut each other. I hope that hemopneumo is not bleeding inside. One strangulated hernia with subnormal temp.

They gave a 9 yr old boy 1500 units of A.T.S. and he had serum reaction in 1.5 hrs. on the wards I gave a cardiac 1/50 gm hyacine to let him rest Lacerated heads galore. Remember to catch and ligate intercostal – arteries in stab wounds of chest – and the blood pressure near the heart is high after ligating blood vessel. Apply adhesive strip as for pleurisy. Woman with eczema of the ear – I thought of erysipelas because of her age but she had no temperature.

Sunday July 8. Slow but steady was the service.

–a baby girl age 5 weeks with abscess of breast

–Plenty of stab wounds for surgery

–a man walking on a split fracture of femur

–a stab wound of the abdomen with intestines and omentum protruding

–a woman in labor

–an acute abdomen – to surgery

–Woody Lloyd with his neck aching from a blow and 3 of his friends with lacerations of the skull
–a woman with her lip cut inside out from a fall
And a few others – caught it about improper filling out of xray requests
–a won with suspected fracture of metatarsals. Sleepy now.

July 9. Everything is quiet now and not many heads to sew so I'm reading physical diagnosis. Skipped one day and I nearly forgot all activities. Visited by Bro. Alexander from Murfreesboro. One guy almost was scalped got his hair sewed on – like a .cap.

July 10 Monday. Still slow. The longest cut is on a guy's leg and thigh about 2 feet long. Too bad I missed that spurting carotid a while ago. Dr. Hale was on duty while I ate the mid nite meal – he ligated, and the man walked away saved .Little girl with tendon severed. (Can't read the rest of the paragraph).

July 11 Tuesday/Wednesday. Of all things, the receiving physician on day watch must give all the saline and glucose. I gave a man with incresed intracranial pressure glucose (50ccof 22%) as ordered - his BP continued to fall – he passed out!! Which goes to show that glucose administration should be dictated by the blood pressure!! And not first ordered because it sounds big. Little girl had epitaxis, she has rhinitis with ulceration of the septum a big B.V. (blood vessel) eroded because adrenaline would not stop it.I sent for the senior to put a packing in the nares.... Dr Rollins stopped that epistaxis by packing the nostril with cotton soaked in ferric chloride sol.
nothing much in the door except that every man I sewed up fainted and applied ammonia.

July 12 Thursday. Gee but it is hot today. Last night was a bear for learning things. Hemiplegia – the BP differed in the two arms.
Little girl came in with coma, air hunger, dilated pupils, we called it TB because she complained of her stomach for 3 days but her urine said diabetes. Always examine urine in doubtful cases. This is the value of routine.
–Old __?____ with a gash halfway around, stood the sutures better than I thought!!
–Poor old fellow is up there bleeding to death with perforations perhaps because he is afraid of an operation – it's too bad that was frail and so drunk.
Two women on GYN. Morphine for one and lamictal for the other. I hope their pain are eased

Friday, July 13. The wards really kept me going last night – one dead on A-1; ___ to the TB patient. Bromides to the demented woman. I inserted my first nasal tube – it was real easy for me. I did not catharize – because I wanted to see it close the ___ way. That poor one legged fellow was in a heck of a shape - some lousy guy cut him under his crutch arm disengaging the axillary space – the scar will make his arm unfit for a crutch for years to come. I sent a case to GYN that I was doubtful about – calling it fibroids and pelvic inflammation. note later. I expected a letter today will check later. Gee but its hot. I can't sleep. Note: No letter and no sleep either.

July 14 Tell Burton about the Epitaxis. What a night and am I tired! Pronounced 4 dead on the wards. Intestinal obstruction came in that had been given morphine by a tyro (?). It is too bad that the young must go it does not matter about the aged, however as much. I stopped a nosebleed with epinephrine and cotton – I wonder if I messed up by not tying a string on the cotton? Dr. Allen checked me on my request – most unusual case – suturing a man's eyelid to his eye. I surely hope I get a letter today – am beginning to get lonesome. Dr. "Hots" Weathers came by yesterday - quite a friendly chap. My my but Ms. Hancock can cuss!! – and so to bed.

July 15 Tell Burton about epistaxis!! I saw a most beautiful case of early diptheria on foot Temp =101.1 first like Dr. Neil said. That was a terribly necrotic throat with a man of stinking tissue hanging on a pedicule and threatening asphyxia – the nurse saved the patient by clamping a hemostate on it so that the patient could breathe. House surgeon excised it _a smear showed Vincents spirellae.I think it is a gumma of the esophagus– I am waiting on the Wasserman. Gave intramuscular injection of MgSO to the kid with spasms. The woman with intestinal obstruction was operated on and had bands of adhesions – after 14 years mind you. She died – no colostomy was done. Perhaps that accounted for her death.

Monday July 16. Not much doing last night but I'm tired from loss of sleep. I need a letter to prepare wife.
Pronounced two last night. Picked up a case of asthma this morning. Lost a 2-1/2 mo fetus brought in a slop bucket. Mother was 17 and not married. Another shot of mag sulphate to that spasm kid. I wish they would find out the cause of his trouble and quit palliating - it is deplorable. The diabetic kid is looking better. Only sewed ____ and head last nite. Hoping for a letter today. And so to bed.

July 17 Tuesday. The most outstanding case last night was that of a ruptured eyeball due to one grand smash - we sent her up. Next time

I'm going to try adhesive strips over wounds of the face a-la-Cristopher. Sutured a cut throat. Hard to feel buried sutures in the facsia colli Extracted one long splinter from a huge finger about 2 in. long extending down along the lateral margin of the nail. Rx ATS 1500 units. A most beautiful case of aortic regurgitation ,too bad since he is young – no pronouncing last night. One brick hat hit,with fracture of the outer table - I don't know what x ray revealed. Auto accident fractured ribs in a woman _man......treatment

Wednesday July 18. Last night was the quietest on the floor so far. I don't see how in the world a Dr. can mistake poison ivy for erysipelas, especially when the former is typical. Too bad I missed seeing last night. With the forehead split open the outer table was incised. The first payday is here!!! I'm sending Layzinka $2.00 of my first $5.00 since I've become Dr. Quig. If I can divie up with with her 40:60 all along she should be made happy some day -n she deserves a 40% split anyway.
Auto accident - _____ 14 yr old girl thought her 1 hip was busted but there was no deformity – no immobility no crepitus no loss of function so I called it sprain of hip – Dr. Payne turned out to be professor Payne's brother. Removed a bug from a kid's ear by gentle use of a hemostat.

July 19 Thursday
Well, I was so sleepy this morning that I failed to write in my diary. Last night was one of oddities. A man came in a rat had bit him on the penis. Another with an ice pick wound in the shoulder and a bite on the hand. A woman went to sleep and rolled over on a crochet needle she had stuck in her hair. It did not penetrate her skull. There came in one fighting bull. He had been crowned with

a bottle. Blood was squirting from the superficial temporal like water from a fountain. He fought ie a bull and bled like a hog – I ligated and sutured, they sent him up - you jut can't bleed these negroes to death! I change this afternoon.

July 20 Friday. Can you imagine a child age 15 mo with pediculosis pubis (body lice)in her eye lashes – they would not believe my diagnosis til Walker saw this kid. Criminal attack on a child age 3 yrs by a 40 yr old moron who used his finger. Dr Townsend_____came in after a case I admitted as cirrhosis of the liver, but the man remained in hospital because Townsend was so long answering the call. Early case of carcinoma. ? with circumscion.urethritis_____ and prostatitis. 3 car_____ and same and missed sewing. Those left over dressings gave me hail Columbia comin in late. The guy with the sinuses following the removal of tumors of the breasts for a check with iodoform(gauze)Dermatitis hypertrofica(?) from insufficent diathermy

July 21 Saturday A Little early. HOT HOT!!! 109F. I thought I would pass out from the heat today. Today or yesterday day was Fisk day – marked by lots of patients coming in with thrush in their throats – extraction was easy under visual control in one as – in another Dr. Sheen pushed the bone on down with his finger. Heat stroke and heat exhaustion. Stroke = high temp; exhaust with low temp. Plenty of it today. Pay day came and tonight I have $150 which I think is very good.
I hope to get a letter tomorrow I need one badly.
Colles fracture from a fall over a stone. Early pregnancy. One big tumor. I stuck my finger sewing up that boy's finger. I hope I don't

have syphilis.

July 22 Sunday. Yesterday afternoon was the hardest of them so far. They came in steadily. A heat stroker and heat exhaustion. One pleurisy strapped and later sent up. A piece of plastic surgery on a woman's nose that was ground off. Lead poisoning. He gave symptoms of an early case but he would not stay in the hospital. Numerous babies – I just sent them up. I did not know what else heck to do with them.. There was one with a week old, covered with lanugo jaundiced and emaciated The kid with history of eating ham(?) I wonder what the end will be in her case. One stab wound in the abdomen.

July 21 Monday.
Gee but last night was a whang doodle for work. We sent up about 14 heat cases – in addition to the usual Sunday night cuts and bruises. One heat case died a respiratory death on the examining table in spite of all we could do. A child broke both bones of his leg. Pronouned a man who had been shot by his wife . No spectacular cases - one boy stabbed in the gluteal region. One thyrotoxicosis lesion sent up - she thought it was the heat – more hot babies. Examined one girl for intercourse but questioning her mother we find that she has had a kid!! The man with suspected lead poisoning came for ck – I lanced one felon after infiltration with novocaine Heat cramps = hear exhaustion. Guy came in with epilepsy and they through it was the heat.

July 24, Tuesday
Not much doing last night – much to my relief. Sent up lots of heat cases. The lousey babies are still with us – still nothing spectacular

on the afternoon shift. I am still waiting on a letter. Doggonit – I forgot that treatment for thrush. Rx for__(?)____1% or boric acid (weak sol) swabbed and cleanliness. These pediatric cases are continuing to puzzle me. It is still hot as blazes. Ho hum! I guess I shall take another nap before time to go to work. Guy came in with iodine poisoning (?) abut when he vomited the starch water it was till white!!! I think he was lying but we gave him the hail Columbia with a stomach tube.I think he was despondent. ok have the ......home

July 25 Wednesday

Let us hope that the heat wave is broken for good and for all – more _____ cases of heat stroke today. The cool breeze is about to cut down the morbidity – let us hope we get more medical cases in the 3-11 shift – but it is not near as interesting as 11-7 Doggonit – I wish I could spell SHOULDER!!! I'm always messing up a good day by bad spelling. Most interesting case = appendicitis in a kid 12 years old they are watching him to operate now. Not many to suture these days – its' too hot to fight. I guess – I must read some more. I'm not so hot on the spelling. A patient asked me today if I was the doctor – was my face red?? I wrote a long letter today – let's hope I get a long one tomorrow. It's almost mid-nite and I am hungry.

July 26 Thursday. I missed writing and now Ive forgotten ? I know darned well that I'm leaving out something important too – oh yes, we sent a kid up - thinking it was appendicitis – but I wonder? Ill 4 days – loss of appetite anorexia – vomiting of bile stained material, pain in abdomen scaphoid T= 101. Gurgling sound over the cecum. Age 12 years.

July 27 Friday

Pretty busy – the morning shift did bot have them out of the way so that left me in for a plenty to do from the beginning – I was not feeling too well either, but it was cool – no unusual cases except that _psychosis with the wig on – she was big, fat and yellow. Bottles , blankets, stimulated to bring him out of it , I' sleepy now. I remember now some points about that kid that should have made me think of typhoid.

July 28 Saturday. Began with a bang!! A guy came in scalped! He had a cut on his forehead inflicted by a man he cut two days ago. Then came that 14 year old frightening girl – I had to sew up her shin. Then came a guy with his testicles shot off by an angry wife. If he has no kids up to now he is in a heck of a fix for descendants. With both cords cut and one testicle _____ a big hole shot through his thigh. The kid we sent up for appendicitis had typhoid!!! Just as Dr. Neil said. A heat exhaustion came in today with a sub normal temperature. He is in a heck of a shape – sure hot water

July 29 Sunday – Lazinka's Birthday Aug 12

Well one Democrat is going to have me thrown out because I could not dress his wound Saturday evening – but he was drunk. This man brought a kid in in whom he had diagnosed worms the kid had a temp of 104 – he took it back home – there is plenty of pelvic inflammation abroad all right. I must keep up with my load better as I have forgotten half or 2/3 of what I did yesterday.

July 30 Monday

Not so bsy today but some good cases nevertheless. There was that man with his arm crushed in a concrete mixer it was pitiful but it had to be cut off. There was also a heart case – some irregularity but mostly nerves –like mine. There was the kid with the ring on her finger her lousy Pa would rather take her away with it still on than to to have her finger pinched– we have some fools in this race of ours. I think a case of diptheria came up. _Name___. mask I must follow it up at isolation to see if my batting average go up or down. Pelvic inflammation – plenty of it A felon lanced by Dr. Sheen was well circumscribed but later came back with lymphangitis.

July 31 Tuesday. I forgot to write I diagnosed facture of the radius in a boy– and the x-ray report came back negative. Did my face turn red!!! A woman came in stinking like hell – granuloma inguinale x T.B.

That was the most peculiar case of tetanus I've ever seen, He took cramps while delivering _____. He could walk with difficulty when they took him—. I thought of "Jake"leg paralysis but Smith said TET. And they took him to isolation where it was again pronounced TET. Where and how he got it – nobody knows.

August 1 Wednesday Lazinka's birthdat August 12th

I did not write - a girl came in cut all over just as we were about to go off duty but I was busy strapping, a case of pleurisy, and did not get in on it. Boy hit by a car – bruises that's all.

Woman fell or jumped from a second floor winder. She landed on her gluteas maximus and hurt her back – Guy with his finger cut off referred to have it sutured – it was hanging only by skin.

August 2 Thursday

Things moved along quietly. Sheen lanced an abscess in the

gluteal region. I lanced a finger. Another guy came in cut to the last notch at 10:55 p. and made us late.

Plenty of nails in feet. Sewed up girl's leg - a longgash.

I sent up a Bartholin abscess.

Man cut on the scrotum but not badly . Still more P.T

August 3, Lazinka's Birthday August 12th

(No entries until August 14)

August 14

I did not write much for the lat week or so – very few extraordinary things happen in the day time, but I've been dressing some wounds that it would be bad to write about – for instance, the fellow with the tuberculosis sinus in his sacral region – when he came in and begin to stink nothing short of ammonia will kill the odor. There is also the follow who had the operation for _____ - he has been draining for years – and the woman who had the salpingectomy – she was operated on some years ago and is still draining. I have lanced a many finger – and gotten splinters out of many feet. The boy came in today with a superficial collection of pus under the bottom of his foot, but I would not be satisfied. I went deeper and found more pus – a pint in an indoform drain – I guess it should have been rubber tissue however. The famous Pearl Johnson went home today – I took many a stitch in his jaw – and he left without a bandage - trusty negroes are fools as a lot. Gosh they have quit using knives and started shooting each other. A guy caught a man with his wife and killed the man – having used all the bullets – he beat his wife over th head with the pistol. Only today a 20 years old fellow came in claiing he shot himself – just below the heart because he could ot find a job. He was shot with a Wincheter – rumor has it that a man caught him in bed with his wife and let him have it – he was sot through and through with fractured ribs and hemothorax. The guy who was stabbed in the neck by his common law wife finally died – how a guy can survive a trip to the hospital even withi his carotid spurting is beyond me – and if he had received a transfusion I think he could have pulled through.

Now for some not quite so bad – take the guy who had his first metacarpal broken with little deformity today – I almost missed getting my cre_____.

They are really wearing me out on this day shift. Well – I'll stop and eat now.

End of Entries

GALLERY

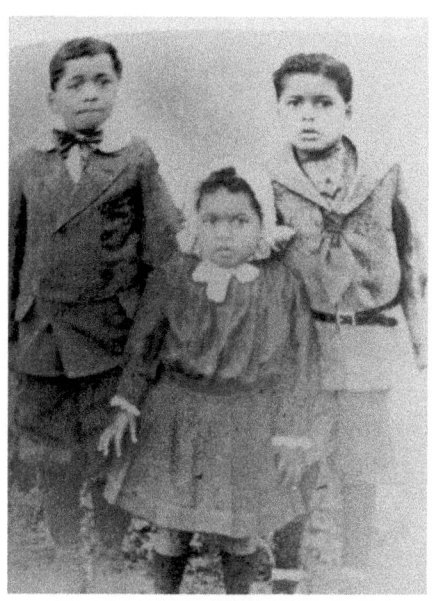

The 3 children: Brother Johnny,
Sister Thelmas and Milton

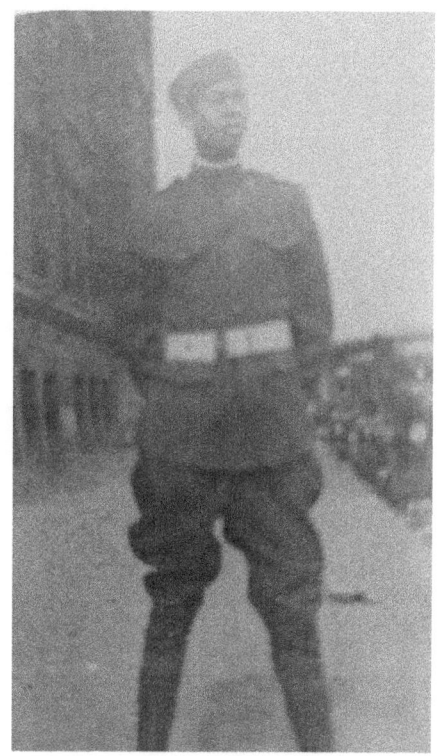

Dr. Q in ROTC uniform

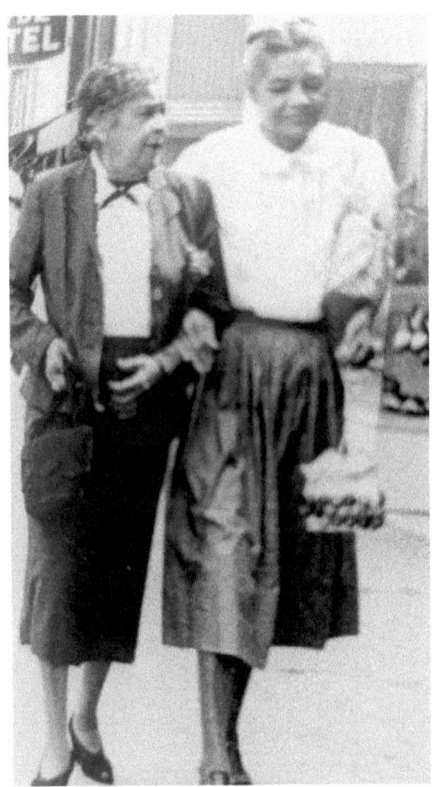

Mother Agnes Quigless
with daughter Ruby

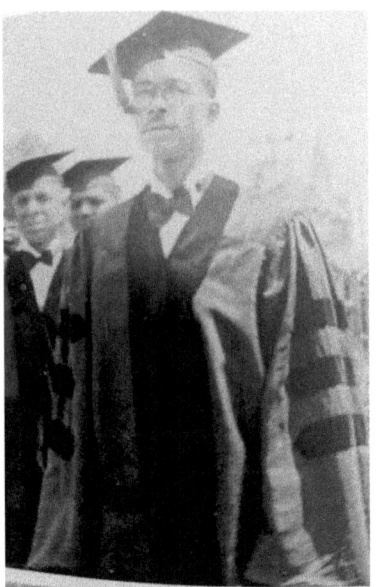

Dr. Q's Graduation at
Meharry Medical School

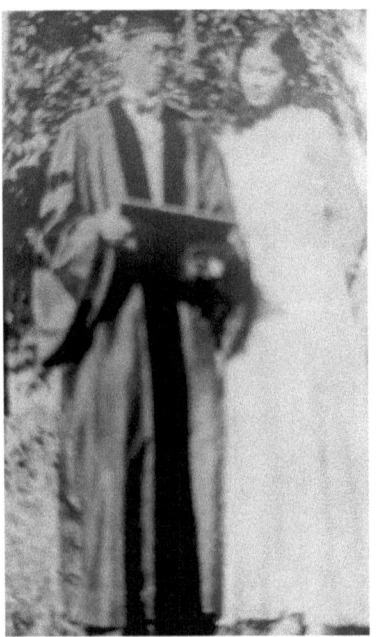

Dr. Q Looking at Diploma
with Lazinka

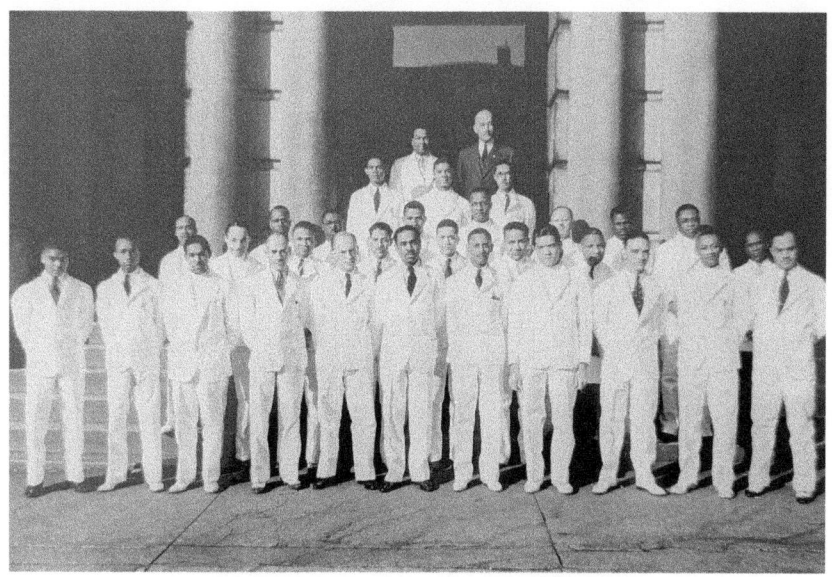

Medical Residence at St. Louis Hospital #2
(Quigless is in 2nd top row on right)

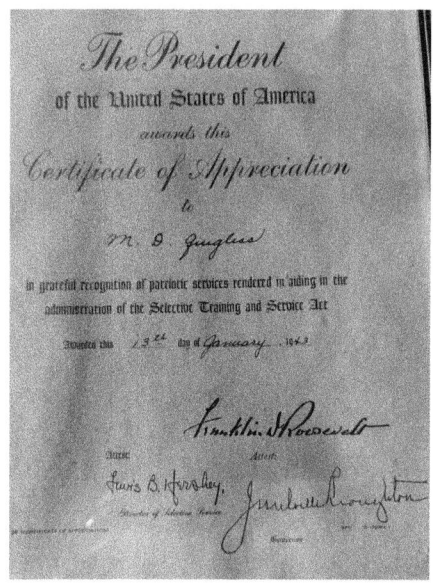

Commendation for Service by President Roosevelt

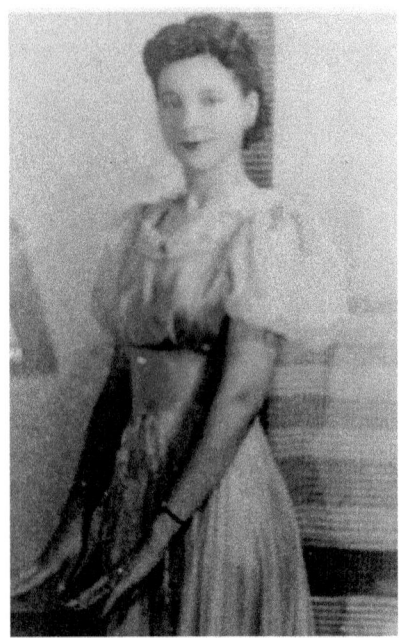

The Young Future Mrs. Quigless

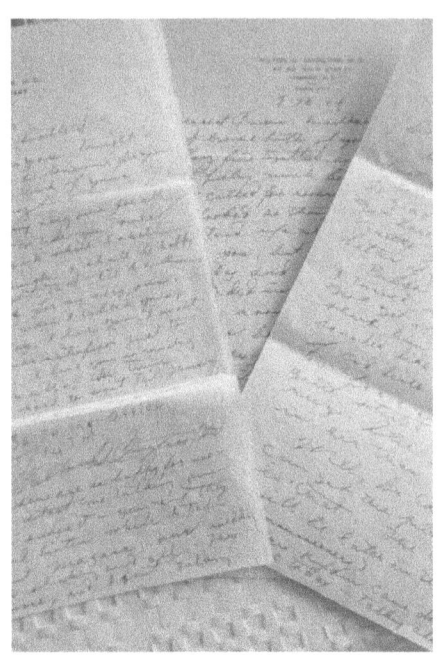

Love Letters

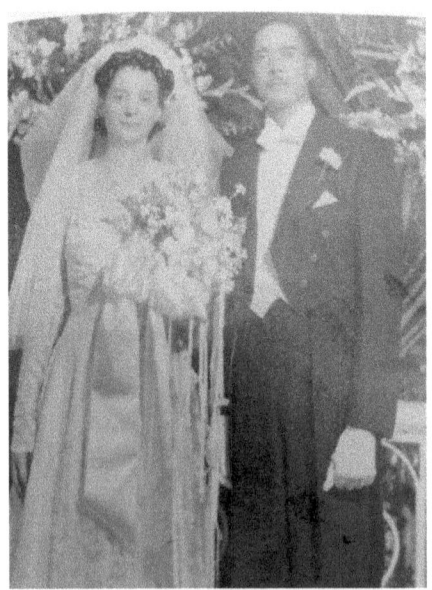

Wedding Day

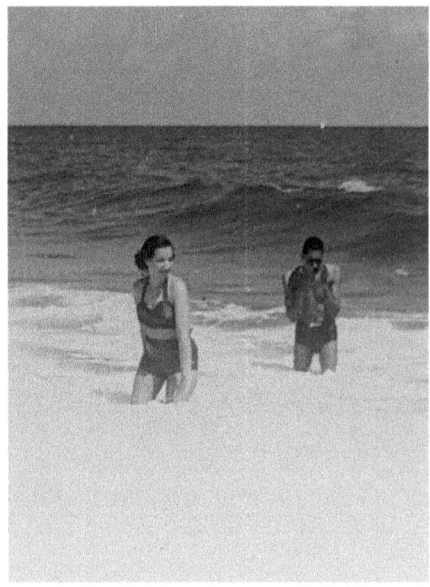

Scenes from Topsail Beach

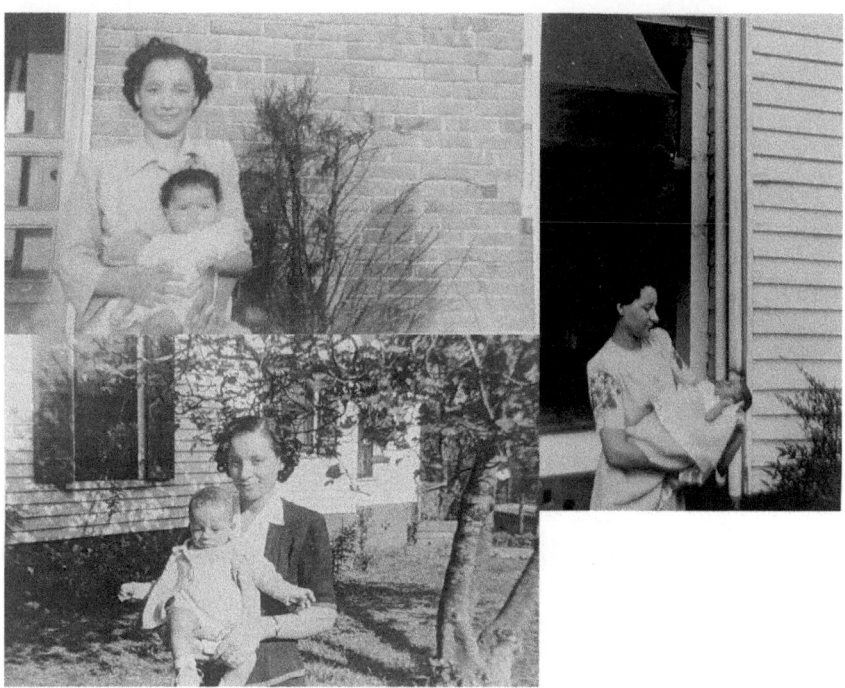

Babies Helen Jr., Milton Jr., and Carol

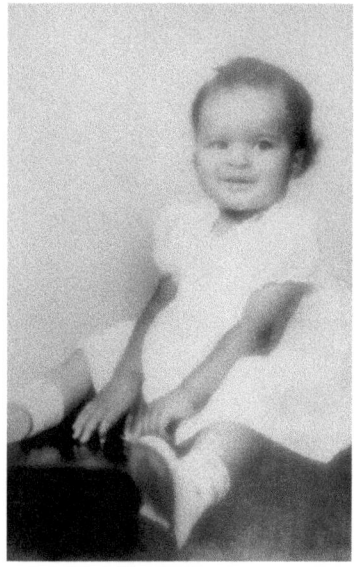

Baby Carol

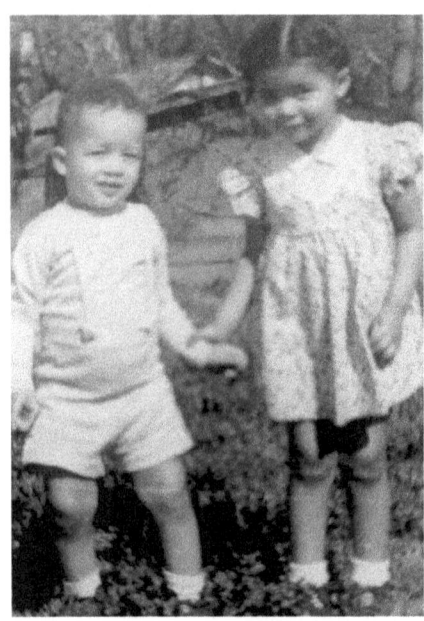

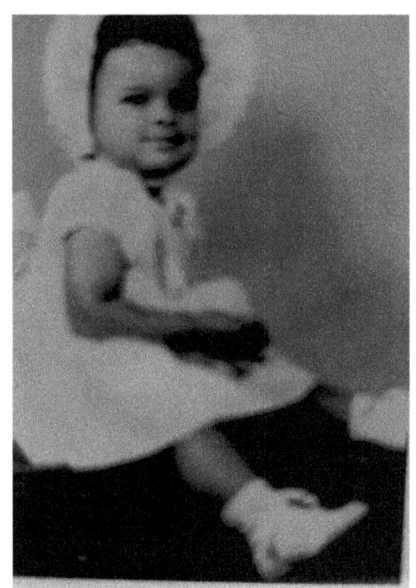

Milton Jr. and Helen Jr.

Baby Carol

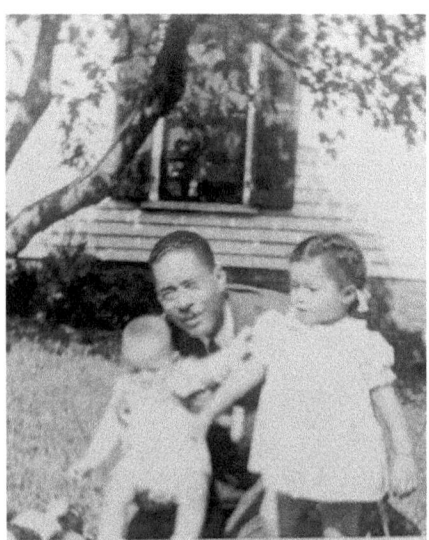

Dr. Q with Helen Jr., and Milton Jr.

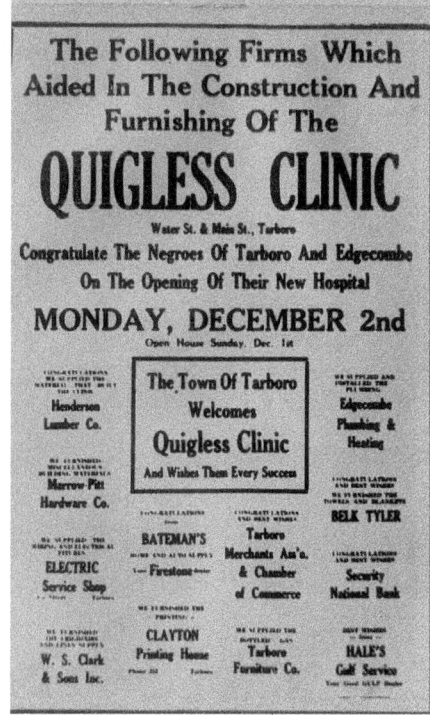

Announcement of Clinic Opening

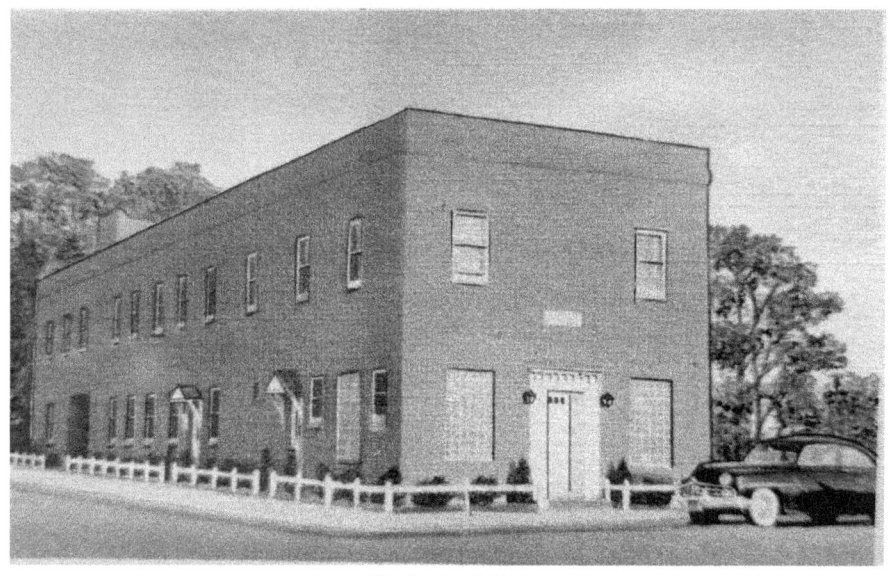

Clinic Building

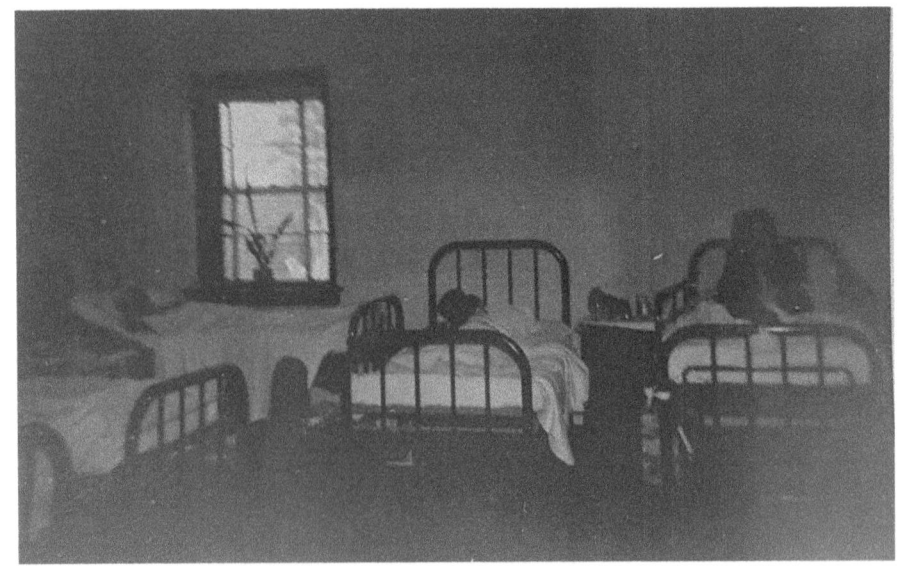

Women's Ward

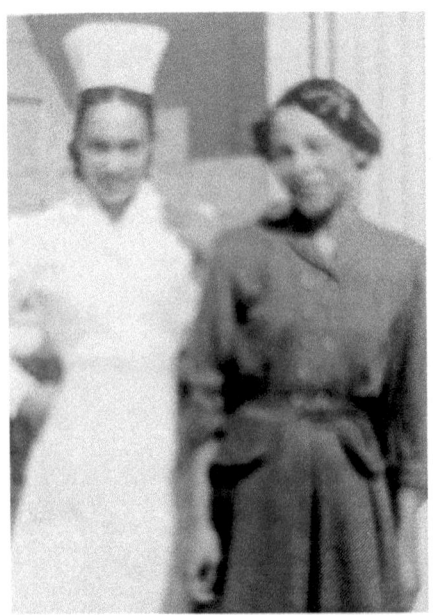

Nurse and Administrative Staff

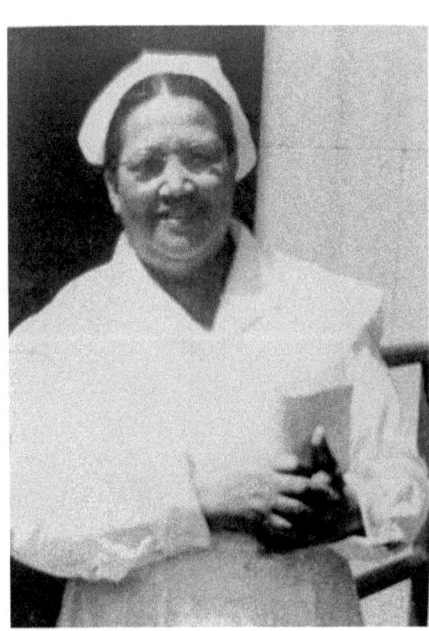

Nurse

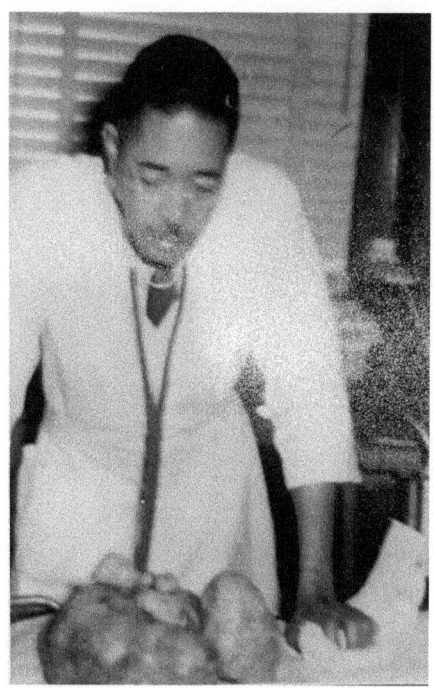

Dr. Q with Benign Tumor He Surgically Removed

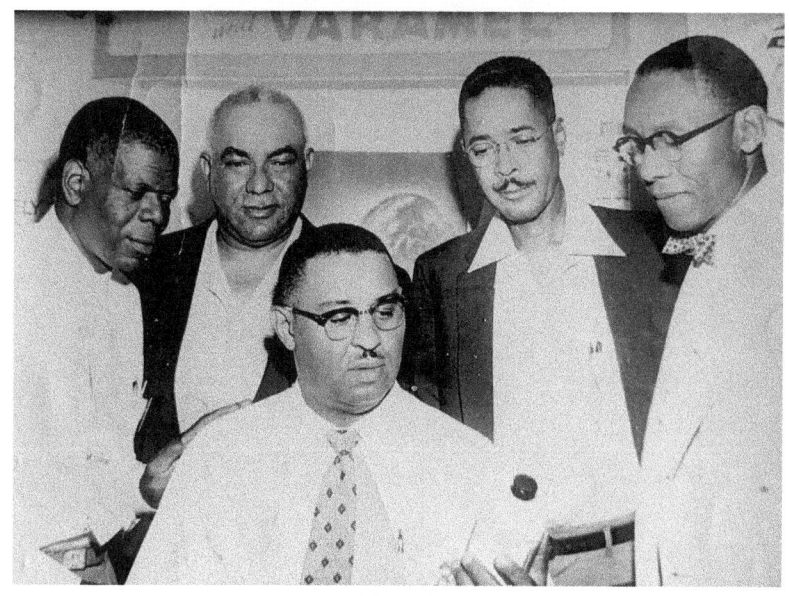

Dr. Q with Colleagues

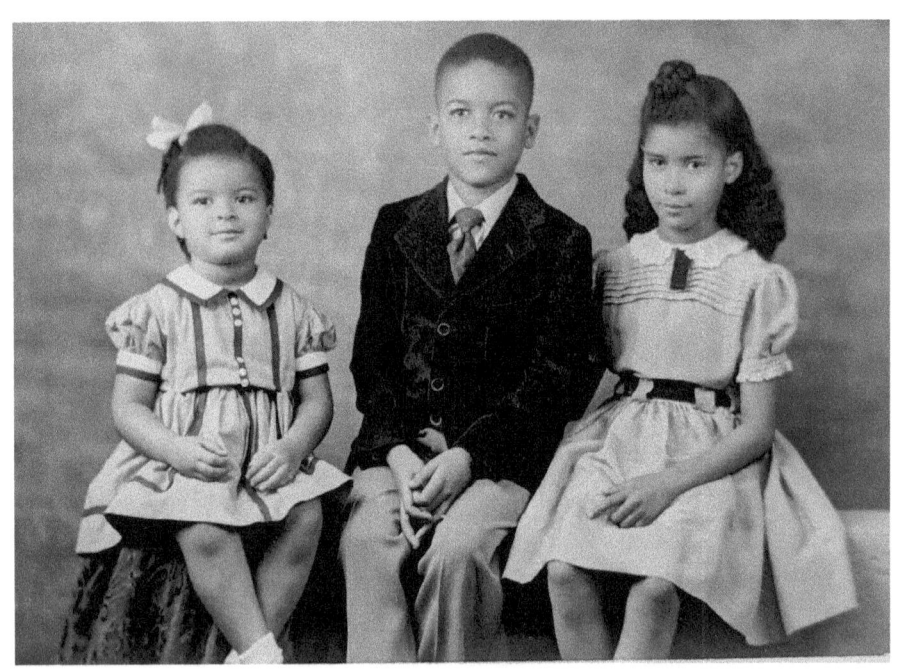

The Children Helen Jr., Milton Jr., and Carol

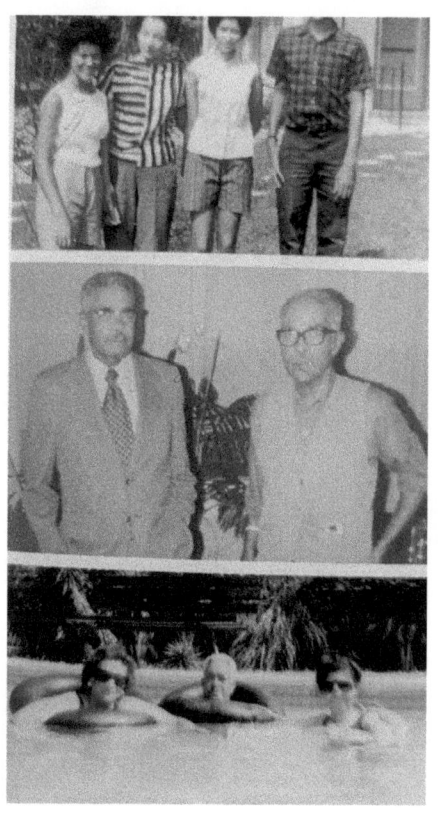

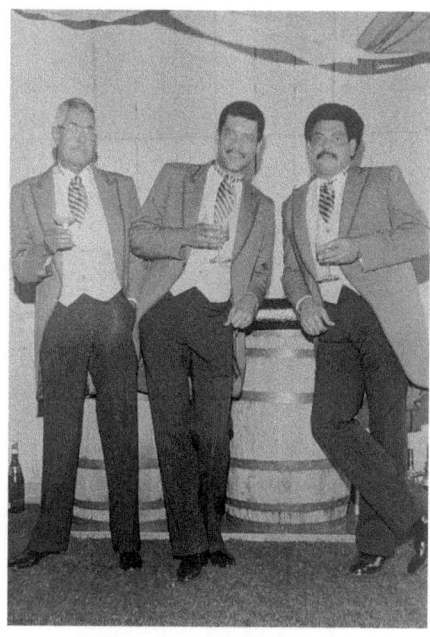

Milton Jr.'s Wedding Day
with Dr. Quigless Sr. and
Wilbur Finks, Father-in-Law

Father-in-Law, Brother Charlie, Dr.
Q, Mrs. Q and Helen Chilling

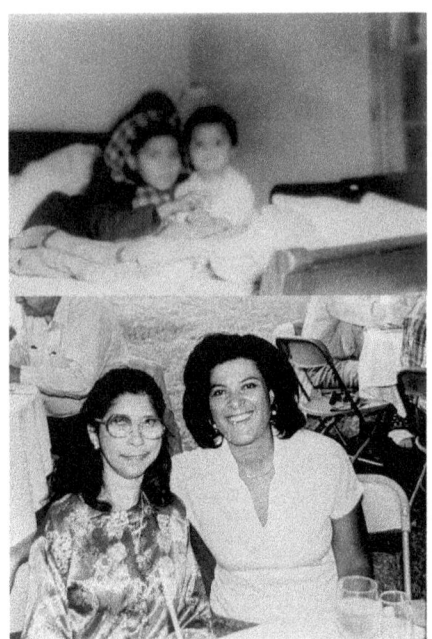

Helen and Carol

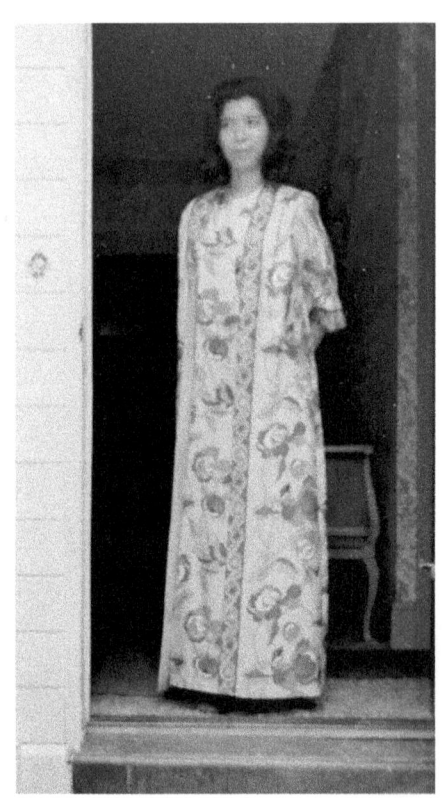

Helen

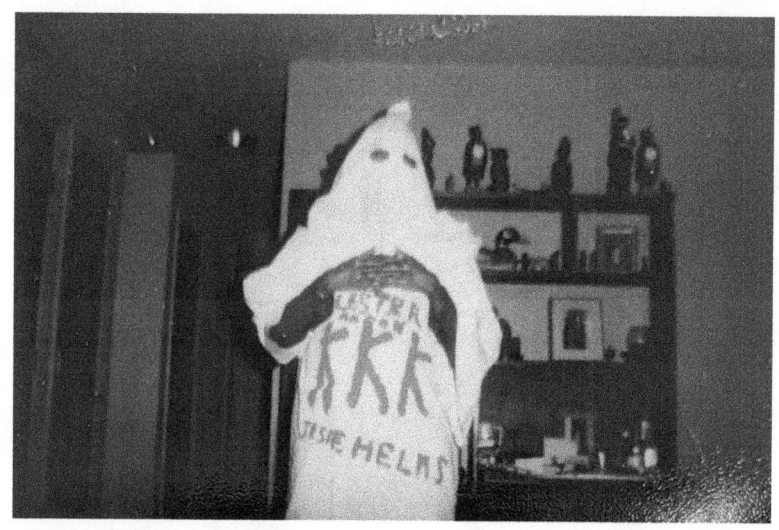

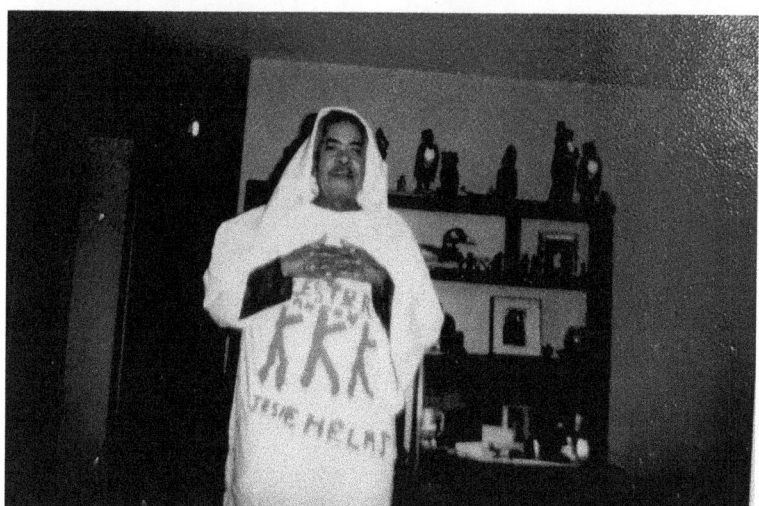

Dr. Q's Halloween Costume for Party at Edgecombe General Hospital

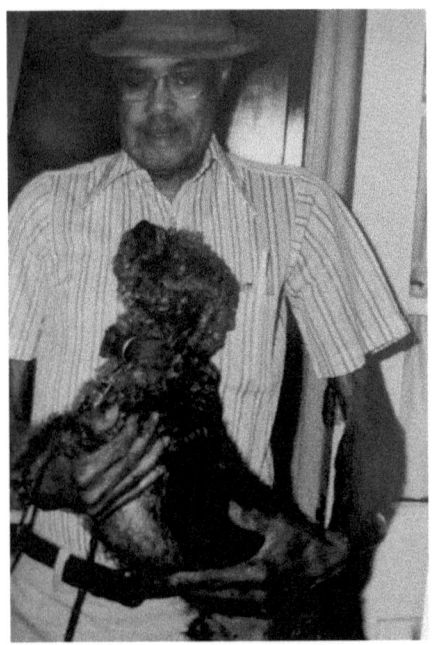 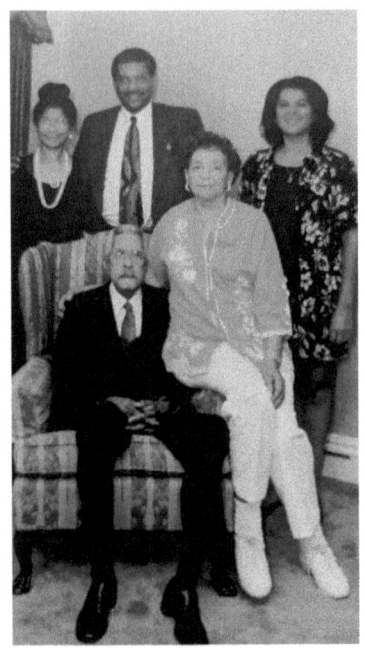

Dr. Q and His Dog. He Loved His Dog

The Quigless Family Shortly before
Dr. Quigless's Death at Age 94

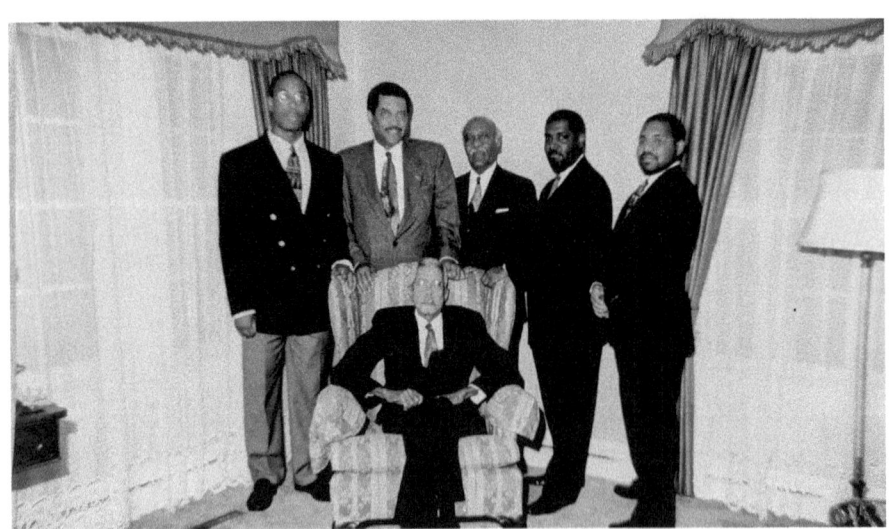

The Quigless Men

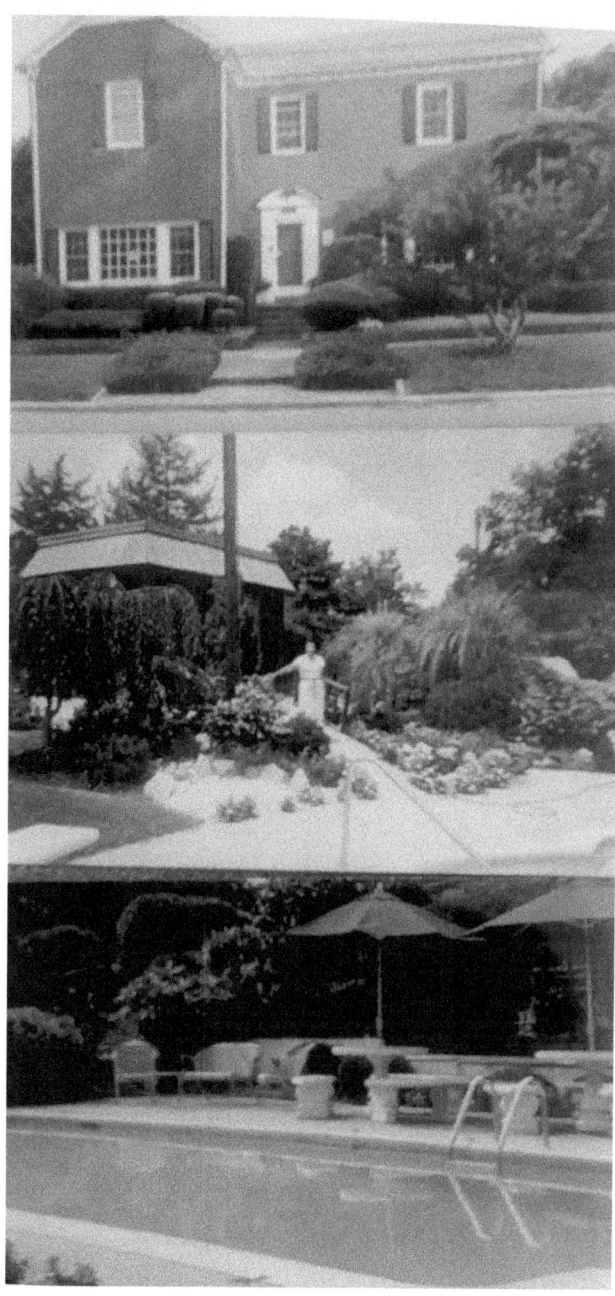

Mrs. Quigless spent over 50 years developing an extraordinary home of beauty for the family.

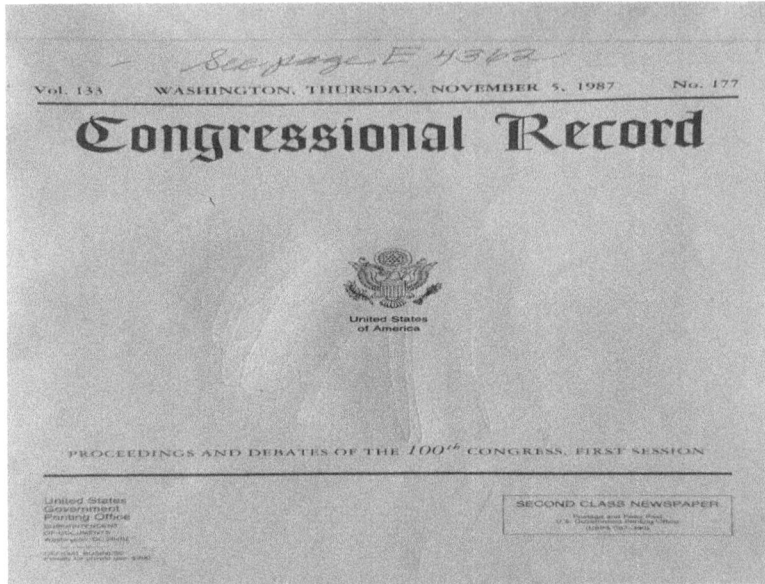

Congressional Record Face Page

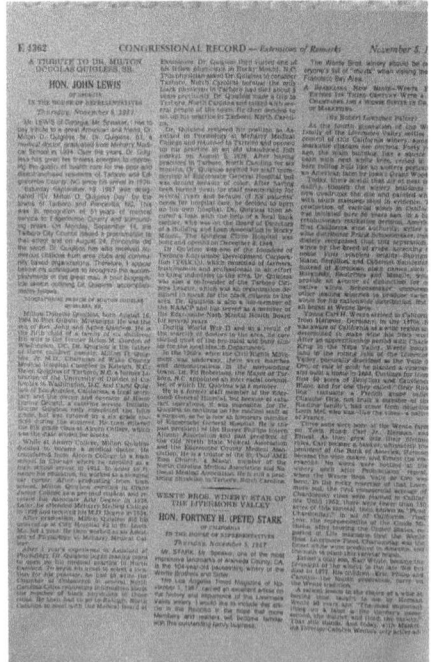

Congressional Record Citation Regarding
Dr. Quigless by John Lewis

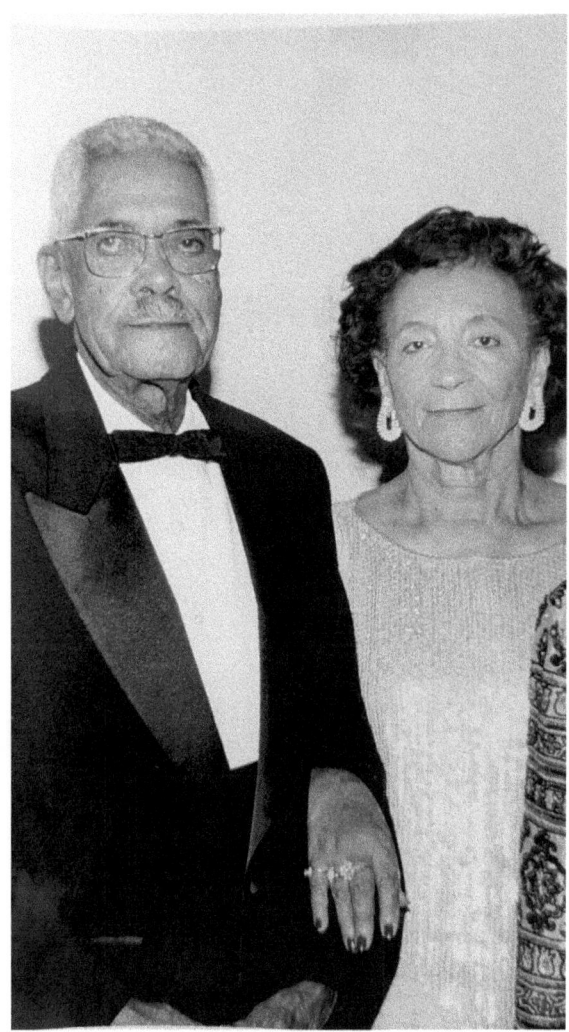

Dr. and Mrs. Quigless, Ages 88 and 75 Respectively

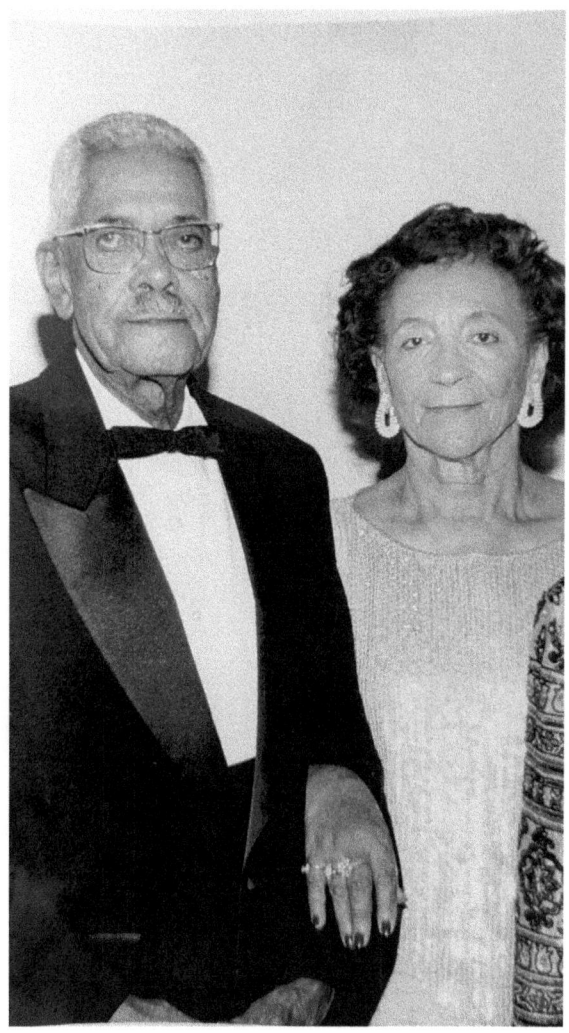

Dr. and Mrs. Quigless, Ages 88 and 75 Respectively

www.ingramcontent.com/pod-product-compliance
Lightning Source LLC
Chambersburg PA
CBHW051129120626
46547CB00012B/734